THE WORLD FOOD PROBLEM

THE WORLD FOOD PROBLEM

Tackling the Causes of Undernutrition in the Third World

THIRD EDITION

Howard D. Leathers
Phillips Foster

LYNNE
RIENNER
PUBLISHERS

BOULDER
LONDON

Published in the United States of America in 2004 by
Lynne Rienner Publishers, Inc.
1800 30th Street, Boulder, Colorado 80301
www.rienner.com

and in the United Kingdom by
Lynne Rienner Publishers, Inc.
3 Henrietta Street, Covent Garden, London WC2E 8LU

Library of Congress Cataloging-in-Publication Data
Leathers, Howard D.
   The world food problem : tackling the causes of undernutrition in the
Third World / Howard Leathers and Phillips Foster.— 3rd ed.
   Foster's name appears first on the earlier edition.
   Includes bibliographical references and index.
   ISBN 1-58826-250-2 (hardcover : alk. paper)
   ISBN 1-58826-275-8 (pbk. : alk. paper)
   1. Food supply—Developing countries. 2. Poor—Developing countries—
Nutrition. 3. Malnutrition—Developing countries. 4. Food supply—
Government policy—Developing countries. 5. Nutrition policy—
Developing countries. 6. Food supply—Developing countries—International
cooperation. I. Foster, Phillips, 1931– II. Foster, Phillips, 1931-
World food problem.   III. Title.
HD9018.D44F68 2004
363.8'09172'4—dc22

                                                       2004003785

British Cataloguing in Publication Data
A Cataloguing in Publication record for this book
is available from the British Library.

Printed and bound in the United States of America

          The paper used in this publication meets the requirements
⊗   of the American National Standard for Permanence of
          Paper for Printed Library Materials Z39.48-1992.

5   4   3   2   1

CONTENTS

PREFACE

In the twelve years since the first edition of this book was published, the world food problem has grown less severe, but is still a long way from solution. Our understanding of the causes and policy solutions continues to evolve. The third edition of this book incorporates material on the growing debates over globalization and genetically modified food and includes new chapters on the history of famines and the feasibility of solving the world food problem through redistribution alone. It incorporates up-to-date statistical information and references to recent analyses of the causes and effects of undernutrition and related policies. This edition also attempts to provide a more solid understanding of how economic principles can be applied to these issues. Real-world examples are presented to illustrate the general points.

Despite these changes, the principal messages of the first edition remain as valid today as they were in 1992. Undernutrition remains a problem for hundreds of millions of people in developing countries. Poverty, income inequalities, population growth, and illness continue to be important causes of undernutrition while increasing agricultural production will be an integral part of any strategy to reduce world hunger.

The Plan of the Book
We begin with an emphasis on definitions and facts. As the material develops, our emphasis shifts to behavioral models of society (for example, economic, demographic) and how these models relate to undernutrition. In the last section, we discuss how these models can be applied in evaluating nutrition policy alternatives.

In Part 1, malnutrition is found to be a leading killer throughout the world, with undernutrition in the developing world the main nutrition problem. Before considering the causes of undernutrition and policy alternatives to alleviate it, we examine the facts and provide answers to questions such as: What is malnutrition? How do we measure it? Who is malnourished?

vii

What are the trends?

In Part 2, we look at the main causes of undernutrition and attribute these causes mainly to economic, demographic, agronomic, and health variables.

In Part 3, we explore public policies that will have an impact on undernutrition. The final chapter contains some speculations about the future.

We have attempted to integrate knowledge from a number of disciplines, taking as a central premise, well articulated by Beatice Rogers (1988b) of Tufts University, that "the solution to the world hunger problem will be achieved only through the integration of knowledge from the whole range of relevant scientific disciplines." Thus, we have drawn on nutrition science, economics, demography, biology, chemistry, health science, geography, agronomy, history, anthropology, philosophy, and public policy analysis.

To a large extent, this book is data driven. From the tables on foreign assistance in the opening chapter through the data on malnutrition in Part 1, and the numbers on elasticity and population in Part 2, to the future projections about production, consumption, and prices in the last chapter, the text is larded with illustrative tables and figures. It is our hope that the data themselves will, in large measure, back up our arguments. The text set in numerous boxes serves not only to provide visual variety, but to bring the reader's attention to interesting related material and examples.

The second edition of this text acknowledged our debt of gratitude to, among others, Professor Leslie Whittington, who taught the course from which this book was developed after Professor Foster, and before Professor Leathers. We dedicate this edition to the memory of Professor Whittington, who was murdered, along with her husband and children, on September 11, 2001.

Howard D. Leathers
Phillips Foster

1

Introduction

Hunger. It was prevalent everywhere. Hunger was pushed out of the tall
houses in the wretched clothing that hung upon poles and lines; Hunger
was patched into them with straw and rag and wood and paper; Hunger
was repeated in every fragment of the small modicum of firewood that the
man sawed off; Hunger stared down from the smokeless chimneys, and
started up from the filthy street that had no offal, among its refuse, of anything to eat. Hunger was the inscription on the baker's shelves, written in
every small loaf of his scanty stock of bad bread; at the sausage-shop in
every dear-dog preparation that was offered for sale. Hunger rattled its dry
bones among the roasting chestnuts in the turned cylinder; Hunger was
shred into atomies in every farthing porringer of husky chips of potato,
fried with some reluctant drops of oil.

—Charles Dickens, *A Tale of Two Cities*

A newspaper headline on starvation may conjure up in your mind the image
of an emaciated infant, the victim of an Ethiopian famine. And if you are a
history buff, places such as Bengal or Ukraine may spring to mind. News
photographs and television images of families migrating in search of food,
or babies with bloated bellies and spindly arms and legs, and of bodies too
weak to sit up, have flooded our consciousness with the horror of hunger.
Every decade has provided horror stories of its own. Famine in North
Korea reached such an acute stage by late 1997 that there were reports of
people eating grass and tree bark. Southern Africa was the subject of an
international effort to avoid widespread death from famine in 2002. One
estimate puts deaths from starvation worldwide during the 1990s at
100,000 to 200,000 per year (Kates 1996). Another study estimates that as
many as 576,000 Iraqi children have died since the end of the Gulf War in
1991 because of economic sanctions against the country and resulting food
shortages (Fawzi et al. 1996).

What happens when you die from hunger? Describing famine-related
death, an anonymous author writing for *Time* magazine put it eloquently
and succinctly:

The victim of starvation burns up his own body fats, muscles, and tissues

1

for fuel. His body quite literally consumes itself and deteriorates rapidly. The kidneys, liver, and endocrine system often cease to function properly. A shortage of carbohydrates, which play a vital role in brain chemistry, affects the mind. Lassitude and confusion set in, so that starvation victims often seem unaware of their plight. The body's defenses drop; disease kills most famine victims before they have time to starve to death. An individual begins to starve when he has lost about a third of his normal body weight. Once this loss exceeds 40 percent, death is almost inevitable. (Anonymous 1974)

Although the drama of famine tends to capture our attention, most hunger-related deaths do not occur in famines. They happen daily—quietly, largely unchronicled—all around the world. Figures vary, but one conservative estimate, using data provided by the World Health Organization of the United Nations, is that some 6 million children die annually from hunger. This amounts to one death every five seconds.

In previous editions of this book, we have tried to emphasize the enormity of the problem as follows: "Another way to put this number into perspective is to imagine the newspaper coverage that would occur if a 747 jet crashed, killing all 220 children on board. The deaths attributable to hunger are equivalent to 75 of these jet crashes every day." After the terrorist attacks on September 11, 2001, in New York City and Washington, D.C., we no longer have to imagine the newspaper coverage, or the grief, or the universal determination that every effort should be made to prevent a recurrence. The tragedy of undernutrition fails to stir such outrage or determination. The world hunger problem is too pervasive, too commonplace, too remote from our own experience, too hopeless.

The world's reaction to widespread undernutrition is reflected in the figures in Tables 1.1 and 1.2. Not one country donates more than 3 percent of its wealth to the poor. And the countries that receive the assistance are likely to be chosen not so much because they are the most in need, but because the donations can help achieve some geopolitical objective of the donor country.

The Food and Agriculture Organization of the United Nations (FAO) estimates that the number of chronically undernourished people in the developing world in 2000 was about 800 million. Bread for the World Institute estimates that the comparable figure for 1997 was 841 million. Based on these numbers, and taking into account that there are some hungry people in the developed world, we can conclude that 13–17 percent of the world's population suffers from chronic hunger.

Of course, as the numbers above make clear, not all of hungry die from it. To visualize the most common scenario, played out again and again in developing countries, picture a loving but poorly educated, poverty-stricken mother with several children. Food is scarce. Her youngest child

Table 1.1   Ranking of Largest Donors of Aid (overseas development assistance), 1998–2002

Ranked by size of aid		Ranked by aid as percentage of GNI	
Country	Average annual aid ($ million)	Country	% of GNI
United States	37,368	Spain	2.90
Spain	16,807	Portugal	2.08
Germany	13,970	Belgium	1.39
United Kingdom	13,222	Sweden	1.33
Japan	13,066	Denmark	1.24
France	8,835	Netherlands	1.19
Italy	7,313	Norway	1.12
Canada	5,257	United Kingdom	0.90
Netherlands	4,553	Switzerland	0.87
Belgium	3,435	Canada	0.84
Sweden	2,996	Ireland	0.82
Switzerland	2,411	Finland	0.77
Portugal	2,208	Luxembourg	0.74
Denmark	2,039	Germany	0.69
Norway	1,849	Austria	0.69
Australia	1,528	France	0.65
Austria	1,376	Italy	0.64
Finland	942	Australia	0.42
Ireland	706	United States	0.39
Greece	227	New Zealand	0.31
New Zealand	152	Japan	0.30
Luxembourg	133	Greece	0.19

Source: OECD. http://www.oecd.org/dataoecd/52/9/1893143.xls Table 3.

has not been growing for months because of undernourishment and the baby's resistance to disease has fallen to a very low level. He drinks from the family's unsanitary supply of water; the older members of his family can handle the microorganisms in the water, but the baby develops diarrhea. He loses interest in eating. He seems more willing to take liquids, so the mother removes solids from his diet. Because he is unable to obtain sufficient nourishment from the liquids to conquer his illness, his diarrhea continues. Finally, in a desperate but seemingly logical attempt to stop the diarrhea, his mother removes the liquids. Although the child by now is feverish, limiting liquids accelerates the baby's loss of fluids. Severe dehydration follows, with death not far behind.

Whereas adult males do die of hunger during a famine, the majority of deaths, whether from famine or from chronic undernutrition, occur among preschoolers. Pregnant and lactating women are also at substantial risk, although less so than children. Children suffer malnutrition in a multitude

Table 1.2   Largest Recipients of Foreign Aid, 1998-2002

Ranked by average annual receipts ($ million)		Ranked by average receipts per person ($)		Ranked by average receipts as a percentage of GNI (percentage)	
China	1,906	Montserrat	5,351	Sao Tome & Principe	74.0
Indonesia	1,571	Tokelau	4,084	Marshall Islands	50.5
India	1,555	Wallis & Futuna	3,215	Micronesia,Fed. States	44.5
Egypt	1,482	Palau	2,282	Timor-Leste	39.9
Vietnam	1,404	St. Helena	2,208	Guinea-Bissau	37.9
Pakistan	1,316	Niue	1,914	Mozambique	34.5
Mozambique	1,142	Marshall Islands	1,169	Palau	32.6
Tanzania	1,103	Micronesia,Fed. States	896	Eritrea	29.3
Bangladesh	1,097	Mayotte	697	Sierra Leone	29.1
Serbia & Montenegro	1,032	Tuvalu	677	Kiribati	25.2
Ethiopia	884	French Polynesia	608	Mauritania	24.8
Palestinian Adm. Areas	849	New Caledonia	603	Malawi	24.6
Bosnia	782	Nauru	528	Mongolia	20.6
Uganda	698	Turks & Caicos Islands	346	Rwanda	20.2
Nicaragua	657	Palestinian Adm. Areas	275	Cape Verde	18.9
Ghana	644	Dominica	262	Palestinian Adm. Areas	18.8
Bolivia	617	Cook Islands	256	Vanuatu	16.9
Philippines	604	St. Kitts-Nevis	242	Laos	16.6
Côte d'Ivoire	601	Cape Verde	238	Burkina Faso	16.1
Thailand	599	Netherlands Antilles	233	Burundi	16.0

Source: OECD, . http://www.oecd.org/dataoecd/52/9/1893143.xls Table 16.
Notes: Receipts per capita are average receipts divided by 2001 population. Receipts as percentage of GNI are average receipts divided by 2001 GNI.

of ways. They may be crippled by vitamin D deficiency, blinded by vitamin A deficiency, or stunted by protein deficiency. But the most common form of child undernutrition results simply from a lack of sufficient calories, with disease and death too often the result.

The purpose of this book is to provide an introduction for the general reader to the world food problem, its causes, and possible ways of addressing it. Our intention is to encourage the reader to be objective and analytical. We try to avoid a process of grabbing on to a point of view and turning a blind eye to inconvenient facts. As the past few paragraphs foreshadow, the pages that follow are replete with data and with inferences drawn from data. We invite the skeptical reader to contend with us; to point out other inferences that can be drawn, or other data that lead in a different direction.

Part 1 of the book presents some factual background. What is undernutrition? How does being undernourished affect a person? How can we determine whether a person is malnourished? What information do we have about the extent of undernutrition in different periods of time and in different geographical areas?

■ Factors Influencing Food Supply and Demand in the Future

Part 2 of the book identifies factors that influence the extent of undernutrition. The framework we use to outline these factors is the framework of economics: supply and demand. As we look to the future, the quality of life worldwide will depend critically on whether the world food supply will grow faster or slower than world food demand. If food supply grows faster than demand, then almost certainly the average quality of life in the world will improve. If supply outpaces demand, food prices will fall; this makes it easier for poor people to afford an adequate diet; for richer people, it frees up income to spend on other goods and amenities. In a similar fashion, if demand grows faster than supply, quality of life may deteriorate.

In analyzing future prospects for food supply and demand, there are four critical factors, which we refer to as the "four P's":

- Population
- Prosperity
- Pollution or environmental quality
- Productivity in agriculture

The impact of population growth on food demand is obvious. More mouths to feed means more demand for food. The question of whether food production can grow as fast as population was posed by Thomas Malthus in his "Essay on the Principle of Population."

Widespread economic prosperity means that more people can afford adequate diets, and that people are more likely to have access to health care, a sanitary water supply, and education. Prosperity as measured by income per capita also affects food demand. As people attain higher income levels, they tend to buy more food, and to buy a wider variety of food including meat and animal products. So 6 billion relatively affluent people require significantly more agricultural production than do 6 billion relatively poor people.

Pollution (or more appropriately—except it does not begin with a P—environmental quality) and the availability of land and water resources needed for agricultural production are critical factors in the future of agricultural production. To what extent can we expand the area devoted to agricultural production? Will soil erosion or water pollution leave us with less arable land, or less irrigable land? In addition, global climate change may influence agricultural production.

Agricultural productivity measures our ability to increase food production without increasing the amount of agricultural land. No matter what happens to environmental quality and land and water resources, the future food supply will continue to grow if productivity grows fast enough.

Productivity per acre can increase because farmers apply more fertilizer, or use more labor, or use more of other inputs per acre. Productivity per acre can also increase because of new technology, such as new seed varieties.

These four factors interact with each other in complex ways. Some examples of these interactions are:

- As population grows, urban and industrial water users compete with agriculture for scarce water
- Population growth slows as people become more prosperous
- As agricultural productivity increases, economic prosperity improves for the entire economy
- Increased use of agricultural chemicals may improve productivity while harming the environment

The above discussion suggests some of the ways that government policies can influence the long-term supply-and-demand balance of food. However, this complexity of interactions illustrates how difficult it can be to decide among various policy alternatives. Appropriate policy changes are the subject of the last part of this book.

■ The Main Nutrition Policy Alternatives

Part 3 of the book will focus on policy interventions that may help alleviate the world hunger problem. For the most part, the policy interventions we examine are aimed at the factors identified in Part 2. Undernutrition can be reduced by reducing the price the hungry must pay for food, or by increasing their ability to pay.

Policies that reduce the rate of population growth lead to less pressure on available food supplies, lowering food prices. Policies that increase average incomes through faster economic growth, or policies that redistribute income to the hungry, increase the ability of the poor to obtain an adequate diet. Some policies may be targeted at reducing the price paid for food by undernourished people, without attempting to reduce the general level of food prices. Policies may drive down consumer food prices by increasing the quantity of food produced; this can be done through government subsidies that pay farmers more than the market price, or by programs that lower farmers' costs of production, permitting them to produce more at lower prices.

PART 1

Malnutrition: What Are the Facts?

Malnutrition is a leading killer. In high-income countries one variant of malnutrition—overnutrition—is the main problem. In the third world another variant—undernutrition—is the main problem. The problem of third world undernutrition is exacerbated by secondary malnutrition—malnutrition stemming from causes such as disease.

Before considering the causes of undernutrition, and policy alternatives to alleviate it, we must examine the facts and provide answers to these questions: What is malnutrition? What are its effects? How do we measure it? Who is malnourished? What are the trends?

2

Famines

Famines get the spotlight. The TV specials and the historical controversies and the sad Irish songs are about famines. But famine is a fairly small part of the world food problem. If through some magical intervention we could end famines, we would still have an enormous problem of widespread, pervasive, and permanent undernutrition. Although most of this book is focused on this pervasive and permanent condition, this chapter discusses famine.

Famines are localized, temporary, and severe food shortages. They are almost always the result of a confluence of forces that include natural disaster and poor policy response. Of course, there is a connection between the permanent state of widespread undernutrition and the crisis of famine: in countries where undernutrition is a serious and common problem, it does not take much of a natural disaster to create a famine.

Brief descriptions of present and historical famines illustrate how natural disasters and policy responses have interacted to create or exacerbate famines. These examples also illustrate some of the ways that economists have studied famines and policy approaches to famine.

■ The Irish Potato Famine

The Irish Potato Famine of the late 1840s is fairly well known in the West because it spurred a wave of Irish emigration to the United States, transforming U.S. culture in ways that continue to be seen, especially on St. Patrick's Day, and because the famine became emblematic of the British repression of Ireland.

Ireland of the 1840s was a country of deep and widespread rural poverty. Seventy-two percent of the Irish people were illiterate (Abbott 2003), and 37 percent lived in mud houses with a single room (Abbott 2003; Donnelly 2001:2). Per capita income in Ireland in the early 1840s was only about 60 percent of the level in Britain (Mokyr 1985).

Poverty was especially prevalent in rural areas. About two-thirds of the Irish population depended on agriculture for their livelihoods (Kinealy

2002:18), and 40 percent of these were landless laborers (Donnelly 2001:9). Much of the land in the Irish countryside was owned in large tracts by landlords. Landless laborers acquired plots of land from the landlord and in return either worked in the landlord's fields (primarily growing grain or linen for export, or producing butter for sale in urban areas) or paid a rent to the landlord. A social structure that trapped Irish labor in the agricultural sector caused labor productivity in that sector to be about half that of British agricultural workers (p. 9).

In this environment of poverty, a third of Irish households depended almost exclusively on potatoes for food. (A farmer in pre-famine Ireland might have consumed twelve or more pounds of potatoes per day.) Potatoes have a number of advantages as a low-cost food source in Ireland: (1) they can be grown in relatively poor soil; (2) they yield a high number of calories per acre; and (3) they are rich in protein, carbohydrates, vitamins, and minerals. A diet of potatoes and buttermilk (a by-product of producing butter) provides better nutrition than a diet consisting primarily of wheat or maize.

Because of the potato-based diet, and despite the widespread poverty, "the Irish poor were amongst the tallest, healthiest and most fertile population in Europe" (Kinealy 2002:32). The cheap and nutritious potato diet served as a foundation for low-wage agriculture; cheap food exported from Ireland in turn fueled the industrial revolution in Britain. In addition, the low-wage labor provided a cushion protecting some landlords from the consequences of their inefficient farming practices.

The potato blight—a fungus that causes potatoes to turn black and rotten as they grow in the ground—had appeared in small areas prior to 1845. But the blight hit about half the crop in 1845, and destroyed nearly the entire crop in 1846, 1848, and 1849. (The 1847 crop was partially successful.) Estimates of famine-related deaths range from 290,000 to 1,250,000 compared to Ireland's pre-famine population of about 8 million (Abbott 2003).

Once the severity of the potato blight was understood, a tremendous amount of attention was devoted to the appropriate "policy response": what can or should the government do? Throughout the nineteenth century, Ireland was governed by Great Britain. The choices made by the British government, and the criticisms of these choices, illustrate a philosophical or ideological debate about the appropriate relationship between government action and private action. The policy decisions fall into three categories (identified here with today's nomenclature): technology policy—what the government should do to encourage better scientific understanding of the causes and consequences of the potato blight; trade policy—what the government should do to increase food imports or reduce food exports during a time of famine; and poverty alleviation policy—what the government should do to help the poor.

The British government recognized the possibility of ending the famine with a technological fix, but their efforts never came to fruition. The government instituted a board of scientific experts to draw conclusions about how to save potatoes that had been infected by the blight. The board's recommendations involved complex chemical procedures requiring materials and training unavailable to the starving Irish masses. Even if followed, the program promised little hope of success. The government also appealed to the private sector by promising to purchase and donate to all farmers any treatment that would kill the blight. No successful antifungal treatment was discovered until years after the Irish famine.

Trade policy in the mid-nineteeth century was the subject of intense ideological debate. The individuals in power during much of the famine were ardent proponents of free trade, or laissez faire—a policy of minimal government intervention in markets. The Irish famine put pressures on both sides of the debate over free trade. On the one hand, the famine provided the impetus for repeal of the Corn Laws that restricted imports of food into Ireland. On the other hand, exports of food from Ireland continued. The rigidity of the position in favor of free trade is reflected in an exchange between Randolph Routh, an official in Ireland administering food distribution, and Charles Trevelyn, the permanent head of the treasury for the British government:

> Routh: "I know there is great and serious objection to any interference with these [food] exports, yet it is a most serious evil."
> Trevelyan: "We beg of you not to countenance in any way the idea of prohibiting exportation. The discouragement and feeling of insecurity to the [grain] trade from such a proceeding would prevent its doing even any immediate good; and there cannot be a doubt that it would inflict a permanent injury on the country" (quoted in Donnelly 2001, p. 69).

Some scholars point to evidence of substantial reductions in grain exports to conclude that "even if exports had been prohibited, Ireland lacked sufficient food . . . to stave off famine" (Gray 1982:46). Kinealy notes that exports of other food commodities remained high, and concludes: "The Irish poor did not starve because there was an inadequate supply of food within the country, they starved because political, commercial, and individual greed was given priority over the saving of lives" (2002:116).

If trade policy illustrates the role of ideology in policy, poverty assistance or relief policy illustrates the law of unintended consequences. Policies to help the poor during the famine were under constant discussion and revision. The government policies included such aspects as:

- Importation of grain from the United States
- "Work houses" where poor families could live
- Public works programs to provide incomes to the jobless
- Soup kitchens distributing prepared food

The cost of these programs was financed in large part through a tax on Irish landlords. The amount of the tax depended on how many poor households or tenants lived on the landlord's property. Landlords realized that they could reduce their tax burden by evicting tenants from their farms and destroying the tenant cottages. In this way, the policy intended to help the poor actually ended up separating many poor people from their shelter and from their means of growing food.

The evictions had the impact of consolidating land holdings into larger farms. Between 1841 and 1851, the number of small farms (5 acres or less) dropped from over three hundred thousand to less than a hundred thousand. The number of large farms (30 acres or more) tripled (Abbot 2003). Many landlords, having lost their rent-paying tenants, went bankrupt. Over the next decades, the landlord-tenant system died out, and it became commonplace for Irish farmers to own the land that they worked.

Some of the better-off tenants who lost their homes to eviction had sufficient resources to emigrate to the Americas. During the 1840s, an estimated 1.3 million Irish people emigrated. The conditions of their voyages were harsh: perhaps as many as 40 percent of the emigrants died during the passage to the Americas (Abbot 2003).

■ Famines Created by Government Policies

Two of the worst famines in the last century occurred in centrally planned economies: the Ukrainian famine of the 1930s and the Chinese "Great Leap Forward" famine of the 1950s. If the Irish potato famine can be blamed in part on a laissez-faire ideology, these two famines illustrate that state socialism is not immune to poor policy choices that cause or exacerbate famine conditions.

The Ukraine Famine, 1932–1933

By the early 1930s, the urban industrial regions of the Soviet Union had been transformed into a collectively (or state-) owned, centrally planned system. In 1929, Stalin introduced a policy of compulsory collectivization of agriculture. Under the collectivization plan, all of the productive assets—land, machinery, cattle, and so forth—of 25 million farmers were to be aggregated into 250,000 collective and state farms.

Even if collectivization had been enthusiastically embraced by Soviet farmers, the process of reorganization would no doubt have been awkward and aggregate agricultural production may have dipped. There were difficulties obtaining agricultural machinery and managing the transportation of agricultural goods, as well as inexperienced managers of the new large farms.

In addition to these problems, the collectivization process was resisted by farmers. For example, farmers slaughtered their horses and cattle rather than surrender them to the collective. This resistance was especially strong in the Ukraine, where peasants had always cultivated their own land, and therefore "had a much stronger sense of private ownership and deeper feeling of freedom and independence" compared to Russian peasants (Dolot 1985:xiv).

The objectives of the central Soviet government during the early 1930s were therefore to maintain ample food supplies for the urban industrial sector while completing the transformation of agriculture to a collective system. In the Ukraine, these objectives were pursued by giving farmers a quota of grain that had to be shipped. Farmers who resisted joining the collectives were forced to ship their entire crops:

> Stepan Schevchenko was a poor farmer . . . like the rest of us [, different] from us in only one way: he had categorically refused to join the collective farm. He paid off all his taxes for the year 1932, and apparently thought that the government would leave him alone. . . . But he was overly optimistic. One day he received a requisition order demanding him to deliver 500 kilograms of wheat to the state. He delivered it in full. But no sooner had he done so when he received another order. This time they demanded twice as much wheat, . . . [even though] he had none left. . . . The officials . . . threatened him with Siberia, . . . [and] he was forced to sell everything he had of value, including his cow, to buy the order of wheat. . . . He soon received the inexorable third order: 2,000 kilograms of wheat immediately! . . . The Bread Procurement Commission paid him a visit. . . . He and his family were ordered to leave their house. . . . All that belonged to the Shevchenkos was confiscated and [became] "socialist property" (Dolot 1985:146).

The seizure of all available stocks of food in the Ukraine caused widespread starvation among the very people who produced the food in the first place. The most extreme famine conditions were suffered in the Ukraine for several reasons: the more active resistance to collectivization in the Ukraine, a nationalistic or ethnic bias against Ukrainians on the part of the Russo-centric decisionmakers in Moscow, and a desire to hide evidence that the agricultural collectivization experiment was less than perfectly successful.

An estimated 6–8 million Ukrainians died during the famine (of a pre-famine population of about 34 million) (see Mace 1984:vi). This leads some historians to compare it to the holocaust of the Nazi concentration camps. (See Table 2.1 for a historical perspective of famines in Europe.) James Mace draws these sobering conclusions: "The Great Famine of 1932–33 is unique in the annals of human history in that it was wrought neither by some natural calamity nor even by the unintentional devastation created by warring armies. It was an act of policy, carried out for political ends in peacetime. It was deliberately man-made" (p. i).

Table 2.1 Largest Famines in Europe

Area Affected	Date	Excess Deaths (in thousands)	Area Affected	Date
Ukraine	1946–47	2,000	England	1321
Greece	1941–43	400	England, Ireland	1314
Lower Volga	1932–34	5,000	England, Scotland	
Ukraine[a]	1921–22	3,000	Ireland	1302
		9,000	England	1294
Eastern Urals	1911–12	8,000	England	1257–59
Ukraine	1905–06		England	1235
Western Plains,			Russia	1230–31
Russia	1897–98		Ireland	1227
Volga Valley	1891–93		Novogorod, Russia	1215
Ireland	1845–50	1,500	England, France	1193–96
Russia	1833–34		England, Wales	1183
Ireland	1822		England	1124
Poland	1770		Ireland	1116
Bohemia	1770		England	1093
Scotland	1766		Rostor-Volyn', Russia	1070–71
England	1740–41		England	1069
France	1661		England	1042–48
Ireland	1650–51		Suzdal, Russia	1024
Moscow	1601–03	500	England	1004–05
England	1594–95		England	976
Ireland	1588–89		Bolobereg	971
England, Ireland	1586		England, Wales,	
Hungary	1586		Scotland	954–58
England	1549		Scotland	936–39
England	1527		England	310
England	1521		Scotland	306
Hungary	1505		Scotland	228
Ireland	1497		Ireland	192
Ireland	1447		Rome	185
England	1437–39		Italian Peninsula	79–88
Ireland	1410		England	54
England	1392–93		Rome	23
England	1353		Rome	AD 6
Europe[b]	1346–50	40,000	Rome	385 BC
England, Scotland[c]	1341–42		Rome	436 BC

Source: Mabbs-Zeno 1987.
Notes: a. Estimates from two different sources.
b. Most deaths not due to malnutrition.
c. No record of excess deaths exists prior to this date.

Table 2.2   Largest Famines in India and Bangladesh Since 1700

Area Affected	Date	Excess Deaths (in thousands)
Bangladesh	1974	1,000
Bengal	1943	1,500–3,000
Punjab, Central Provinces	1899–1900	2,500
Bengal, Bombay, Central Provinces	1885–97	5,000
Orissa, Ganjam	1888–89	1,500
Madras, Bombay, Hyderabad	1876–78	5,000–8,000
Punjab, Deccan	1868–70	2,500
Orissa, Hyderabad[a]	1865–67	1,900
		10,000
Madras, Deccam	1853–55	
North	1837–38	800
Southeast	1833–34	
Madras	1832–33	
Sind, Rajasthan, Madras	1812–13	1,500
West	1802–03	
Bombay, Hyderabad	1790–93	
Mahratta	1787	
Bihar, Madras, Mysore	1781–83	
Afgot, Chingleput, Madras	1780–82	
Bengal, Bihar	1770	10,000
Chingleput	1733	
Madurai	1709–21	
Decca	1702–04	2,000

Source: Mabbs-Zeno 1987.
Note: a. Estimates from two different sources.

The Chinese Great Leap Forward Famine: 1959–1961

The most destructive famine in terms of human lives lost occurred in China during Mao's "Great Leap Forward." During this period, a large number of social and economic changes were being instigated by the central government. In the agricultural sector, collectivization began in 1952 and was successful in increasing agricultural output through 1958. Beginning in 1958, the government insisted that farmers undertake untested production methods based on unorthodox (and as the Chinese experience was to prove, flawed) science. The government forced a reorganization of smaller group or cooperative farms into larger communes (see Box 2.1). In addition, a commitment to an ideology of regional self-sufficiency led to a program that forced farm workers to divert some of their working hours to industrial production such as small-scale steel plants. China was also seeking to establish its economic independence from the Soviet Union, so food exports were increased during 1959 and 1960 to repay debts.

Simultaneously with these changes in government policies, poor

Box 2.1 Incentives in Chinese Agricultural Communes.

One of the changes that accompanied the Great Leap Forward campaign was a change in the way group farms were organized. Economist Justin Yifu Lin (1990) has examined the details of farm organization and concludes that the changes in the rules of these organizations contributed to the famine of 1959–1961.

After the revolution of 1949, many Chinese farmers voluntarily formed cooperatives of different types. In "mutual aid teams," a handful of neighboring families would share tools and draft animals and would help on each other's plots when needed. Each farm household continued to own land, tools, and animals; each family made its own decisions about what crops to plant; each family received the output from its land for consumption or sale. In "elementary cooperatives," twenty to thirty households agreed to combine into a single farm. Here, each family continued to own land, tools, and animals, but the decisions were communal, and output was shared. The sharing of output depended on how much land, tools, and animals the household contributed to the cooperative, and on how much work each household contributed. In "advanced cooperatives" the cooperative itself owned the land, tools, and animals, and members shared in output based solely on their labor contribution.

Each of these three kinds of organization provided an incentive for people to work hard: the harder you work, the more you earn. Even in the most "communal" of these organizations—advanced cooperatives—each farm household received a bigger share of the commune's output if it contributed more labor. What is more, Lin points out, the fact that membership was voluntary created an additional reason for families not to be laggards. If one family became known as a lazy household, the other hardworking households could form a new cooperative the following year, leaving out the lazy household. The initial collectivization effort in China was quite successful; agricultural output increased 28 percent from 1952 to 1958.

In 1958, the central government disbanded existing agricultural cooperatives and forced all farmers to join large communes of about 5,000 households and 10,000 acres. As well as being larger than previous cooperatives, the rules of organization were different in two important respects. First, peasants were paid "based mainly on subsistence needs and only partly on worked performed" (p. 1236). Second, membership in the communes was no longer voluntary, and peasants were forbidden from withdrawing from the commune. With this change, it became "impossible to use withdrawal [from the commune] either as a way to protect onself or as a means to check the possibility of shirking by the other members. . . . Since supervision in agricultural production is extremely difficult, . . . incentives to work in a compulsorily formed . . . collective must be low. A peasant will not work as hard as on the household farm. Therefore the productivity level of a collective will be lower than the level reached on the individual household farm" (p. 1242).

Lin notes that the downturn in production coincided exactly with the adoption of these new rules for cooperatives. The rules were abandoned in 1961, again coinciding exactly with the rebound in agricultural production.

Table 2.3   Largest Famines in China Since 1800

Area Affected	Date	Excess Deaths (in thousands)
China	1958–60	30,000
Honan	1941	3,000
Northwest	1929–32	5,000
Central	1925	
North	1920–21	500
North	1892–94	
Honan	1887–89	2,000
North	1876–79	10,000
China	1846–49	5,000
China	1810–11	20,000

Source: Mabbs-Zeno 1987.

weather conditions occurred in the years 1959–1961; conditions were especially poor in 1960 and 1961, with 15–20 percent of agricultural land being hit by natural calamity. Agricultural production, which had risen by 28 percent from 1952 to 1958, fell back below 1952 levels. A paper by Houser and Sands (2000) looks at regional data to see whether higher mortality rates were uniform throughout the country (as we would expect if policy caused the famine), or whether there were geographical differences (as we would expect if weather problems caused the famine). They conclude that about two-thirds of the famine-related deaths are attributable to policy mistakes, and about one-third to poor weather.

An estimated 30 million people died prematurely as a result of the Great Leap Forward famine. (See Tables 2.2 and 2.3 for a historical perspective on other famines in Asia.) The enormity of the problem emboldened political leaders in the provinces to abandon the policies imposed by Mao's central government. The famine can be said to have had political as well as demographic consequences, as power devolved to the provinces until the Cultural Revolution in the late 1960s reasserted the primacy of the central government.

■ Recent Famines: North Korea and Southern Africa

The famines described above were in a sense "national" problems. In none of the cases was there a discussion about how the world community could or should respond to the famine. Recent experiences with famine illustrate an evolving internationalist perspective.

North Korea

Since the 1990s, North Korea (the Democratic Peoples Republic of Korea) has suffered from famine conditions of varying intensity. The roots of this famine are found in the Cold War. During the Cold War, North Korea was closely allied with the Soviet Union and China, often playing one of those superpowers off against the other to get increased aid. With the breakup of the Soviet Union and the end of the Cold War, this aid dried up. Not only did food donations dwindle, but domestic agriculture in North Korea, which had been designed to utilize subsidized imports of energy and fertilizer, now required radical restructuring. Drought struck in 1995, and an estimated 2–3 million people (about 10 percent of the population) died from famine-related illness in the 1994–1998 period. (See Box 2.2.)

The response of the Korean government undoubtedly made things worse. Prior to the famine, nearly all grain in Korea was produced on state or communal farms. The workers on these farms were given a grain ration out of the harvest that was nutritionally sufficient. As grain yields began to fall because of poor weather and insufficient inputs, the central government cut peasant worker rations by over a third. The intention was to preserve more of the grain harvest for shipment to hungry urban areas. The unintended impact was to reduce the grain harvest even further, for two reasons (Natsios 1999): (1) Farm workers secretly "preharvested"—taking grain out of the communal fields before it was ready for harvest—and hid the grain for their own consumption. Because the grain was harvested before it was fully ripe, the grain yield was lower than it would have been if harvested according to plan; (2) farmers diverted effort from communal fields to legal and illegal private plots. These private plots were often in poor terrain and the yields lower than on the collective farms, but the output did not have to be shared.

Box 2.2   A Diet of Grass, Trees, and Children

Starving people resort to extreme behavior. Reports from North Korea illustrate this in striking ways. In 1997, Oxfam, a leading hunger-related nongovernmental organization, reported "people in North Korea are eating 'wild' foods like bark, leaves and grasses, in their desperation to survive the famine that is presently sweeping the country."

In 2003, in a macabre echo of Jonathan Swift's "Modest Proposal," reports emerged of a particularly horrible form of cannibalism in North Korea. "Aid agencies are alarmed by refugees' reports that children have been killed and corpses cut up by people desperate for food. . . . Anyone caught selling human meat faces execution, but . . . one refugee said: "Pieces of 'special meat' are displayed on straw mats for sale. People know where they came from, but they don't talk about it. . . . If a funeral takes place during the day and the burial is performed that evening, the grave may be dug open and the body stolen before morning," said one refugee (Nicol 2003).

The international response to the famine was substantial. Shipments from all sources averaged over 1 million metric tons per year from 1995 to 1998 (Natsios 1999). (To put this in context, the World Food Programme estimated that in 2001, North Korea would produce 3 million metric tons of food, but would require 4.8 million metric tons to feed its population [Struck 2001].) Reliance on food donations from abroad has created pressure on the North Koreans to bring their foreign affairs and military policies into conformance with demands by countries that make the food donations. For example, in 2002 the United States suspended food aid to North Korea (see Dao 2003). Observers suspected that the suspension was a reaction to North Korea's refusal to halt its nuclear weapons program, although U.S. officials denied that this was the reason. Support for aid to North Korea was also undermined by reports of corruption in the aid distribution system and fears that the aid was not helping those most in need.

Southern Africa

International response also played a major role in ameliorating the impacts of famine conditions in southern Africa in the years 2002–2003. By June 2002, it was obvious that poor weather conditions (a drought followed by heavy rains during the harvest season) would devastate crop production in a large part of southeastern Africa, affecting Zimbabwe, Zambia, Lesotho, Malawi, Mozambique, and Swaziland.

The situation in Zambia was one of unusually poor weather occurring in an extremely poor country where much of the population suffers from undernutrition during "normal" or nonfamine times. Production of Zambia's staple crop—maize—fell in 2002 to a level about half that of the average output over the previous four years. Between mid-2002 and early 2003, the World Food Programme directed shipments of 130,000 metric tons of food to Zambia, helping to feed 1.7 million people. The weather conditions improved considerably for the 2003 crop, with maize production double that of 2002. Zambia faces ongoing problems of poverty, AIDS, and undernutrition, but the acute crisis of the 2002 famine has ebbed.

The weather situation in 2001–2002 in Zimbabwe was similar to that in Zambia. But in Zimbabwe food output was suppressed further by a government program to redistribute agricultural land. During Zimbabwe's period as a colony of Britain (when it was known as Southern Rhodesia) prime agricultural land along the railway line was given over to white commercial farmers. After independence in 1980, these farmers continued to farm the land, but the government was under increasing pressure from its supporters to seize the white-owned land and distribute it to indigenous supporters of the ruling party.

In the first eighteen years of independence, less than one-quarter of the land in commercial farms was acquired by the government and reassigned to black Zimbabwean families. In 1998, the land reform process was accelerated, and in 2000 a new law was passed authorizing the government to force white farmers to give up their farms. In addition, white farmers were forced off their farms by "farm invasions" that were not legally authorized. The area planted with maize on large commercial farms fell from 163,000 hectares in 1998 to 74,000 hectares in 1999, and to 61,000 hectares in 2000. Much of the land remained in cultivation in smaller parcels by the recipients of the land reform, but yields dropped precipitously. Zimbabwe cereal production in 2002 was less than one-quarter of the peak production of 1996.

The Zimbabwean government purchased substantial amounts of food, but additional help was needed from the international community. The ruthlessness of the land reform activities and the impression that the Zimbabwean government was turning a blind eye to lawless farm invasions created a reluctance on the part of developed-country donors to provide assistance. Ultimately, the World Food Programme did make substantial amounts of food aid available (in 2002–2003 amounting to about 500,000 metric tons of food). However, as of the summer of 2003 nearly half of Zimbabwe's population continues to face the specter of famine.

These historical examples illustrate the difference between famine and the problem of permanent undernutrition. Famine is a shock or a disaster— it is a disturbance to the normal condition. There is both good news and bad news in this. The good news is that the needed policy response to famine is a temporary (though urgent) response. The bad news is that existing institutional frameworks (laws, power structure, social mores) often lack the flexibility to respond, and thus exacerbate the impact of the natural disaster.

■ Famine and Disaster Relief

In times of famine, international disaster relief agencies respond as best they can to get food into the hands of the starving. But sometimes the relief can be a mixed blessing.

Reutlinger and his colleagues (1986:27) list the groups most likely to fall victim to a famine:

- Small-scale farmers or tenants whose crops have failed and who cannot find other employment in agriculture (the Wollo in Ethiopia in 1973)
- Landless agricultural workers who lose their jobs when agricultural production declines (Bangladesh 1974) or who face rapidly rising food prices and constant or declining wages (the great Bengal famine of 1943)
- Other rural people, including beggars who are affected by a decline in real income in the famine regions (almost all famines)

- Pastoralists who get most of their food by trading animals for food grains; their herds may be ravaged by the drought, or animal prices may collapse relative to food-grain prices (the Harerghe region of Ethiopia in 1974 and the drought-stricken Sahel in 1973)

The authors of a well-documented and detailed OXFAM report warn that poorly supervised or uncontrollable distribution of food aid can do more harm than good. To quote one example, a field worker helping out in a drought-relief food aid program (where the food handouts were supposed to be free of charge to the recipients) wrote:

In Haiti we had . . . a problem of theft and mishandling. In [a] town . . . fairly near to us and very badly hit by drought, the magistrate [appointed mayor] was known to sell PL480 [international relief] food for $7.00 a 50 pound bag. At other times the CARE food distributors were so desperate that they would just throw bags of food off the truck and drive on, so that the food would go to the strong and the swift (Jackson and Eade 1982:9).

When disaster has created the need for assistance, but the local food supplies are adequate, supplying emergency food relief can be counterproductive. It depresses the local price of food, in turn depressing the income of the local farming community, and may lead to other socially undesireable results (see Box 2.3).

Martin Ravallion (1997) did a thorough review of the economics literature regarding famines. He cites examples of failed policy responses to famine: "The British government's . . . non-intervention in food markets during [nineteenth-century] famines almost certainly made matters worse. . . . At the other extreme, . . . food procurement policies implemented [by] . . . the Soviet Union . . . resulted in severe famine in the Ukraine in the 1930s" (p. 1225). Ravallion draws the following lessons for policies in response to famine:

- *Better governance.* Greater democratization and freer flow of information in a society make it more difficult for a government to ignore famines.
- *Early warning and rapid response.* Policy interventions are likely to be more effective if they take place before famine conditions are firmly entrenched.
- *Increased aggregate food availability.* Policies to increase the total amount of food available in famine areas include food aid, policies to discourage hoarding in private or public storage, and policies to encourage domestic food production.
- *Distribution policies.* "Although the case is often strong for increasing aggregate food availability during a famine, food handouts need not be the best form of intervention from the point of view of minimizing

Box 2.3   When Food Aid Is Not Needed

Tony Jackson and Deborah Eade

Imported food may not be necessary at all, despite a major disaster, and its arrival may do more harm than good. The classic example of this comes from Guatemala where the earthquake in 1976 killed an estimated 23,000 people, injured over three times as many and left a million and a quarter homeless. The earthquake occurred in the middle of a record harvest. Local grain was plentiful and the crops were not destroyed but left standing in the fields or buried under the rubble but easy to recover.

During the first few weeks, small consumer items—salt, sugar, soap, etc.—were in short supply and temporarily unavailable in the shops. Some of these small items, such as salt, were lost when the houses collapsed. People expressed a need for these food items in the short period before commercial supplies were resumed. However, during that year, about 25,400 tons of basic grains and blends were brought in as food aid from the US. A further 5,000 tons of US food aid already stored in Guatemala were released and supplies were also sent in from elsewhere in the region.

Catholic Relief Services (CRS) and CARE both received reports from their field staff saying food aid was not needed. The Director of CARE's housing reconstruction program visited the disaster area soon after the earthquake. In a US Government report he stated:

"Another thing I was really concerned with was whether there was any need to import food or seed. But I saw no indication of that whatsoever. First of all, the earth was not damaged, and there was no reason why the crops couldn't be harvested on time, and I believe it was a good crop that year. Also, in a few places I visited, I asked people if they could pull the food they had in their houses out of the rubble, and they said they certainly could."

CRS field staff objected to the importing of food aid but they were over-ruled by their headquarters in New York. Two weeks after the disaster, the League of Red Cross Societies asked national Red Cross societies to stop sending food. As early as February (the same month as the earthquake), the Co-ordinator of the National Emergency Committee of the Government of Guatemala asked voluntary agencies to stop imports of food aid. On 4 March, the Assistant Administrator for the Latin America Bureau of the United States Agency for International Development (AID), the Hon. Herman Kleine, testified before a House of Representatives Sub-Committee. "I should like to add here, Mr. Chairman, that the Guatemalan Government has requested officially to all donors that further contributions not be of food and medicine but roofing and building materials."

Finally, the Government of Guatemala invoked a presidential decree to prohibit imports of basic grains from May 1976 onwards. Yet after this decree, quantities of food aid were still imported in the form of blended foodstuffs. One article refers to these blends as "basic grains in disguise."

Field staff and local leaders identified three negative results. Firstly, they considered that food aid contributed to a drop in the price of local grain that occurred soon after the earthquake and continued throughout 1976. As to the need for basic grains, a peasant farmer explained: "There was no shortage.

continues

Continued

There was no need to bring food from outside. On the contrary, our problem was to sell what we had."

After an extensive survey of towns and villages in the worst-hit areas six weeks after the earthquake, an OXFAM–World Neighbors official reported: "Virtually everyone in the area is selling more grain this year than he does normally. Furthermore, emergency food shipments have drastically curtailed demand for grains. Thus the prices of the farmers' produce have plummeted."

Later, the then Director of CRS in Guatemala was to tell the *New York Times:* "The general effect was that we knocked the bottom out of the grain market in the country for nine to twelve months."

This last view may be overstated as other factors, such as the excellent grain harvest, would usually have led to a fall in prices anyway. Nonetheless, the basic fact remains: $8 million of food aid was sent into a country with plentiful food-stocks of its own. Any food that it was necessary to distribute to earthquake victims could have been bought in Guatemala (as the World Food Programme did).

The second negative effect of the continuing supply of free food was to encourage the survivors to queue for rations instead of engaging in reconstruction or normal agricultural work.

Thirdly, it brought about a change in the quality and motivation of local leadership. The OXFAM–World Neighbors official, quoted above, noted:

"Immediately after the earthquake, we tended to see the same leaders whom we'd seen before the earthquake—people [with] a high degree of honesty and personal commitment to the villages. But gradually . . . I began seeing fellas who I knew were totally dishonest. They'd go into the different agencies and . . . say that theirs was the most affected village in the Highlands, and they'd get more food. So largely because of the give-aways, the villages started to turn more to leaders who could produce free things like this, whether they were honest or dishonest, rather than to the leaders they'd been putting their trust in for years.

With larger and larger quantities of free food coming in, there are increased incentives to corruption. . . . Groups that had worked together previously became enemies over the question of recipients for free food."

Source: Extracted from Jackson and Eade 1982:9–11.

---

mortality. Cash or coupon payments to potential famine victims can provide more effective relief than the usual policy of importing and distributing food" (p. 1230).

• *Stabilization policies.* "An effective but affordable . . . stabilization policy in famine-prone economies . . . will probably combine buffer stocks and . . . a relatively open external trade regime" (p. 1233). Buffer stocks are programs in which the government purchases food in periods when it is plentiful and sells food out of their stocks when shortages occur.

  • *Other policies.* Ravallion argues that there are potential synergies between policies to address famines and other policies to spur economic development, including credit programs, improved infrastructure, and assignment of property rights.

3

Malnutrition Defined

One common definition of malnutrition is "overconsumption or underconsumption of any essential nutrient." This chapter will be devoted to exploring this definition.

■ Four Types of Malnutrition

The internationally famous nutritionist Jean Mayer (1976) identifies four types of malnutrition: (1) overnutrition, (2) secondary malnutrition, (3) dietary deficiency or micronutrient malnutrition, and (4) protein-calorie malnutrition.

Overnutrition

When a person consumes too many calories, the resulting condition is called *overnutrition*. Overnutrition is the most common nutritional problem in high-income countries such as the United States, although high-income people in low-income countries also suffer from this type of malnutrition. The diet of the world's high-income people is usually overladen with calories, saturated fats, salt, and sugar. Their diet-related illnesses include obesity, diabetes, hypertension, and atherosclerosis. This is a serious problem, and is being addressed through an international effort coordinated by the World Health Organization (WHO 2002); however, it is not the focus of this book.

Secondary Malnutrition

When a person has a condition or illness that prevents proper digestion or absorption of food, that person suffers what is called *secondary malnutrition*. It is called "secondary" because it does not result directly from the nature of the diet, as do the other types of malnutrition, which are termed *primary*. Common causes of secondary malnutrition are diarrhea, respiratory illnesses, measles, and intestinal parasites. The following mechanisms cause secondary malnutrition:

- *Loss of appetite (anorexia)*
- *Alteration of the normal metabolism.* For example, when the body shifts some of its attention to fighting infection, among other things, production of disease-fighting white blood cells may be increased and body temperature raised.
- *Prevention of nutrient absorption.* For instance, diarrheal infections irritate the lining of the gastrointestinal tract, creating difficulty in absorbing nutrients and at the same time causing it to shed contents before full digestion has had time to occur.
- *Diversion of nutrients to parasitic agents.* Parasites such as hookworms, tapeworms, and schistosome worms rob the body of nutrients it would otherwise retain (Briscoe 1979; Martorell 1980).

Public health measures such as providing sanitary human-waste disposal and clean water are especially important in reducing secondary malnutrition. Low-income people in developing countries are at risk for undernutrition (insufficient calories), which is commonly exacerbated by secondary malnutrition (e.g., a diarrheal infection that robs the body of nutrients). Because of the strong link between the two, undernutrition and secondary malnutrition are commonly grouped together and called, simply, *undernutrition.*

Dietary Deficiency or Micronutrient Malnutrition

A diet lacking sufficient amounts of one or more essential micronutrients, such as a vitamin or a mineral, results in dietary deficiency. Although a deficiency of any micronutrient can become a serious problem, most nutritionists are primarily concerned about deficiencies in vitamin A, iodine, and iron.

Vitamin A. Deficiency of vitamin A can cause "xerophthalmia," or night blindness. It is also associated with increased mortality from respiratory and gastrointestinal disease. One study suggested that vitamin A supplements could reduce deaths of children aged between six months and five years by 23 percent. Recent research suggests that vitamin A plays a role in maintaining the immune system and in fighting cancer.

Iodine. Iodine deficiency causes goiter and leads to a reduction in mental abilities. Babies born to iodine-deficient mothers can suffer from "cretinism," which can result in learning disabilities in children. One study indicates that even mild iodine deficiency can reduce intelligence quotients (IQ) by 10–15 points. Iodine deficiency is the greatest single cause of preventable brain damage and mental retardation. The WHO estimates that one-third of the world's people live in "iodine-deficiency environments."

Iron. Iron deficiency, or anemia, causes reduced capacity to work, diminished ability to learn, increased susceptibility to infection, and greater risk of death during pregnancy and childbirth. More than 40 pecent of people in developing countries are estimated to suffer from iron deficiency.

Other micronutrients. In recent years, nutritionists have become concerned about zinc deficiencies. Zinc now appears to be effective in increasing the growth of very young children; it also reduces the incidence of diarrhea and assists in absorption of other micronutrients. Other diseases caused by micronutrient deficiencies include rickets (soft bones), caused by vitamin D deficiency; scurvy, caused by vitamin C deficiency; and beri-beri and pellagra, caused by deficiencies in B vitamins. Some research (Tang et al. 1993) indicates that the risk of contracting AIDS is substantially lower among those who consumed very high levels of niacin (a B-vitamin), vitamin A, and vitamin C.

When compared with underconsumption of proteins or calories, the problem of underconsumption of micronutrients appears relatively easy to solve. The missing elements are inexpensive, and programs to provide them are relatively easy to initiate. In the United States, "iodized" salt (salt to which iodine has been added) protects us from iodine deficiency, specially fortified milk provides vitamin A (and vitamin D), and iron pills (or multiple vitamins with iron) are a common source of iron. Examples of successful interventions in the developing world are as follows:

- In Guatemala, dietary anemia was greatly reduced in a rural community after the inhibitants were persuaded to substitute iron cooking pots for aluminum pots.
- Also in Guatemala, fortification of sugar with vitamin A has been effective, and experiments are now under way to fortify sugar with iron.
- In Brazil, a school's drinking water was fortified with iron, creating a noticeable improvement in students' iron levels at a cost of about 15 cents per student per year.
- In China, iodine deficiency was treated by dripping potassium iodate solution into the water of an irrigation canal. The amount of iodine excretion by people in the area increased two-and-a-half times.

Other interventions to combat micronutrient malnutrition include making vitamin pills available to the population and cultivating plants that contain one or more micronutrients. The World Bank (1994) estimated that it would cost about $3 per year to meet a person's entire needs for vitamin A, iron, and iodine. By comparison, an antioxidant formula of vitamin E, beta-carotene, and vitamin C may cost $60 per person per year.

Despite the apparently easy solution to these vitamin and mineral deficiencies, the problems have remained surprisingly persistent. In the mid-1990s, the World Bank launched a "Micronutrient Initiative" to reduce these types of deficiencies. Under this initiative, in 2002, 300 million children under the age of five were given a high-dose vitamin A supplement. This remains an important policy because of the huge impact on public health that relatively small expenditures can have. As we shall see in the next chapter, the health impacts of micronutrient deficiencies are significant. However, the solutions to these deficiencies are more likely to come from fortification programs such as those described above, and less likely to come from additional food consumption and production.

Protein-Calorie Malnutrition

The underconsumption of calories or protein—known as *protein-calorie malnutrition* (PCM) or *protein-energy malnutrition* (PEM)—is a problem that can only be solved by increasing the amount of food that an individual eats. A person suffering from PCM is short of the protein or calories needed for normal growth, health, and activity. PCM hardly ever occurs in families with enough income to satisfy their basic needs for food, shelter, clothing, and heat; PCM is found predominantly in low-income countries where poverty is widespread.

In extreme forms, PCM manifests itself as the potentially fatal nutritional disorders known as *kwashiorkor* and *marasmus* (see Boxes 3.1 and 3.2). Kwashiorkor is most likely to be encountered among populations where the diet is heavily based on cassava (as in West Africa) or on plantains (as in parts of Latin America and southern Uganda). These particular plant foods are almost completely devoid of available protein, and children who are weaned on them are at high risk for severe protein deficiency. Marasmus is most likely to occur under conditions of extreme poverty in which children are weaned onto a gruel that contains modest amounts of protein, but where available food is nutritionally inadequate. Marasmus is thus more common among the poorest populations of the world, such as those of Ethiopia, Nepal, and Bangladesh. Without warmth, loving care, and expert medical attention, children with marasmus or kwashiorkor can die quickly.

Calories and Protein

Because PCM is a major source of nutrition-related disease, and because reducing PCM requires increasing food consumption, much of this book

Box 3.1 Kwashiorkor

Eleanor Whitney and Eva Hamilton

The word kwashiorkor originally meant "the evil spirit which infects the first child when the second child is born." It is easy to see how this superstitious belief arose among those Ghanaians who named the disease. When a mother who has been nursing her first child bears a second child, she weans the first and puts the second on the breast. The first child soon begins to sicken and die, just as if an evil spirit had accompanied the new baby into the world and set out to destroy the older child. What actually happens, of course, is that protein deficiency follows soon after weaning, for while breast milk provides these children with sufficient protein, they are generally weaned to a protein-poor gruel.

Millions of children in the world are affected by kwashiorkor. It typically sets in around the age of two. By the time children with kwashiorkor are four, their growth is stunted; they are no taller than they were at two. Their hair has lost its color; their skin is patchy and scaly, sometimes with ulcers or open sores which fail to heal. Their bellies are swollen with edema; they sicken easily, and are weak, fretful, and apathetic.

The swollen belly of the kwashiorkor child is due to edema; blood protein is so low that fluid leaks out into the body. Since the child is too weak to stand much of the time, the fluid seeks the lowest available space—in this case the belly. The picture of such a child is one of skinny arms and legs and a greatly swollen belly. On first glance you might think the child is fat, but if the fluid could be drawn off, his true condition would be revealed: he is actually a wasted skeleton, just skin and bones.

The body follows a priority system when there is not enough protein supplied to meet all its needs. It abandons its less vital systems first. When it cannot obtain amino acids enough from dietary sources, the body switches to a metabolism of wasting, and begins to digest its own protein tissues in order to supply the amino acids needed to build the most vital internal proteins and keep itself alive. Hair and skin pigments (which are made from amino acids) are dispensable and are not manufactured. The skin needs less integrity in a life-and-death situation than the heart, so its maintenance ceases and skin sores fail to heal. Many of the antibodies are also degraded in order that their amino acids may be used as building blocks for heart and lung and brain tissue. Children with a lowered supply of antibodies cannot resist infection and readily contract dysentery, a disease of the digestive tract. Dysentery causes diarrhea, leading to rapid loss of those nutrients—including amino acids—which these children may be receiving in food. Thus dysentery worsens the protein deficiency, and the protein deficiency in turn increases the likelihood of a second or third or tenth attack of dysentery.

The water loss in diarrhea increases losses of the water-soluble B vitamins and vitamin C. The children's inability to manufacture protein carriers for the fat-soluble vitamins makes them deficient in vitamins A and D as well. Their inability to manufacture protein carriers for fat often leaves them with fat accumulated in the liver tissue, from which it would normally be carried away. As the liver clogs with fat, its cells become unable to carry out their other normal functions, and gradually they atrophy and die.

Source: Reprinted from *Understanding Nutrition* by Whitney, Hamilton & Rolfes, copyright 1990 by West Publishing Company. Used by permission of Wadsworth Publishing Company.

Box 3.2   Marasmus

Eleanor Whitney and Eva Hamilton

When children are almost totally deprived of food, they cannot obtain the energy necessary to maintain their body systems, much less that necessary for growth. Marasmus, a wasting disease, results. Invariably, protein deficiency occurs with this condition, as available protein is used not to build body protein but to supply energy (which takes priority). As a result, the marasmic child has many, though not all, of the same symptoms as the child with kwashiorkor.

Marasmic children are wizened little old people in appearance, just skin and bones. They are often sick because their resistance to disease is low. Their hearts are weak, and all their muscles are wasted. Their metabolism is slow. They have little or no fat under their skin to insulate against cold. Their body temperatures may be subnormal. The experience of hospital workers with victims of this disease is that their primary need is to be wrapped up and kept warm. They need love, since they have often been deprived of maternal attention as well as food.

Unlike the kwashiorkor child, who is fed milk until weaning, the marasmic child may have been neglected from early infancy. The disease occurs most commonly in children from six to eighteen months of age in all the overpopulated city slums of the world. Since the brain normally grows to almost its full adult size within the first two years of life, marasmus impairs brain development and so may have a permanent effect on learning ability.

Marasmus also occurs in adults in countries where calorie deficiency is prevalent.

Source: Reprinted by permission from Understanding Nutrition by Whitney, Hamilton & Rolfes, copyright 1990 by West Publishing Company. Used by permission of Wadsworth Publishing Company.

will focus on PCM. These two elements—calories and protein—are both derived from food and are both necessary for growth, health, activity, and survival. But their nutritional roles are different. More important, calories and proteins are derived from foods in different ways, and a diet must be carefully planned if it is to be adequate in both.

Nutritional Role of Calories and Proteins

Calories are a measure of the energy contained in food (see Box 3.3). The body gets energy from carbohydrates (e.g., sugar and starch) and fats (e.g., corn oil and butter). Calories are used by the body to provide energy needed for

- The "involuntary functions" such as breathing, blood circulation, digestion, and maintaining muscle tone and body temperature

- Physical activity
- Mental activity
- Fighting disease
- Growth

The human body makes the millions of different proteins that it needs from some twenty amino acids, which are the building blocks of the body's proteins. Proteins function in ways other than providing a source of calories:

- They are necessary for building the cells that make up muscles, membranes, cartilage, and hair.
- They carry oxygen around our bodies.
- They carry nutrients into and out of cells and help assimilate food.
- They contribute to the development of antibodies that fight disease.
- They work as enzymes that speed up the digestive process.

Simple organisms such as yeasts and algae can synthesize almost all of the amino acids they need. But humans cannot synthesize some amino acids; we make insufficient quantities of others for our requirements. To

---

Box 3.3   Calories and Kilocalories

In physics, chemistry, and engineering, a calorie is the amount of heat energy required at sea level to raise the temperature of one gram of water one degree centigrade. A kilocalorie (abbreviated Kcal) is the energy it takes at sea level to raise the temperature of 1,000 grams of water (a kilogram—also a liter) one degree centigrade.

Nutritionists always quote their data in kilocalories, but unfortunately commonly shorten the word to Calories. Usually people capitalize the word Calorie when intending to indicate a kilocalorie as distinguished from calorie. But the convention is not always observed. At any rate, when you are reading nutrition literature and see the word *calorie* (note the lower case c), it is safe to assume that it means kilocalorie.

There is another thing to bear in mind when comparing nutritional calories to those in the physical sciences. The energy value of foods found in the standard handbooks, such as *Agricultural Handbook* no. 8, represents the energy available after deductions have been made for losses in digestion and metabolism. The system for determining these energy values was developed through the classic investigations of W. O. Atwater and his associates at the Connecticut Agricultural Experiment Station.

For more information on this subject, consult U.S. Dept. of Agriculture 1963.

live, therefore, we must consume enough *essential amino acids* (those which the body cannot produce in sufficient quantities). Of the approximately twenty amino acids needed, nine are essential or "indispensable." Because the body cannot manufacture them, we must consume them as part of our diets. All of these amino acids are found in eggs, milk, and meat— proteins from these dietary sources that contain all the essential amino acids are referred to as *complete proteins.*

Proteins from vegetable sources tend to be deficient in at least one of the essential amino acids and are therefore "incomplete proteins." To understand the importance of this for diet, we need to understand the way that the human body takes the amino acids from protein in food and constructs protein for the body's use. Protein molecules in food are composed of fixed proportions of amino acids. A balanced protein is one in which the essential amino acids appear in the same ratio to each other as the body needs them for constructing its protein molecules. (This ratio is shown in Table 3.1, which also lists the dietary reference intakes for a healthy adult.)

If you consume more amino acids than you need, your body cannot use them for making proteins; instead, it burns the amino acids for energy. If you consume less of an amino acid than you need, a portion of other amino acids goes to waste for want of the "matching" part needed to manufacture protein molecules. Whitney and Hamilton (1977:92) provide a delightful analogy:

> Suppose that a signmaker plans to make 100 identical signs, each saying LEFT TURN ONLY. He needs 200 L's, 200 N's, 200 T's and 100 each of the other letters. If he has only 20 L's, he can make only 10 signs, even if all the other letters are available in unlimited quantities. The L's limit the number of signs that can be made. The quality of dietary protein depends

Table 3.1 Estimated Average Requirement (EAR) and Recommended Daily Allowance (RDA) for Essential Amino Acids for Adults (expressed in mg/day for each kg of bodyweight)

Essential Amino Acid	EAR in mg/kg/day	RDA in mg/kg/day
Histidine	11	14
Isoleucine	15	19
Leucine	34	42
Lysine	34	38
Methionine + cysteine	15	19
Phenylalnine + tyrosine	27	33
Threonine	16	20
Tryptophan	4	5
Valine	19	24

Source: National Academy of Science 2002, pp. 10-65–10-66.

first on whether or not the protein supplies all the essential amino acids, and second on the extent to which it supplies them in the relative proportions needed.

You can get balanced protein from animal products such as meat, milk, eggs, and cheese, but not from isolated grain or vegetable products. You can, however, get balanced protein by combining different *types* of grains and vegetable products (see Figure 3.1). Consuming a certain quantity of beans provides you with more than your needs for the amino acid lysine, but leaves you short on methionin and cystine. Consuming a certain quantity of wheat leaves you short of all the amino acids, especially lysine. A 50-50 mix of beans and wheat provides a reasonably balanced mix.

The Chemical Process of Producing Dietary Calories and Protein
The energy that our bodies use comes from the sun; but our bodies cannot absorb solar energy directly and use it for physical growth and activity. The chemical process by which plants transform solar energy into a form of energy (in plants) that can be absorbed by humans or animals is known as *photosynthesis:* carbon dioxide plus water plus radiant energy from the sun

Figure 3.1 Protein Complementarity Between a Cereal and a Pulse

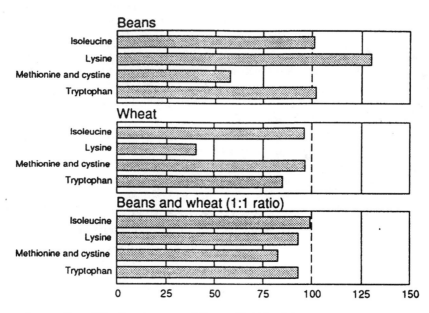

yields (in the presence of chlorophyll) a carbohydrate plus oxygen plus water. Written as a chemical equation:

Chlorophyll
$$6CO_2 + 12H_2O + \text{Light energy} \rightarrow C_6H_{12}O_6 + 6\ O_2 + 6\ H_2O$$

Using enzymes, a plant can rearrange the carbon, hydrogen, and oxygen atoms of the carbohydrate, or sugar ($C_6H_{12}O_6$), as shown in the above equation, to form starch or fat.

The conversion of sugar to starch is energy-efficient: practically all the energy in the original sugar can be released in burning the starch made from it. The conversion of sugar to fat, however, is about 77 percent energy-efficient, so we can say that most of the energy in the original sugar can be released in burning the fat that is made from it.

Making amino acids is not so easy. Like carbohydrates and fat, amino acids contain carbon, hydrogen, and oxygen, but they also contain nitrogen, and nitrogen in the form that can be used to build amino acids is scarce. In the process of photosynthesis, plants can use carbon dioxide (CO_2) straight from the atmosphere. But in making amino acids, nitrogen cannot be used as N_2, the form in which it is found in the atmosphere. It has to be converted to more complex forms, such as ammonia (NH_3), before the plant can use it.

Converting atmospheric nitrogen to usable nitrogen is called *nitrogen fixation*. It can be done in a commercial fertilizer plant, where energy is combined with some raw organic stock such as naptha. Or it can be done by nature, which provides three other ways of fixing nitrogen: (1) lightning storms, (2) nitrogen-fixing bacteria, and (3) blue-green algae. By and large, the nitrogen fixed by blue-green algae is not available to plants useful to man. Leguminous plants, such as beans, peas, and alfalfa, provide a suitable environment on their roots for nitrogen-fixing bacteria and thus have an extra boost of nitrogen available.

The fixed nitrogen taken up by plants becomes available in the food chain to make amino acids, and ultimately, proteins. Plants and animals must spend energy (use up sugar) to synthesize amino acids. They spend still more energy to recombine these amino acids into enormous molecules of protein. As a result, the energy available from burning a protein is substantially less than the energy used to produce that protein. By contrast, the amount of energy released in the burning of a carbohydrate or fat is closer to the amount of energy it took to make it in the first place.

Which Is the Bigger Problem:
Protein Deficiency or Calorie Deficiency?

The chemistry involved in producing calories and proteins helps explain why proteins are scarce relative to carbohydrates and fats. The relative scarcity implies that putting adequate protein into our diets is going to be more expensive than consuming adequate calories. And, generally speaking, we do pay a premium for protein-rich foods. For instance, you probably know that hamburger is a richer source of protein than rice and that hamburger costs more per pound than rice (and you can get about twice as many calories from a pound of rice as you can from a pound of hamburger).

Because protein is more expensive than carbohydrates, the question arises: Should we show more concern about the protein intake of poor people than we do about their calorie intake? Until the 1970s, nutritionists believed that protein was the central concern.

No doubt, protein deficiency can and does occur. However, the experience of the past thirty years demonstrates that calorie deficiency is a more widespread problem. For example, a study of 15,000 Indian preschool children in the 1960s found that 35 percent showed evidence of both calorie and protein deficiency, 57 percent showed evidence of calorie deficiency but not protein deficiency, but virtually none showed evidence of protein deficiency without an accompanying calorie deficiency.

Recent data on food availability also indicate that calorie deficiency is likely to present a bigger problem than protein deficiency. Food and Agriculture Organization of the United Nations (FAO) numbers for 2001 show that in sub-Saharan Africa, food available per capita would provide 2,229 calories and 53.9 grams of protein per person per day. If we compare this to the average requirements in Table 3.2 for adults, we see available protein is substantially higher than requirements for any group, but available calories are less than requirements for most adults (and substantially less than requirements for adult men and pregnant and lactating women). Similarly, numbers from the FAO's Sixth World Food Survey for 1990–1992 show that among the least-developed countries, food supplies provide 50 grams of protein per capita per day, but only 2,040 calories per capita per day.

Nevin Scrimshaw, a renowned advocate of the importance of protein in the diet, puts it like this: "It is true that adult protein needs are met by most traditional developing country diets when they are consumed in sufficient quantity to meet normal energy needs" (1988). A review of studies of protein intake in developing countries reached the same conclusion: "At the habitual levels of intake, only 75 to 80 percent of the . . . requirement for energy is satisfied, while more than the current safe level for dietary protein is supplied" (Rand, Uauy, and Scrimshaw 1984: section 5.1).

■ How Much of a Nutrient Is Enough?

Before describing what can happen when a person does not get enough of a nutrient, we need to explore what "enough" means. Of course, no single standard applies to everyone. Each person is different. Growing children

Table 3.2 Dietary Reference Intakes for Calories and Protein (by age, sex, and condition)

Category	Age (years) or Condition	Estimated Calorie Requirement (kcal per day)	Protein (grams per day) Estimated Average Requirement (EAR)	Protein (grams per day) Recommended Daily Allowance (RDA)
Males	0–0.5	570	9.1[b]	9.1[b]
	0.5–1	743	9.9	13.5
	1–3	1,046	10.6	13
	4–8	1,742	15.2	19
	9–13	2,279	27.4	34
	14–18	3,152	44.5	52
	19–30	3,012[a]	46.2	56
	31–50	2,852[a]	46.2	56
	51+	2,607[a]	46.2	56
Females	0–0.5	520	9.1[b]	9.1[b]
	0.5–1	676	9.9	13.5
	1–3	992	10.6	13
	4–8	1,642	15.2	19
	9–13	2,071	28.1	34
	14–18	2,368	38.3	46
	19–30	2,345[a]	37.6	46
	31–50	2,253[a]	37.6	46
	51+	2,081[a]	37.6	46
Pregnant	1st trimester	+0	+12	+25
	2nd trimester	+300	+12	+25
	3rd trimester	+300	+12	+25
Lactating	1st 6 months	+500	+22	+25
	2nd 6 months	+500	+22	+25

Sources: Protein RDA: National Academy of Sciences 2002. Protein EAR: National Academy of Sciences 2003, summary table 1. Calories EAR: Thomson-Wadsworth (developed from NAS 2002).

Notes: a. Figure for 19-year-olds is 3,067 for males and 2,403 for females. For each year above 19, subtract 10 for males or 7 for females. The numbers shown are for individuals 24.5 years old, 39.5 years old, and 65 years old for the three age groups.

b. For infants under 6 months, adequate intake of protein is reported.

have different nutritional needs than mature adults. Men have different nutritional needs than women. Active people have different nutritional needs than sedentary people. Box 3.4 describes how energy requirements can be different for two people of the same sex and age. And some people are just different for unexplainable reasons. For example, we all know someone who can eat and eat yet never gain weight; that person has a higher metabolism, or a higher daily need for calories, than the rest of us.

Nutritionists have several different ways of describing the nutritional needs of a group. The RDA (or recommended daily allowance) shows the

---

Box 3.4   How Many Calories Do I Need Each Day?

Table 3.2 shows the dietary reference intakes for people in different groups. But not everyone in each group is the same. To get an absolutely accurate calculation of how many calories you burn each day, you would need to undergo a complicated and expensive clinic assessment. But you can get a good estimate by using the following formulas (applicable to people over age nineteen who are not excessively fat or thin):

For men
661.8 – 9.53 x AGE (yrs) + PAC x [15.92 x WEIGHT(kg) + 539.6 x HEIGHT (m)]

For women
354.1 – 6.91 x AGE (yrs) + PAC x [9.36 x WEIGHT (kg) + 726 x HEIGHT (m)]

Plug in your age, weight (1 pound = .4536 kg), and height (1 inch = .0254 m). The Physical Activity Coefficient (PAC) takes on one of four values, depending on how active you are.

Category	PAC	Example of daily exercise done by people in this category
Sedentary	1	None
Low Active	1.12	30 minutes of moderate walking
Active	1.27	30 minutes of moderate walking, 25 minutes of moderate bicycling, and 40 minutes of tennis
Very Active	1.45	45 minutes of moderate cycling, 25 minutes of jogging, and 60 minutes of tennis

You can see how there can be a wide range of calorie requirements for different people in the same category. Consider two twenty-one-year-old men. One is 5 feet 3 inches, weighs 104 pounds, and has a sedentary lifestyle. His daily calorie requirement is about 2,000. The other 6 feet 3 inches, weighs 199 pounds, and has an active lifestyle. His daily calorie requirement is about 4,000.

---

nutrient level at which 97–98 percent of the group will be adequately nourished. These are useful as targets for an individual: An individual who gets his/her RDA of a nutrient can be quite confident of obtaining an adequate level of that nutrient. However, "RDAs are not useful in estimating the prevalence of inadequate intakes for groups" (NAS 2002: p. 13-7). Nor are they appropriate as targets for the *average* intake of a group. For these purposes, a better measure is the estimated average requirement (EAR) (for calories, the EAR is often referred to as the estimated energy requirement). The EAR is the daily intake amount that will be adequate for half the individuals in the group. Thus, the EAR is always lower than the RDA.

(Compare the EAR and RDA for protein shown in Table 3.2.) The RDA for calories is no longer reported, since it might encourage people to consume too many calories (Trumbo et al. 2002).

The difference between the EAR and the RDA is shown in Figure 3.2. The normal (bell-shaped) shows the distribution of people in a certain group (say men between the ages of nineteen and twenty-two) according to how much of a certain nutrient (say calories) each person needs. Some men in this age group need few calories (near point A); some need a lot of calories (near point G). On the curve, point D is the mean (or average) requirement. This is the EAR. The degree to which the bell curve is spread out around the mean is measured by a statistic called the *standard deviation* (SD)—a large standard deviation means that the curve is a relatively flat spread-out bell; a small standard deviation means a tall, skinny bell. An intake level at point F is calculated by taking the standard deviation, multiplying it by two, and adding the result to the mean. Statisticians have shown that point F calculated in this way will show the following characteristics: nearly all (97.5 percent) of the people in the group will have a

Figure 3.2   Distribution of Nutrient Requirements in a Typical Population of Healthy Individuals

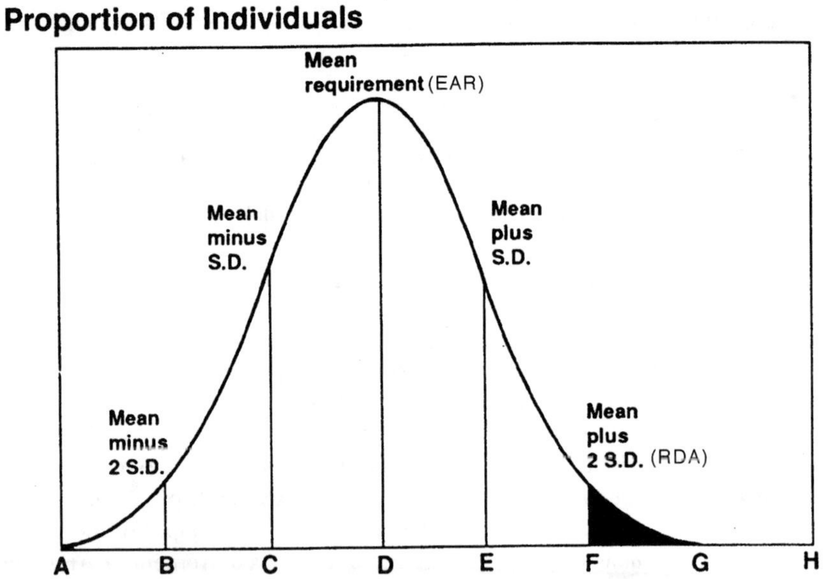

Proportion of Individuals

Note: The curve is bell-shaped. S.D. = standard deviation.

requirement that is less than F; only 2.5 percent of the population will have a requirement greater than F. The RDA for a nutrient in a given age-sex group is set at point F by adding two standard deviations to the mean requirement for the group.

RDAs and EARs for micronutrients (vitamins and minerals) can be found in National Academy of Sciences (2003).

4

Measuring Undernutrition

In the last chapter, we identified underconsumption of calories, protein, and micronutrients as the most serious types of malnutrition. Next we turn to the question of how we can measure the extent of undernutrition in a group. In this country, or city, or village, is undernutrition rare or is it commonplace? Because resources for coping with undernutrition are scarce, they must be spent wisely, and that requires that we accurately identify where the problem is the most serious.

■ Measuring the Nutritional Status of the Individual

Measurements of undernutrition in a group will be based on determinations of nutritional status individual by individual. The common methods of direct assessment of the nutritional status of an individual are: clinical, biochemical, dietary, and anthropometric. Each method has shortcomings and each may result in a somewhat different assessment of the nature and extent of nutritional disorders.

Clinical Assessment

Clinical assessment of nutritional status relies on the examination of physical signs on the body that are symptomatic of nutritional disorders (Jelliffe 1966). Kwashiokor, for instance is accompanied by loss of pigment in the hair (it often turns reddish) and by edema (swelling) of the ankles. Examples of clinical assessment can be found in a national Philippine nutrition survey that examined schoolchildren for goiter (a generalized swelling at the base of the neck above the collarbone) and found that 3.1 percent of children over the age of nine suffered from iodine deficiency. More recently, researchers examined the extent of vitamin A deficiency among preschool children in Mali by giving eye tests and diagnosing xerophthalmia (Schemann et al.).

Correct identification of nutritional disorders using physical signs depends not only on the training and skill of the clinician but on how well the signs are manifested in the particular individual. Clinical signs are diffi-

41

cult to quantify and are usually obvious only in the advanced stage of the disease; for this reason, clinical assessment can be used in only the most severe and specific types of nutritional disorders.

Biochemical Assessment

Biochemical assessment requires examination of bodily fluids such as blood or urine for the complex metabolic changes that accompany nutritional disorders. In the Philippine nutrition survey, over 14,000 blood samples were drawn and analyzed. From these samples and from using standards of the World Health Organization, 27 percent of the population were found to be anemic. The highest rates of anemia occurred in those under one year (51 percent) and in pregnant women (49 percent).

Biochemical tests provide an accurate indication of short-term nutritional problems, but their complexity and expense are an impediment to their widespread use in field surveys. Imagine the problems associated with persuading a sample of over 14,000 individuals living all over the Philippines to submit to having blood drawn—then transporting these samples to appropriate laboratory apparatus for analysis before they deteriorate in the heat!

Dietary Assessment

Dietary surveys are often employed to assess nutritional status. Two approaches are used: (1) dietary recall, in which the subject is asked to remember what he or she ate, say during the past twenty-four hours or the past seven days; and (2) dietary record, in which someone records the amount of food consumed at mealtimes, often by weighing it. Both methods have their advantages and drawbacks.

Dietary recall (see Box 4.1) has the advantage of researchers' being able to interview the subjects when they are not expecting to be surveyed; they are less likely to adjust their consumption because of the survey. Yet it is often difficult to remember exactly what you or members of your family ate during the past twenty-four hours, much less during the past week. And estimates of quantity consumed are particularly prone to error in recall surveys.

When keeping food records, especially if every portion of food must be weighed, the cook tends often to simplify the diet to make record keeping easier (Quandt 1987). Subjects in the food record-keeping survey are especially likely to adjust their diets so that things will "look better" to the surveyor, especially if the surveyor is in the household for the sole purpose of making and recording the measurements.

In both types of surveys, measuring the quantity of food consumed by breast-fed babies presents difficulties. And in both cases, seasonal variation in consumption may confound the data unless appropriate adjustments are

---

Box 4.1 Use of a Dietary Recall Survey to Evaluate Nutrition in Indonesia

A study (Hartini et al. 2003) of the prevalence of undernutrition among pregnant women in Indonesia used a dietary recall survey. Four hundred and fifty women in their second trimester of pregnancy were interviewed repeatedly (up to six times) and asked to recall their food intake in the twenty-four hours preceding the interview. The results were averaged to get for each woman an estimate of her normal average dietary intake of food. From this, daily nutrient intake (how many calories, how many grams of protein, etc.) was estimated using coefficients about the nutritional composition of the food items. The daily nutrient intake for each woman was compared to the estimated average requirement for the nutrient for Indonesia. The study ran from 1996 to 1998, spanning the Indonesian financial crisis that began in 1997. Therefore the study was able to analyze the impact of the crisis on nutrition. Before the economic crisis, 40 percent of women in the study were at risk for inadequate calories and protein, and 70 percent were at risk for inadequate iron, vitamin A, and calcium. The economic crisis caused a decline in most nutrients for poor women living in cities.

---

made. For instance, the Philippine survey was done from February through May, a time when access to the countryside is easier because of the relative absence of monsoon rains and typhoons. The retail price of tomatoes, for example, is typically 250 percent higher in November than it is in April. Similarly, the price of rice tends to be low during the survey period, while the price of corn tends to be high (Philippines Ministry of Agriculture 1981a, 1981b). The unadjusted survey data thus sometimes overestimate annual consumption of tomatoes and rice, which are in abundant supply during the survey period, and to underestimate the consumption of corn.

In either case (dietary recall or record), results of the survey can be used to determine amounts of various nutrients consumed; these amounts can then be compared to a dietary standard appropriate to the particular country being observed, to determine nutritional status.

Dietary assessment is useful in studies relating consumption and income, or in determining food allocation patterns within the family. But care must be taken in interpreting the results of such surveys. Food intake is not always a good index of nutritional status. For instance, secondary malnutrition can substantially degrade the nutritional status of an otherwise appropriately fed individual.

Anthropometric Assessment

Anthropometry is the science of measuring the human body and its parts. It serves as the most commonly used measure of nutritional status. To understand how anthropometric assessment works, we must first understand how human physical growth and development are responsive to nutritional status. We will then turn to a fuller explanation of anthropometric assessment.

■ Impact of Undernutrition on Physical Growth and Development

Because calories and protein are necessary for the growth of the human body, the most obvious physical manifestations of undernutrition are in the individual's size. In considering this impact, we should discriminate between *acute undernutrition* and *chronic undernutrition*. Acute undernutrition is short-term, severely inadequate food intake, such as one might see during famine or war. The human body can recover from a relatively short bout of acute undernutrition; people who lose weight in a famine can gain it back when the famine ends. In some cases, children whose growth has slowed during a famine will regain their normal size when the famine ends. Chronic undernutrition refers to long-term inadequacy of protein and/or calories. Chronic undernutrition causes physical effects even when it is moderate. The physical effects of undernutrition include the following.

Low Height-for-Age, or Stunting

An individual whose height is low for her age is said to be *stunted*. Such a person may have suffered from chronic undernutrition at some time during the growth years. Low height-for-age is a symptom of past undernutrition; the person may or may not be undernourished today. We find evidence of the link between nutrition and height in a variety of places.

The first kind of evidence shows that the average height of people in a country increases through time, as nutritional status improves. During the period from 1889 to 1950, the populations of northern Europe and North America were growing taller at the rate of approximately one centimeter per decade. The trend has stopped in most well-off sections of these countries, but continued in Japan into the 1970s (Tanner 1977:349). Similarly, in the Indian village of Bagbana, 61 percent of adult sons were taller by an average of 3.1 centimeters (1.25 in.) than their fathers. Presumably, these secular trends in height of populations during the past one hundred years is largely the result of better health and nutrition.

Studies in a variety of countries indicate the same trend: average height of adults increases over time. Strauss and Thomas (1998) present data on this for the United States, Côte d'Ivoire, Brazil, and Vietnam. In the United States, the average man born in 1930 was 4 centimeters taller than the average man born in 1910, reflecting a marked improvement in nutrition; but the increase from 1930 to 1950 was only 1 centimeter, because there was less room for improvement in nutritional status. In Vietnam, average height increased with birth year from 1920 to the late 1950s, when the Vietnam War started. From the late 1950s through the 1970s there was little change in height, reflecting the impact of war on nutritional improvement. In what amounts to a kind of naturally occurring controlled experiment, Alderman et al. (2003) examined the impact of the drought in Zimbabwe in the period 1982–1984. They compared the height-for-age of children at the beginning and after the end of the drought period, and conclude: "Exposure to the . . . drought resulted in a loss of stature of 2.3 cm."

Low Weight-for-Height, or Wasting
People who are currently undernourished are thin. In scientific jargon they exhibit low weight-for-height, or *wasting*. This fact is known to anyone who has tried to lose or gain weight by changing their food intake. Low weight-for-height is a symptom of current undernutrition.

Low Weight-for-Age, or Underweight
Low weight-for-age is a symptom of either past or present undernutrition. Individuals with low weight-for-age are referred to as *underweight*.

Fat Composition of the Body
The human body stores excess calories as fat. In periods when calorie intake exceeds requirements, fat is added, and in periods when calorie intake is deficient, fat is depleted. No single part of the body represents the fat content of the whole body. Even a careful calculation of total body density (by weighing people and then comparing their weights to the weight of the water they displace when submerged in a tank) may not estimate accurately the percentage of the entire body that is fat. Nevertheless, the mid-upper arm is considered to be fairly representative of the body as a whole and is used as an indicator of nutritional status.

Nature Versus Nurture, or Heredity Versus Environment
Of course, nutrition is not the only determinant of body size. We observe differences from country to country, or ethnic group to ethnic group. Figure 4.1 shows variations of body weights in seven Latin American countries and the United States. Boys in all eight countries start life with similar weights, but by adulthood, we see considerable variation among countries.

In Figure 4.2, the height of the U.S. population is contrasted with that of an Indian village (Bagbana) surveyed by Foster in 1981 (unpublished data). The U.S. data here and elsewhere in the chapter are from a survey by the U.S. National Center for Health Statistics (NCHS) (U.S. Department of Health and Human Resources 1981). Both males and females in the village are at about the fifth percentile of height observed in the United States. A plotting of weights comparing Bagbana villagers to the U.S. population shows a similar picture: by age seventy, the village females' weight is only slightly over 50 percent of the weight of U.S. females of the same age. Are the Indian women underweight? Are the U.S. women overweight? Are the weight and height differences attributable to nutrition?

Some ethnic groups have reputations as being unusually small or unusually large. Weiner (1977:419–420) reports a number of different studies of these kinds of groups indicating that protein composition of the group's diet may explain size. The meat-eating Sikhs of northern India are noticeably larger than the vegetarian Madrassi of southern India. In Kenya, the farming Kikuyu tribe lives on cereals, tubers, and legumes. The Masai tribe—also in Kenya—are nomadic cowherds. Their diet includes meat and milk; in addition, Masai get high-protein nutrition from blood drained from living cattle. On average, Masai men are 3 inches (7.5 cm) taller and 22 pounds (10.75 kg) heavier than Kikuyu men.

Stephenson, Latham, and Jansen (1983:53) compared growth data from U.S. children, privileged African children, and underprivileged African children, and concluded that ethnic differences were less important than other factors as determinants of growth in children: "Poverty, poor food

Figure 4.1   Median Male Weight-for-Age in Seven Latin American Countries and the United States

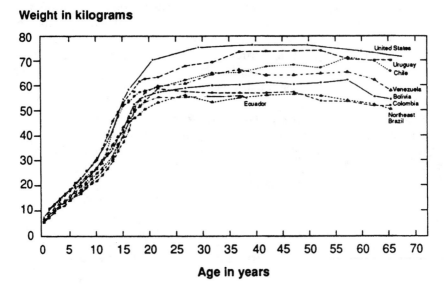

Weight in kilograms

Age in years

Source: Adapted from U.S. white House, President's Science Advisory Committee 1967:37.

Figure 4.2   NCHS (U.S.) Median Height-for-Age vs. Median Height-for-Age, Bagbana Village, India

Male

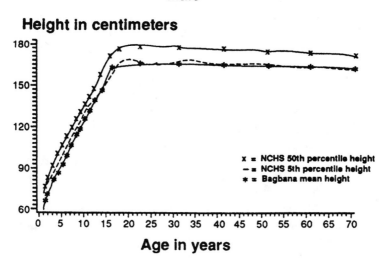

Female

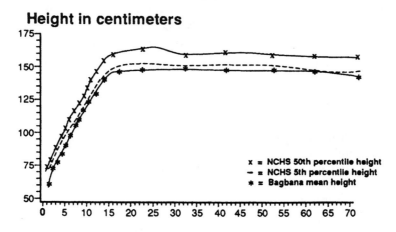

Source: Adapted from Dever 1983:71.

intakes, infectious and parasitic diseases, and other environmental factors combine to prevent children from realizing their growth potential. There are, of course, genetic influences that lead to differences of body size, and especially of stature, but it seems that in pre-pubertal children, heredity is a much less significant cause of below-average growth than are other factors.

Environmental influences are major determinants of the body-size characteristics of a population. This will provide a basis for anthropometric measurement of malnutrition. But we must bear in mind that, especially for a particular individual, body size is the product of both heredity and environment. Note also that, despite substantial genetic variation in height and weight within any population, the growth trajectories of infants and very young children are much more uniform than those of older children.

■ Anthropometric Assessment of Nutritional Status

As discussed in the previous section, human physical growth and development are responsive to variations in calorie and protein intakes. Because of this, measurements of the human body, when compared to a reference standard, provide clues as to protein and calorie nutrition. This is especially true during youth, when growth is so rapid, but to some extent also true during adulthood, when various dimensions change gradually with aging. Thus anthropometry can be used to suggest the protein and/or calorie nutritional status of adults as well as children.

An anthropometric assessment of an individual's nutrition status has three steps: (1) take measurements of the individual; (2) compare that individual to a "reference group"—the measurements of other individuals of the same age, sex, and ethnic group, for example; and (3) make a determination of nutritional status based on that comparison.

How Is Anthropometry Used?

As noted above, nutrition is not the only influence on bodily growth and development. Growth and development can also be affected by such variables as genetic disposition, health, hormonal abnormalities, or deficiencies in micronutrients (e.g., zinc deficiency is associated with poor growth). Because anthropometry does not provide particularly useful clues as to dietary deficiencies (micronutrient shortages), it is not normally used to measure them. Nevertheless, because nutritional status is by far the most common variable influencing bodily growth and development, and because deficiencies in calories and/or protein are by far the most important causes of subnormal growth and development in the developing world, anthropometry is generally assumed to provide strong clues as to protein and calorie nutrition.

In developed countries, anthropometry is used most often as a measure of overnutrition, which is the most common nutritional problem among high-income people. Adults who are trying to keep their weight down are using the anthropometric measure weight-for-height as a reference standard, although they seldom think of their activities in such technical terms.

Since 1966, when the WHO published a monograph by D. B. Jelliffe titled *The Assessment of the Nutritional Status of the Community,* which provided a set of standardized anthropometric measurements useful in nutritional assessment, anthropometry has become the most widely used tool in nutritional assessment. The most common measures used for anthropometric assessment of nutritional status are height, weight, and a combination of arm circumference and skin-fold thickness. They are usually used in conjunction with sex and age (as in weight-for-age or height-for-age) and sometimes in combination with each other (as in weight-for-height).

Low cost and a relatively high degree of accuracy combine to make this method so popular. Training time of field surveyors is cut to a minimum. The measurements are relatively easy to take, and the tools required are simple to use: scales, tape measures, measuring boards, and skin-fold calipers. Intelligent amateurs can be trained in a matter of days to take accurate measurements. By contrast, training technicians to recognize and diagnose undernutrition from clinical symptoms can take weeks or months.

Although anthropometric measurements can be made by individuals with little training, length is considerably more difficult to obtain than weight, especially from children under two. The operation requires a special board and two trained surveyors. While one holds the baby's legs straight and moves the baby's feet close against the footboard, the other moves the headboard against the top of the baby's head, taking care to hold the head in the prescribed position. Needless to say, when two strangers, no matter how gentle they try to be, hold a baby tightly in the prescribed position on this new contraption for the first time in her life, a certain amount of kicking and screaming, and occasionally urinating and defecating, can be expected. The exercise can be traumatic for all concerned.

From the point of view of accuracy, age data may be the biggest problem in using anthropometry. Adults in developing countries often have only a vague idea of how old they are, and illiterate mothers sometimes have difficulty telling the age of their children.

Capital requirements for anthropometry are minimal. Compared to the laboratory apparatus involved in biochemical analysis, anthropometric tools are inexpensive. And anthropometry measures the results of nutrition (the size and shape of the body) rather than nutritional inputs (as in dietary intake). Because of its quantitative nature, anthropometry can be used to judge varying degrees of undernutrition—not just its presence or absence. And by using a mix of anthropometric indices, researchers can make judgments about a nutritional disorder (protein or caloric) as well as the time dimension of the disorder (past or present).

Reference Groups

A person's size can only be evaluated by comparing it to the sizes of other people (the *reference population*). These comparisons lead to statements such as "Tommy is shorter than average," meaning that "Tommy is shorter than the average person in the reference population." Or we might say, "Adele is in the ninety-fifth percentile of height," meaning "95 percent of people in the reference population are shorter than Adele."

The purpose of a reference population is to provide a standard against which the growth and maturation of particular individuals can be judged. By observing how much one person deviates from others of a similar status (age and sex, for example), we can draw inferences about the subject's nutritional status.

Similarly, whenever you try to guess someone's age, you use (as at least some of your clues) the person's body size and configuration. That is, your life experience teaches you what to expect in the way of variations in height, weight, and even fatness as people grow and develop, and from this (and other clues, such as amount of gray hair and wrinkled skin) you deduce age.

In setting up a reference population, it is important to control for as many variables as possible that might influence the observed variables. For example, if an individual is much shorter than the reference group, we don't learn much if the individual is four years old and the reference group is composed of teenagers. Therefore, reference groups are chosen so that we can compare persons of approximately the same age and sex.

The curves in Figure 4.3 show how the reference population can be described. The top part of this shows the distribution of height (length) among girls age three years and younger. The curves in the bottom half of Figure 4.3 describe the weight-for-age of the same reference group. A twenty-four-month-old girl who weighs 12 kilograms is at the fiftieth percentile (or 12 kilograms is the "median weight" for girls this age). A twenty-four-month-old girl who weighs 10.2 kilograms is at the fifth percentile—about 95 percent of girls in the reference population weigh more than she does. A similar set of curves can plot weight against height and serves as a description of the reference population for the measure weight-for-height.

Because third world populations often track well below the European and U.S. data (review Figure 4.2), there is a strong motivation for third world governments to build their own reference tables. Colombia, India, Brazil, and the Philippines have established their own reference populations. In Table 4.1, the Philippine and U.S. reference standards are compared. The Philippine data track the U.S. data for the first two years, but by the sixth birthday, the Philippine data have dropped to 90 percent of those for the United States.

Figure 4.3 Height-for-Age and Weight-for-Age Percentiles for Girls Age 0–36 Months, United States, 2000

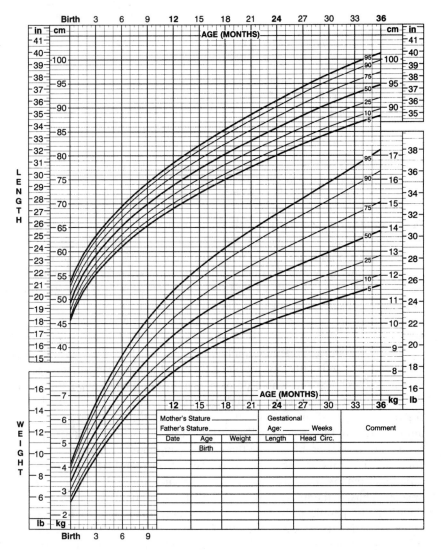

Source: Centers for Disease Control: http://www.cdc.gov/nchs/data/nhanes/ growthcarts/set1clinical/cj411018.pdf.

Classification System for Identifying Undernutrition

Choosing a classification system for undernutrition involves selecting an appropriate anthropometric measure or measures in conjunction with an appropriate set of criteria (deviations from the reference standard) to identi-

Table 4.1   Philippine and U.S. Weight-for-Age Reference Standards for Preschool Children (in kilograms)

Age in Years	U.S. (median weight)			Philippines (4)	Percentage That Column 4 Is of Column 3
	Boys (1)	Girls (2)	Average (3)		
1	11.7	10.7	11.2	11.2	100
2	13.5	12.7	13.1	13.1	100
3	15.4	14.7	15.0	14.7	98
4	17.6	16.7	17.2	16.1	94
5	19.4	19.0	19.2	17.8	92
6	22.0	21.3	21.6	19.4	90

Sources: U.S. Department of Health and Human Services 1987; Philippines National Science and Technology Authority 1984:218.

fy undernutrition, or various levels of it. We have measured the body size characteristics of the individual. We have the body size characteristics of the reference population. Now what can we conclude about nutrition by comparing the individual to the reference group? When is the individual's height or weight so low that it indicates undernutrition? No matter which system is chosen, the aim is to flag those in most need of help, either because they are undernourished or because they are in danger of becoming so.

Table 4.2 shows five commonly used classification systems. The first three can be used with any measure (height-for-age, weight-for-age, or weight-for-height). The whole point of using a reference population is to decide whether an individual's height or weight is roughly "abnormally low for that group." If an individual's height or weight is below a certain amount (referred to as a *cut-off point*), then he or she may be presumed to have a nutritional problem. The three most commonly proposed candidates for cut-off points are each based on deviation from the *median score.* "Median" means that half the reference population is larger and half is smaller. Thus, if the median weight of a reference population is 90 pounds, then half the people in that group weigh more than 90 pounds, and half weigh less. The three candidates for cut-off points are: (1) percentile, (2) percentage of the median, and (3) standard deviation unit. For the purposes of explanation, we use weight as the variable being measured and compared to the reference population. The terms can also be applied to any other variable, such as height.

Percentile measures what percentage of the reference population weighs less than the individual. Thus, if the individual's weight is at the "thirtieth percentile," this indicates that 30 percent of the reference population weighed less than the individual. The fiftieth percentile is the same as

Table 4.2   Anthropometric Classification Systems for Comparing an Individual
to the Reference Group

System	Range	Malnutrition Category
World Health Organization	Z-score of -1 to -2	Mild
	Z-score of -2 to -3	Moderate
	Z-score lower than -3	Severe
RTH [a]	Greater than 80% of median	Normal
	60–80% of median	Mild-to-moderate
	Less than 60% of median	Severe
Gómez	Greater than 90% of median	Normal
	75–90% of median	Mild
	60–75% of median	Moderate
	Less than 60% of median	Severe
Body Mass Index	Greater than 18.5	Normal
	17–18.5	Grade I
	16–17	Grade II
	Less than 16	Grade III
MUAC	Less than 18.5 cm	Moderate
	Less than 16 cm	Severe

Source: Cogill 2003:42, 72–73.
Note: a. *Road to Health.* See Cogill 2003, pp. 42, 72–73

the median. In the discussion of the reference groups' charts (Figure 4.3), we noted that a twenty-four-month-old girl who weighs 10.2 kilograms is at the fifth percentile.

We calculate percentage of the median by dividing the individual's weight by the median weight for the reference population. The 10.2-kilogram girl in our example is at 82 percent of the median weight, since median weight for girls this age is 12 kilograms.

The Gómez classification (Gómez et al. 1956) applied to weight-for-age measures was used to measure the extent of undernutrition in Bagbana village. The results are shown in Figure 4.4. Examination of this figure yields some interesting speculations: Middle-aged to older Indian villagers are mostly moderately to severely undernourished; middle-aged to older people in the United States are overweight; so optimal nutrition must lie somewhere in between. Figure 4.4 also illustrates a phenomenon commonly found in low-income third world populations, namely, that the indicated severe undernutrition rate (look at the line for severe undernutrition) tends to decline during the first six years of life. This is partly because, as the child grows up, he more easily commands his share of the family's food resources (weaning children are notoriously difficult to feed) and partly

Figure 4.4   Gómez Classification by Age, Bagbana Village, 1981

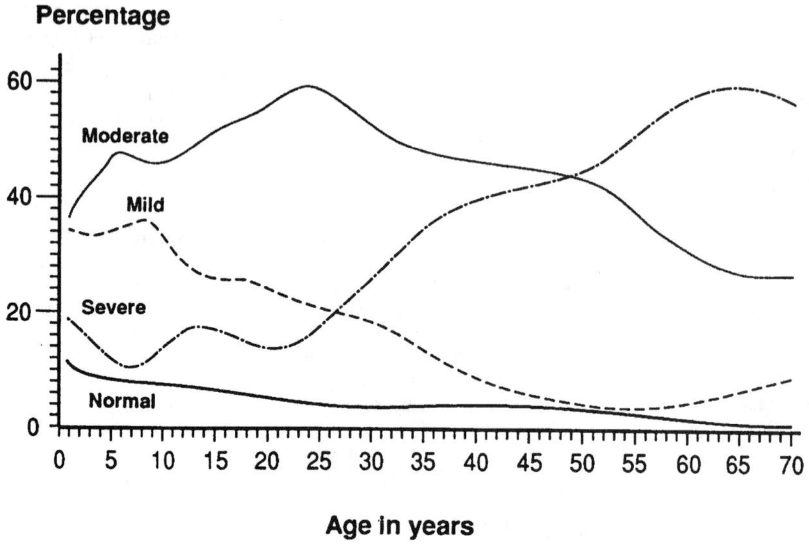

Percentage

Age in years

Source: Adapted from Dever 1983:88.

because the weakest individuals have already succumbed to malnutrition and disease. With their early deaths, the remaining population of older children "looks better."

Standard deviation unit, or "Z-score," is a statistical measure of dispersion away from the mean. An observation that is two standard deviation units below the mean will be approximately on the second percentile—only 2 percent of the reference population will weigh less than this amount. For measures of height and weight, experience shows that two standard deviations below the mean is usually fairly close to 75 percent of the median. Experience also shows that the average weight (and height) of population groups is usually quite close to the median (Krick 1988:326–328). Our reference chart (Figure 4.3) does not tell us the standard deviation of the sample, but an estimate allows us to calculate a Z-score of −1.65 for the 10.2-kilogram girl we have been using as an example. A twenty-four-month-old girl weighing 10.2 kilograms is 1.65 standard deviations below the mean weight for girls of this age.

As mentioned above, these three categorizations can be used for any anthropometric measure. Waterlow et al. (1977) suggests that a more complete picture of a person's nutritional status can be obtained by combining weight-for-height (which identifies present undernutrition) and height-for-age (which identified past undernutrition). The beauty of this system is that it is likely to correctly identify individuals who are presently at risk for undernutrition and eliminate from present consideration those who merely have been undernourished in the past. The other two categorizations are discussed below.

Body Mass Index. As a measure of undernutrition (or overnutrition) among adults, FAO and WHO now regard the Body Mass Index (BMI) as the most suitable. BMI is calculated as weight in kilograms divided by the square of the height in meters. According to the FAO (*Sixth World Food Survey,* 1996c), a BMI below 18.5 is regarded as lower than normal and thus indicative of undernutrition. Twelve-and-a-half percent of adults in China and 48.6 percent in India have a BMI below this critical level. A person 6 feet tall with a BMI of 18.5 would weigh about 135 pounds. In the United States, the National Institutes of Health (NIH) puts the ideal ranges for BMI at from 21 to 23 for women and from 22 to 24 for men.

Estimating body fat from arm circumference. One of the more interesting features of child growth and development is that, while the body of a well-nourished child is gaining in length and weight from one to five or six years of age, his or her mid-upper arm circumference (MUAC) remains essentially the same. Using this observation, Shakir (1975) developed a screening device to identify severely undernourished preschoolers that is simplicity itself. It consists of a tape that is wrapped around the child's mid-upper arm, lightly enough to not compress the skin but firmly enough to fit exactly. The reference standard used is 16.5 centimeters. A circumference of greater than 14 centimeters (85 percent of standard) is considered normal. Between 12.5 and 14 centimeters (76 percent to 85 percent of standard) is classed as undernutrition. Under 12.5 centimeters (less than 76 percent of standard) is classed as severe undernutrition. The tape is inexpensive and can be made by hand, if necessary. If the tape is coded with culturally appropriate colors, even illiterate health workers can do the classification.

The accuracy of the system is good for severe cases and moderate for mild cases. Nevertheless, because of its simplicity and because it works on preschoolers without age data, it has become an important screening tool. As Cogill (2003:12) says,

> Mid-upper arm circumference (MUAC) is relatively easy to measure and a good predictor of immediate risk of death. It is used for rapid screening of acute malnutrition from the 6–59 month age range (MUAC overestimates rates of malnutrition in the 6–12 month age group). MUAC can be used for screening in emergency situations but is not typically used for evaluation purposes. MUAC is recommended for assessing acute adult

undernutrtiion and for estimating prevalence of undernutrition at the population level.

(Table 4.2 shows the nutritional classifications for adults, based on their mid-upper arm circumference measure.)

■ Measuring Nutritional Status in the Aggregate

Above we discuss various ways to determine an individual's nutritional status. Policymakers also need to learn about the nutritional status of large groups. They need to know the extent of undernutrition in a continent or subcontinent, in a country, in a state or region of a country, or among some demographic or ethnic group.

Drawing Inferences from a Sample

Of course, if we can measure the nutritional status of a number of representative individuals in a country or in a group, we can draw inferences about the extent of malnutrition in the whole group. The science of statistics deals with the problem of how to determine the characteristics of an entire population (in this case, the extent of malnutrition in a country or among a group) by observing the characteristics of a sample from that group. So if we have anthropometric evidence categorizing, say, 11,000 children under the age of five in Nigeria, which tells us that 34 percent of these children are undernourished, this might allow us to deduce that 34 percent of all children in Nigeria are undernourished.

Mortality or Disease Rates

A second way of drawing inferences about the incidence of malnutrition in a country or other large group is to examine aggregate data about effects of malnutrition and to draw inferences from that data. For instance, low birth weights or high infant mortality rates in a country or region are assumed to indicate high rates of undernutrition. Aggregate data such as this can provide a pretty good first approximation on where you are likely to find substantial numbers of undernourished people. Because undernutrition and poor health often occur together, aggregate data on morbidity can also provide indirect measures of the incidence of undernutrition in that country or region.

The Philippines does one of the most careful jobs of nutrition surveillance of any developing country. According to the 1982 Nationwide Nutrition Survey (Philippines National Science and Technology Authority 1984), 52 percent of the country's population was afflicted with roundworms (*ascariasis*). Hookworm infection was noted among 19 percent of the male population from thirteen to fifty-nine years of age. Of the 14,785 subjects examined, 69 percent were found to test positive for some kind of parasite. With morbidity data such as this, one could expect to find substantial rates of undernutrition in the Philippines.

As we will see in the next chapter, high infant and child mortality rates or high morbidity rates are suggestive of high rates of undernutrition in a population, but these variables do not measure nutritional status directly. Rather, undernutrition is inferred from the nonnutritional aggregate data.

Food Balance Sheets or Food Availability Measures

Another indirect approach to identifying regions or countries with nutritional problems is to look at aggregate nutrient intake or average per person nutrient intake. These are available on a country-by-country basis in food balance sheets published annually by the FAO. The food balance sheet shows sources and uses of over one hundred separate food items on an annual basis. Sources of food listed include beginning stocks, production, and imports; uses include ending stocks, exports, animal feed, and human consumption. The term "balance sheet" refers to the fact that total supply of each food item equals the total use: sources and uses are in balance. A condensed balance sheet for India in 2001 is shown in Table 4.3. This version aggregates many individual food items into groups, and also aggregates several sources and uses. (For a full version of this food balance sheet, see the FAO website: http://apps.fao.org/page/collections?subset=nutrition.)

Once human consumption is estimated for every food commodity in a country, the food consumed can be converted to calories and nutrients, and per capita consumption figures can then be derived. If a country's per capita consumption turns out to be below amounts recommended by nutritionists, we have good cause to assume that a substantial block of its population is undernourished.

Measures derived from food balance sheets—in particular, calories per capita per day—have become perhaps the most widely used measures of malnutrition. The big advantage of such measures is that they are readily available from the UN's FAO for almost every country for a number of years or time periods. (See FAO's *Sixth World Food Survey*, 1996c, or food balance sheets in FAO 2004a.)

However, the measures are not free of problems. We have emphasized that calories are not the sole nutrient of concern in identifying malnutrition. In addition, as noted in Chapter 3, not a single level of nutrient requirement applies to all people. And if we are looking at national data (for a population that includes infants, children, and adults) we see an especially wide variation in the nutritional requirements of the population. In addition, the information on food availability shows us only the average nutrient intake. Some people in the country or region consume less than the average and some more than the average. So even if average caloric intake is greater

Table 4.3   Food Balance Sheet for India, 2001

	Production	Imports-Exports	Stock changes	Total supply	Feed, seed, nonfood uses	Food	Per capita supply, kg/year	Calories per capita per day	Grams of protein per capita per day)	Grams of fat per capita per day
			(Million metric tons)							
Cereals	196,843.4	−5,333.13	−6,160.47	185,349.9	19,016.02	166,345.8	162.27	1,486.82	35.14	6.66
Starchy roots	30,242.7	−23.43	0	30,219.27	6,306.38	23,916.59	23.33	46.56	0.79	0.07
Sugar and sweeteners	327,832.3	−1,524.63	−863.91	32,5443.7	286,158.7	39,290.07	38.32	255.03	0.25	0.07
Pulses, nuts, oilcrops and oils	48,551.9	6,237.61	109.68	54,899.18	26,445.92	28,481.1	27.78	375.06	7.67	30.38
Fruits, vegetables, and misc.	135,192.8	−1,262.73	0	133,930	14,495.36	119,441.9	116.51	128.77	4.09	1.26
Meat and meat products	8,646.58	−248.51	0	8,398.06	179	8,219.97	8.02	76.25	2.17	7.56
Milk and eggs	86,025.75	−374.93	0	85,650.81	17,277.02	68,718.34	67.03	110.54	6.91	5.27
Fish	5,352.3	−335.27	0.66	5,016.89	473.01	4,544.68	4.44	8.19	1.35	0.26
Vegetal products total								2,292.23	47.93	38.45
Animal products total								194.98	10.43	13.1
Grand total								2,487.21	58.36	51.55

Source: FAOSTAT 2004b

than average caloric requirement, a country can still suffer significant undernutrition. Therefore, comparing caloric intake to caloric requirement does not always give an accurate view of the extent of undernutrition. For example, the FAO reports that during the 1990–1992 period, India and Senegal had virtually the same calories available per person per day (2,310 in India, 2,320 in Senegal). However, anthropometric data for the two countries in the late 1980s found that the percentage of children who are underweight was 63.9 percent in India and 21.6 percent in Senegal.

Aggregate food intake measures can also be used to estimate the percentage of a population that has inadequate food intake. FAO's *Sixth World Food Survey* uses the following method: average caloric intake per capita is calculated from food balance sheets, and an estimate of the statistical variance of caloric intake per capita is derived from studies of individuals. These two statistics (average and variance) give an estimate of the distribution of food intake, for example, what percentage of the population has caloric intake below 2,000 calories per day, what percentage below 2,500, and so on. Once a minimum food requirement is identified for the population, that distribution will then tell us what percentage of population takes in less than the minimum requirement. Minimum food requirements are identified for different age and sex classes (e.g., children under ten, males over ten). Minimum requirements are calculated in two ways. First, we can ask, "What level of calories would give a person of average height a minimally healthy weight?" A minimally healthy weight is determined as a BMI of 18.5. (See above discussion of BMI.) A second method is to determine the *basal metabolic rate* (BMR) for the population. The BMR shows the number of calories needed for survival when the body is at rest. The minimal food requirement is calculated by multiplying the BMR by a constant (1.56 is the constant used in the *Sixth World Food Survey*, for example).

5

Impacts of Undernutrition

In Chapter 4, we examined the impact of undernutrition on height, weight, and fat composition of the body. In this chapter, we discuss other impacts of undernutrition, especially impacts on health, mental capacity, and economic productivity.

■ Undernutrition, Menstruation, and Breastfeeding

Delayed Age of Menarche

The female sex hormone, estrogen, is produced from cholesterol, a fat (Pike and Brown 1984:42). The fatter a woman is, the more estrogen she is likely to produce. An undernourished girl is likely to produce less estrogen than a well-nourished girl of the same age; therefore, the well-nourished girl is likely to begin menstruation at a younger age. Delayed age of menarche (age of first menstruation) is an indicator of low levels of calorie intake. Girls in the United States reach menarche earlier today than they did a century ago because they now produce a higher percentage of fat (and estrogen). Because vigorous exercise reduces body fat, well-fed young girls who are also athletes often reach menarche later in life than do their more sedentary counterparts.

Table 5.1 shows a geographic breakdown of menarche. Notice how much higher the age of menarche is in the developing world populations listed in the bottom half of the table than in the presumably better-nourished industrialized populations in the top half. Not all the advantages lie with the well-nourished populations. Recent research suggests that women who have fewer ovarian cycles (late menarche) are at reduced risk for breast cancer. Evidence also exists that lean women are less inclined to cancer because their lower levels of estrogen may reduce the growth of cells that can start tumors.

Breast-Feeding as Birth Control

In the next section, we will review the importance of breast-feeding to the health of infants. An additional benefit of breast-feeding is that it postpones

Table 5.1   Median Age of Menarche, by Location of Population Studied

Place	Median Age	Year of Observation
Santiago, Chile (middle class)	12.3	1971
Hong Kong (affluent)	12.5	1961–65
Madrid (affluent)	12.8	1968
United States, all	12.8	1960–70
Hong Kong (middle class)	12.8	1961–65
Sydney, Australia	13.0	1970
Hong Kong (lower class)	13.3	1961–65
India, all urban	13.7	1956–65
Baghdad (poor)	14.0	1969
India, all rural	14.4	1956–65
South Africa (Bantu, rural)	15.0	—
Rwanda (Tutsi)	16.5	1957–58
Rwanda (Hutu)	17.0	1957–58
New Guinea (Lumi)	18.4	1967

Source: Evelth and Tanner 1967:table 15.

the recurrence of menstruation after childbirth. The same hormone (pro-lactin) that stimulates the production of breast milk also suppresses ovula-tion. In addition, the production of breast milk tends to use up the body's supply of fat, reducing estrogen production and impeding ovulation. The use of breast-feeding to postpone ovulatory cycles after childbirth is referred to as the Lactational Amenorrhea Method of birth control. The method is at least 98 percent effective if three conditions are met: (1) the mother has not experienced the return of her menstrual periods, (2) the mother is fully or nearly fully breast-feeding, and (3) the baby is less than six months old. Studies in developing countries confirm the effectiveness of breast-feeding as a birth control method: In Chile, only one of 422 breast-feeding women became pregnant during the six months after child-birth; in Pakistan, there was one pregnancy among 391 women; in the Philippines, there were two pregnancies among 485. The experience in Pakistan and the Philippines showed 98–99 percent effectiveness for a full year after childbirth among women meeting the first two of the above three conditions (Family Health International 1997). One study estimates that breast-feeding is by far the most widely used contraceptive method in India—six times more important than the birth control pill, four times more important than sterilizations and intrauterine devices, and nearly twice as important as condoms (Gupta and Rohide 1993).

■   **Undernutrition and Child Health**

Undernutrition is an especially serious problem for infants and children because their immune systems are less fully developed than those of adults.

They are, therefore, more susceptible to diseases than are adults. Undernourished children are especially susceptible, because their bodies are already weakened.

Mothers' Nutrition, Breast-Feeding, and the Health of the Baby

Mothers who are undernourished during pregnancy are likely to give birth to babies with low birth weights. These babies start life malnourished and are significantly more likely to die in the first year of life; in fact, during the period shortly after birth, low-birth-weight babies die at a rate forty times that of normal babies (Samuels 1986; Overpeck, Hoffman, and Prager 1992). Low birth weight for an infant indicates that the infant was malnourished in the womb or that the mother was malnourished during her own infancy, childhood, adolescence, or pregnancy. The malnourishment is typically due to underconsumption of calories and protein; however, it can also result from underconsumption of micronutrients such as iron (Levinger 1995).

Even nutrition early in a girl's life can affect the health of the babies she bears as an adult. One study in Guatemala (Stein et al. 2003) followed the lives of girls who were given nutritional supplements during their early childhoods in the 1960s and 1970s. Some girls were given a high-protein, moderate-energy supplement, and others were given a low-energy supplement with no protein. The girls who received the more nutritious supplement grew up to be larger women, on average, and when they gave birth, their babies were larger on average.

If the baby is breast-fed, her health is significantly improved. Breast milk contains all the nutrients a child needs during the first months of life. Breast milk also helps the baby fight infection. In developing countries, breast-feeding contributes to infant health in two indirect ways. First, breast-feeding provides the baby with a guaranteed food supply; the infant does not have to compete with other family members for scarce food. Second, the breast-feeding assures that the baby will have a clean food supply; babies who do not breast-feed are exposed to diseases caused by unsanitary food and water. According to one estimate, 1.5 million children in the developing world die because they are not breast-fed (Grapentine 1998). Even women who are suffering from mild to moderate undernutrition are able to produce sufficient milk to feed their infants, although severe undernutrition such as that resulting from a famine does compromise a woman's ability to produce breast milk (Prentice, Goldberg, and Prentice 1994).

In the past decade, AIDS has created a new problem with breast-feeding: breast milk is a means of passing the AIDS virus from an infected mother to her child (Coutsoudis and Rollins 2003). But nutrition can also influence the mother-child AIDS transmission. A study in Malawi indicated that women with vitamin A deficiencies were more likely to pass on the HIV virus to their infants. Among pregnant women who were HIV-positive, the transmission rate for those with the highest vitamin A concentrations was 7 percent; for women with the lowest vitamin A concentrations, that rate was 32 percent (Semba et al. 1994).

High Infant and Child Mortality Rates

Death is the most dramatic of adverse effects of undernutrition. As mentioned in Chapter 1, deaths from acute undernutrition—such as those that occur in famines—are not nearly as big a worldwide tragedy as are deaths in which chronic undernutrition weakens the ability of people to resist diseases. This form of fatal undernutrition is an especially large problem among children.

Childhood mortality is a significant problem, as Figure 5.1 illustrates. More than 20 percent of the 52 million people who died in 1995 were between birth and five years old. Yet this age category accounts for about only 11 percent of the population. The only age category with more deaths is seventy-five and older. The death rate is especially high for third world children. The WHO reports: "Defined as the probability of dying by the age of five years, the global average in 1995 was 81.7 per 1,000 live births; 8.5 in the industrialized world, 90.6 in the developing world, and 155.5 in the least developed nations" (WHO 1996b).

Childhood diseases, to which undernutrition contributes by weakening the immune system, are major killers of children in developing countries (Dever 1983). Intestinal disorders that lead to diarrhea are the leading child killers in developing countries, but other diseases associated with malnutrition such as pneumonia, influenza, bronchitis, whooping cough, and measles are also important.

The WHO reports that "malnutrition has been found to underlie more than half of deaths among children in developing countries" (WHO 1997). One study of fifty-three developing countries estimated that 56 percent of child deaths are caused by the "potentiating effects of malnutrition in infectious disease." Eighty-three percent of the nutrition-related child deaths are caused by mild-to-moderate malnutrition; only 17 percent are caused by severe malnutrition (Pelletier et al. 1995). Recently, analysts of health policy have introduced a concept called Disability Adjusted Life Years (DALYs), which measures total amount of healthy life lost, whether from premature mortality or from temporary or permanent disability. A study for the WHO estimates that poor nutrition is responsible for 46 percent of DALYs lost to children (WHO 1996a).

Keilmann and McCord (1978) showed that infant mortality doubles with each 10 percent decline below 80 percent of the median weight-for-age. Figure 5.2 is a graphic representation of their results.

The risk of death from nutrition-related disease in the third world decreases dramatically after the second year of life (Figure 5.3). Differences

Figure 5.1 Death and Population in the World by Age, 1995

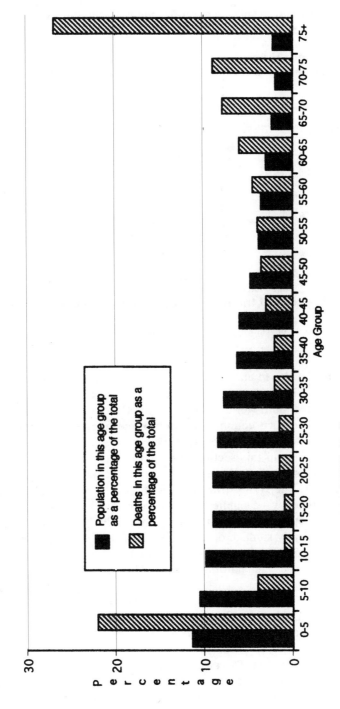

Source: UN, WHO, http://www.who.ch/whr/1997/fig13.gif.

Figure 5.2   Mortality in Children Age 1–36 Months by Nutritional Status, Punjab, India

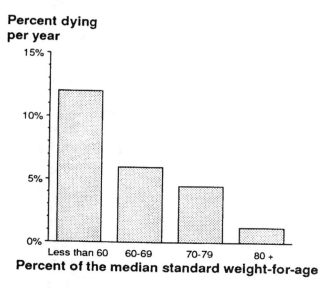

Source: Adapted from Galway et al. 1987:31. Data from Keilmann and McCord 1978

between the developed and the developing countries in death rates among children under five are startling and are dramatized by comparing the data for representative third world countries (top six lines of Table 5.2) with representative developed countries (bottom three lines of the same table). Again, these differences are strongly related to differences in nutrition.

The emphasis in this section has been on deaths caused by disease related to undernutrition. Disease related to undernutrition is not always fatal, or course. The WHO's *World Health Report 1995* states: "As a result of iodine deficiency—a public health problem in 118 countries—at least 30,000 babies are stillborn each year and over 120,000 are born mentally retarded, physically stunted, deaf-mute or paralyzed. A quarter of all children under age 5 in developing countries are at risk of vitamin A deficiency." Interactions between nutrition and health are discussed in Chapter 15.

■ Effects of Undernutrition on Intellect, Education, and Learning

Impact on Intellectual Development

Ancel Keys, working with conscientious objectors during World War II, found that male adults subjected to diets leading to measurable undernutri-

Figure 5.3   Third World, Age-Specific Mortality Rates

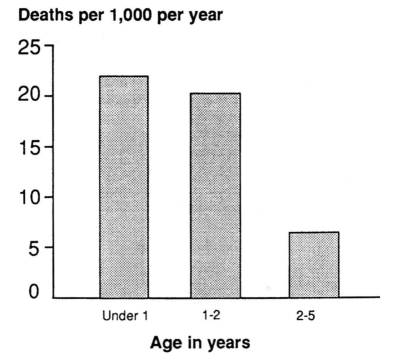

Deaths per 1,000 per year

Age in years

Source: Adapted from De Zoysa et al. 1985:9.

tion first experienced intellectual problems. Later, as their undernutrition continued, the men suffered problems with physical dexterity (Keys et al. 1950). Since then, nutritionists have found in a wide variety of settings that poor nutrition in the first years of life can have a negative impact on intellectual development (Grantham-McGregor, Fernald, and Sethuraman 1999a and 1999b).

More recent research has tended to focus on the potential effect of childhood undernutrition on later intellectual development and achievement. If a mother suffers from undernutrition during pregnancy, her baby can suffer from reduced intellectual capacity and cognitive functioning. When malnourished women were given protein supplements during pregnancy, improvements in their children's cognitive functioning could be observed through age six or seven (Hicks, Langham, and Takenaka 1992). If pregnant women are given adequate calories and protein, the effects on their offspring can be sustained into adolescence and even young adulthood (Pollitt et al. 1993).

Table 5.2   Child Mortality Rates in Selected Countries, 2001

Country	Percentage in age group who die each year		Percentage that die before fifth birthday	Age at Which Same Percentage as in Column 3 have died in the United States
	Under 1	1–4		
Sierra Leone	18.2	3.3	31.6	70
Niger	15.6	2.7	26.5	68
Angola	18.1	2	26.0	68
Afghanistan	16.5	2.3	25.7	68
Liberia	15.7	2	23.5	66
Mali	14.1	2.2	23.1	66
India	6.7	0.6	9.3	54
China	3.1	0.2	3.9	41
Brazil	3.1	0.1	3.6	39
United States	0.7	0.025	0.8	5
Japan	0.3	0.05	0.5	1
Sweden	0.3	0	0.3	1

Sources: UNICEF, *State of the World's Children 2003.*
    U.S. mortality rates: Centers for Disease Control and Prevention, Mortality Rates Table: http://www.cdc.gov/nchs/fastats/pdf/mortality/nvsr52_03t03.pdf.

Chronic malnutrition in children—especially during the first two or three years of life—can impair mental development directly (since brain development is negatively affected) and indirectly (because undernourished children are less active, and therefore their brains are less stimulated) (World Bank 1997).

In a study conducted in Hyderabad, India, children who had previously suffered from kwashiorkor scored an average of 35 points below their matched controls on IQ tests administered up to six years after their recovery. However, the authors note that it was difficult to determine "to what extent this is a result of the episode of kwashiorkor and to what extent it is due to other factors" (Champakam, Srikantia, and Gopalan 1968). Galler (1986), in a longitudinal study in Barbados, matched 183 children who had a history of PEM, or kwashiorkor, with 129 classmates without any such history but of similar age and sex, and from the same socioeconomic group. Both sets of children were followed from age five to eighteen years. By sexual maturation, the previously undernourished children had essentially caught up with the matched group in terms of physical growth, but demonstrated small deficits in IQ throughout the growth period. UNICEF's *State of the World's Children 1998* reports findings that support the conclusion that poor nutrition reduces IQ: iron deficiency during infancy and early childhood was found to reduce IQ by 9 points on average; two-year-old children that are severely stunted (an anthropometric indicator of poor nutrition) have IQs 5–11 points below two-year-olds of normal height; low-birth-weight babies (born to mothers who have been poorly nourished during pregnancy) have IQs 5 points below normal children.

Iodine deficiency is the most significant avoidable cause of mental retardation worldwide. An overview of eighteen studies shows that iodine-deficient groups have IQ levels that are 13.5 points below those of non-iodine-deficient groups (Bleichrodt and Born 1994). To see how important a difference of this magnitude can be, consider that a person with an IQ of 100 is at the median score (half the population gets scores of less than 100, half greater than 100); a person with an IQ of 86.5 has a score higher than only about 20 percent of the population (and lower than 80 percent). Deficiencies in other micronutrients such as iron and vitamin A are also associated with impaired intellectual abilities (Levinger 1994).

Using the Bayley scales for cognitive skills, Gretl Pelto (1987), professor of nutritional science at the University of Connecticut, in a seven-year longitudinal study of nutrition and cognitive development among seventy-eight Mexican preschool children, tested short-term memory, responsiveness to stimulus, attention and distractability, abstract categorization skills, and sedentary passivity. She found that children with little animal food in their diets were short in stature and delayed in cognitive development, and that delays in intellectual development resulted from nutritionally induced growth stunting.

Chavez and Martinez (1982) studied child development among poor Mexican peasant families. They set up a controlled experiment in which one set of families was given supplemental food for the child through three years of age, and for the mother while she was pregnant and lactating. The control group was a set of families matched to the treated group to have similar genetic and socioeconomic characteristics, but given no food supplements. Of the many tests for neurological maturation and mental performance given to each set of children, in virtually every instance—walking, control of bladder, and language development—the control children lagged behind the treated children. The better-nourished children were found to be more precocious in constructing three-word sentences (see Figure 5.4).

Chavez and Martinez stress that it is not possible, at this time, to determine the ultimate significance of the gap between the undernourished and better-nourished children; the undernourished children may catch up later in life. There is some evidence that intellectual impairment is (at least partially) reversible if nutrition is improved. Winick, Meyer, and Harris (1973) tracked severely undernourished Korean orphans and found no signs of mental impairment years after their adoption by U.S. families. A study that

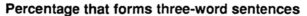

Figure 5.4   Age at Which Child Constructs First Three-Word Sentence, Cumulative Percentage, Mexico

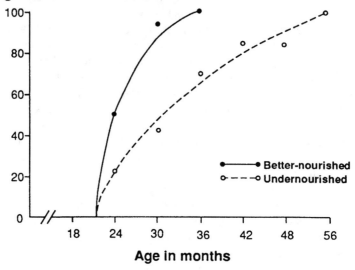

Source: Adapted from Chavez and Martinez 1982:90.

followed Filipino children through the first years of life also found that IQ deficiencies resulting from infant malnutrition persisted in children up to the age of twelve (UNICEF 1998, *State of the World's Children 1998*, panel 3). Lynn and Vanhannen conclude: "Rises in intelligence that occurred in Western populations during the twentieth century are largely attributable to improvements in nutrition" (2002:185).

Impact on Educational Attainment

Not surprisingly, given the discussion in the preceding section, the impact of undernutrition can also be seen in the educational achievements of children.

In the United States, children who had low birth weight were found to have problems succeeding in school. They were more likely to need special education services and more likely to repeat a grade (Levinger 1995).

The Barbados study mentioned above (Galler 1986) found that the most striking difference between the undernourished and well-nourished groups was a fourfold increase in the frequency of attention deficit disorder among the previously undernourished. This syndrome is characterized by decreased attention span, impaired memory, high distractability, restlessness, and disobedience, and was found to reduce educational progress among the previously undernourished children to a far greater extent than the slight deficit in IQ they experienced.

Recent studies in the Philippines (see Box 5.1) and Kenya found a significant relationship between nutritional status and educational attainment as measured by test scores (Glewwe, Jacoby, and King 1996; Bhargava 1996).

Other research shows that if children miss breakfast—if they fast for sixteen hours or more—their school performances suffer. In particular, students suffer from poorer memory and ability to pay attention. World Bank nutrition specialist Alan Berg (1973) points out that education also suffers from missed days of school due to nutrition-related illnesses. He cites the case of four Latin American countries where "illness caused children to miss more than 50 days of school a year."

The study of children born during the 1982–1984 drought in Zimbabwe found that those children started school an average of 3.7 months later than children born in a nondrought period; the children of the drought also finished fewer grades of schooling (Alderman, Hoddinott, and Kinsey 2003).

Recall the discussion of anthropometric results showing that nutrition is positively related to height for age. If nutrition also effects educational attainment, does this mean that we can find a correlation between height of an individual and years of schooling? Strauss and Thomas (1998) show that in fact taller individuals finish more years of schooling, both in the United States and in Brazil.

Box 5.1　The Cebu Longitudinal Study

A current example of nutritional research study is the Cebu Longitudinal Study, led by Professor Linda Adair of the University of North Carolina. This study began as study of about three thousand pregnant women in Cebu, Philippines, who gave birth during the year May1983–April 1984. The original plan was to study the infant-feeding practices of these women (how long did they breast-feed, when did they introduce different kinds of solid food, etc.). In 1991–1992, 2,400 of the families were located and revisited, and both mothers and children were interviewed and evaluated anthropometrically. The younger siblings of the 1983–1984 babies were also measured and evaluated. In 1994 and in 1999, the families were revisited for interviews and tests. Thus the impact of nutritional practices in the first years of life could be traced through the children's first sixteen to seventeen years of life. Studies of the data collected include Glewwe, Jacoby, and King (1996). For a more complete description of the study and analyses of its data, see the website at: http://www.cpc.unc.edu/projects/cebu/cebu_home.html.

■ Effects of Undernutrition on Labor Productivity

In this chapter and the last, we have seen evidence that undernutrition has negative effects on physical growth and development, health, intellectual capacity, and educational attainment. For all of these reasons, we might expect that undernutrition can reduce productivity. A number of studies have analyzed this empirically; a good review of the literature is in Strauss and Thomas (1998).

A study of Chinese cotton-mill workers found that the women were able to do 14 percent more work for each 1-gram increase in their hemoglobin—increases attained by giving the workers iron supplements (Li et al. 1994).

In a study of agricultural workers in Colombia and the United States, Spurr, Barac-Nieto, and Maksud (U.S. Department of State 1976) looked at the relationship between nutritional status and physical work capacity. They concluded that a high correlation exists between the two variables. Among undernourished Colombian sugar cane cutters, physical work capacity was reduced to the order of 50 percent.

Strauss (1968) surveyed smallholder farmers in Sierra Leone and discovered that a 50 percent increase in calories per capita was associated with a 16.5 percent increase in farm output. When nutrition levels are extremely low, the impact of improved nutrition is higher: for families where average intake was less than 1,500 calories per person per day, a 50 percent increase in calories led to a 25 percent increase in farm output.

Again, relying on the anthropometric measure height-for-age as an indicator of poor nutrition, studies have found that smaller adults are less productive workers in many jobs—they cannot lift and carry as much heavy weight, for example, as larger adults. Strauss and Thomas (1998) show that in a test of physical capacity, taller people were more likely to be able to carry a heavy load. The *1995 World Development Report* of the World Bank estimates that this stunting causes an economic loss of $8.7 billion per year worldwide.

The same 1995 World Bank report finds that an increase in a person's height by 1 percent is associated with an increase in that person's wages by 1.38 percent. Strauss and Thomas (1998) show that the positive correlations exist between wages and height and between wages and Body Mass Index (BMI) for Brazil, where undernutrition is fairly widespread, but not in the United States. This is consistent with the explanation that the lower wages are tied to undernutrition. Strauss and Thomas also show that lower wages are not only a result of less education; when they limit the comparison to Brazilians with no education, they still find that wages are higher for taller people or for people with higher BMI.

Paul Schultz (1999) examined the impact of nutrition on wages in Ghana and Côte d'Ivoire. In Ghana, he found a positive correlation: taller people and higher BMIs were associated with higher wages. However, in Côte d'Ivoire, the nutritional indicators were not found to have a statistically significant impact on wages. Schultz concludes that the reason for this disparity is that nutrition was much worse in Ghana than in Côte d'Ivoire during the period studies; the implication is that undernutrition ceases to be a cause of low wages once the problem has been reduced to a certain level. This conclusion is buttressed by the findings in the last paragraph about the lack of correlation between wages and nutrition in the United States.

Finally, Strauss and Thomas (1998) find that poorly nourished people are more likely to be unemployed. Among urban males in Brazil, individuals that were 165 centimeters and taller had average unemployment rates of less than 5 percent. For individuals who were 155 centimeters tall, the average unemployment rate was 10 percent. Likewise, BMIs of 24 and higher were associated with unemployment rates of 4 percent, while average unemployment was 10 percent for individuals with BMI of 18.

In the study cited previously of the impact of the drought on Zimbabweans born between 1982 and 1984, Alderman, Hoddinott, and Kinsey (2003) conclude: "We present calculations that suggest that this loss of stature, schooling and potential work experience results in a loss of lifetime earnings of 7–12 percent and that such estimates are likely to be *lower* bounds of the true losses."

Economic historians have also examined the link between nutrition and productivity. Nobel Prize–winning economist Robert Fogel concluded that food shortages were so severe in Europe in the eighteenth and early nineteenth centuries that "the bottom 20 percent subsisted on such poor diets that they were effectively excluded from the labor force," being too weakened from hunger to work. Fogel estimates the improved nutrition accounts for 30 percent of the growth in income per capita in Britain between 1790 and 1980 (Fogel 1994).

6

Undernutrition: Who, When, Where?

In Chapter 4, we saw a number of ways to measure undernutrition. In addition, some measures are based on somewhat arbitrary cutoff points. Given this situation, we should not be surprised to find that estimates of undernutrition can only be approximations.

Nevertheless, we know enough about what we mean by undernutrition to put the severity of the problem into perspective. In this chapter we consider the following questions: How widespread is undernutrition? What kinds of people suffer from it? When do they suffer (or when have they suffered)? And where do they live?

■ Global Trends in Long-Term Perspective

Table 6.1 presents estimates of the number of people worldwide who are affected by undernutrition-associated conditions. For technically advanced readers, descriptions and criticisms of the method used by the Food and Agriculture Organization of the United Nations (FAO) to measure the extent of undernutrition can be found in Svedberg (1999) or Gabbert and Weikard (2001).

Over time, the number of undernourished people has declined. This is illustrated by Table 6.2. For the developing world as a whole, the number of undernourished people dropped from 918 million in the early 1970s to 906 million in the early 1980s, to under 800 million at the turn of the century. Expressed as a percentage of the population, the drop has been more dramatic; over one-third of the developing world's population was undernourished in the early 1970s; by the turn of the century, the proportion had dropped to 17 percent. However, these declines have not been spread evenly throughout the developing world. Progress in Asia has been remarkable; the number of undernourished people has dropped by over 25 percent (more than 200 million people) since the early 1970s, and the percentage of undernourished people has dropped from 38 percent to 16 percent. These declines offset worsening conditions in sub-Saharan Africa, where the number of undernourished people has increased by over 95 million, and the per-

Table 6.1   World Population Affected by Different Kinds of Malnutrition

Deficiency	Prevalence (millions)
Iodine deficiency disorder	1,989
Vitamin A deficiency	140–250
Iron deficient anemia	2,000
Inadequate caloric intake	798
Stunting from inadequate protein and energy	175

Sources: WHO 1997; UN 1997; SOFI 2003

Table 6.2   Trends in Number and Percentage of People Undernourished, by Continental Area

Area	1969–1971	1979–1981	1990–1992	1999–2001
	Number of undernourished (millions)			
Sub-Saharan Africa	103	148	215	198
Near East and North Africa	48	27	37	41
East and Southeast Asia	476	379	269	212
South Asia	238	303	255	293
Latin America and Caribbean	53	48	64	53
All Developing Countries	918	906	841	798
	Proportion of the population that is undernourished (%)			
Sub-Saharan Africa	38	41	43	33
Near East and North Africa	27	12	12	10
East and Southeast Asia	41	27	16	12
South Asia	33	34	22	22
Latin America and Caribbean	19	14	15	10
All Developing Countries	35	28	20	17

Sources: 1969–1992: FAO 1996c, *Sixth World Food Survey.* 1999–2001: FAO 2003.

centage of population that is undernourished has declined only slightly from 38 percent to 33 percent.

Additional evidence of a long-term trend of an improving food situation is shown in Figures 6.1 and 6.2. These show that worldwide food production per capita increased steadily from 1961 to 2003, and that world food prices fell over the period. Figure 6.2 shows that food prices jumped around quite a bit. They took a huge jump between 1972 and 1974 (see Johnson (1975) for a discussion of the reasons), and then fell sharply. Box 6.1 discusses a situation thousands of years ago when nutrition did not improve.

Figure 6.1   Index of World Food Production per Capita, 1961–2001

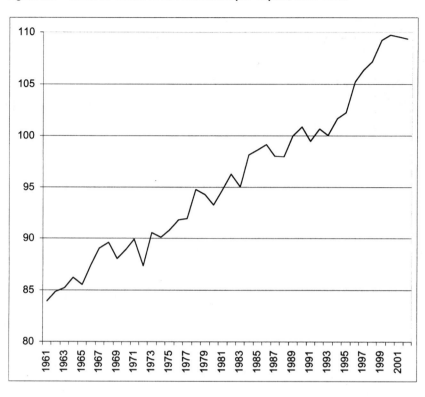

Source: FAOSTAT 2004a
Note: 1993 = 100

■ The Seasonality of Undernutrition

People at risk for undernutrition are not usually at risk all the time; it tends
to come in fits and starts. We are all aware of the periodicity of famine—
the word connotes a time of extreme food scarcity as contrasted with normal times when food is less scarce. But we are less aware that third world
hunger usually follows the rhythm of the seasons. In the third world, a
strong seasonality is usual in the production, price, and availability of food,
as well as in the availability of employment (Sahn 1989). All these factors
can influence the nutritional status of a family at risk for undernutrition.

The seasonality of undernutrition is often linked to the agricultural
year, which in the tropics is usually heavily dependent on rainfall patterns.
In monsoon Asia, for instance, rice is planted at the beginning of the wet
monsoon that typically starts in July. Harvest begins about four months

Figure 6.2   Index of Real Food Prices, 1961–2003

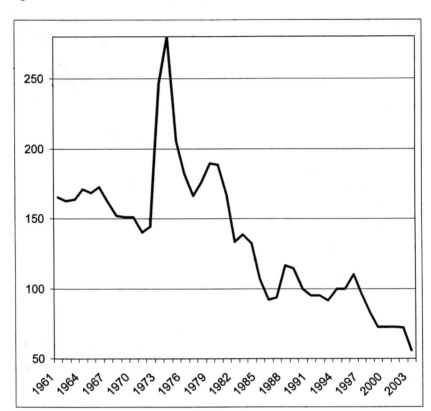

Note: 1995 = 100, figures are the index of food prices (IMF) deflated by the U.S. GDP price deflator.

after planting. With irrigation, farmers can harvest more than one crop per year, but most of the rice starts during the wet monsoon. Likewise, in the Sahel region of Africa (including parts of Chad, Niger, and Mauritania) crops mature in September and October, but the food supply begins to run out in May, and the hungry season can run for four months, from May through August (FAO 1997b).

Consequently, the price of rice is lowest just after harvest and rises gradually as supplies dwindle. During the growing season, supplies may become short and prices may rise more sharply. The pattern of seasonal price variation in the Philippines is shown in Figure 6.3. Compare this with consumption rates in Table 6.3. Consumption is at its lowest in September when the price has been high for three months and picks up during the following months when the price falls below the annual average. Similar sea-

**Box 6.1   Nutrition, the Natural Environment, and the
            Development of Agriculture**

It is tempting to presume that the improvements in worldwide nutrition seen over the past half century are simply an extension of a long history of gradual improvement in human nutrition. But some anthropological evidence indicates that precivilized hunter-gatherers obtained good nutrition with relatively little effort.

Angel (1975) found that thirty thousand years ago—before the birth of agriculture—the average adult male was 177 cm (5'11") tall; but twenty thousand years later average height was only 165 cm (5'6"). Other information from Angel (1984) indicates that residents of the eastern Mediterranean at the beginning of the age of agriculture were taller than modern Greeks. Harris (1977) says that it is "hard to reconcile [a view of starving hunter-gatherers] with the enormous quantities of animal bones accumulated at various Paleolithic kill sites. . . . The skeletal remains of the hunters themselves bear witness to the fact that they were unusually well-nourished" (p. 10). Cohen (1984) notes that skeletal evidence indicates low rates of anemia and infection among hunter-gatherers.

Other evidence that hunter-gatherers had good nutrition comes from studies of modern hunter-gatherer societies. Lee studied the !Kung bushmen of Africa and found that they consumed 93 grams of protein per day, mostly from meat and nuts. The composition of the diet of many hunter-gatherers is varied and more likely to contain sufficient quantities of a broad array of nutrients.

An even more remarkable result from Lee's study of the !Kung (1968b) is that they achieve this nutritious diet with relatively little effort—less than three hours per day per adult, despite the fact that the !Kung live on the edge of the Kalahari Desert. The rest of the time was spent resting, visiting with others, doing embroidery, playing games, etc. The aborigines of Australia work for two days and take the third as a holiday (Sahlins 1968). These observations are consistent with studies of great apes who spend about half their time grooming, playing, and napping, and the other half foraging for food. "As collectors of food . . . [paleolithic populations] were certainly no less effective than chimpanzees" (Harris 1977:10).

Why—if hunting and gathering was so nutritionally efficient—did agriculture ever develop? According to Marvin Harris, the answer is global warming.

"As long as . . . exploitation of [naturally occurring animal and plant resources] is kept relatively low, hunter-collectors can enjoy both leisure and high-quality diets. . . . Then, about 13,000 years ago, a global warming trend [began, and] . . . forests invaded the grassy plains which nourished the great herds [of large animals, known as "megafauna"]. . . . The collapse of the big-game hunting cultures . . . was followed by . . . [a system of] preying on smaller species . . . called . . . "broad spectrum" hunting and collecting. . . . [H]unters then intensified predation of [smaller species], and these too soon became extinct. . . . As they fought their long and futile delaying action against the consequences of the depletion of animal species, [they] . . . shifted their primary subsistence effort away from animals toward plants. . . . It seems clear that the extinction of the Pleistocene megafauna triggered the shift to an agricultural mode of production. (1978:10–25)."

Figure 6.3   Seasonal Price Variation in Rice, Philippines

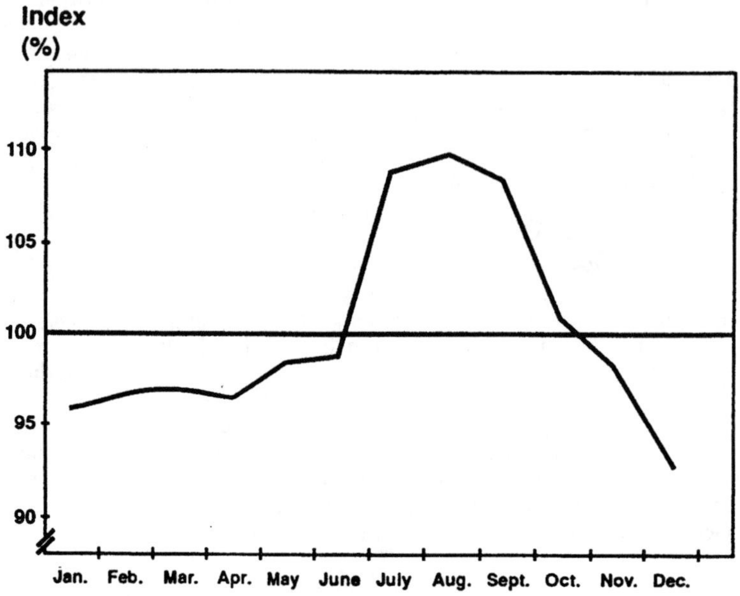

Source: Adapted from Philippines Ministry of Agriculture 1981b.

Table 6.3   Annual Rate of Consumption of Rice and Rice Products, Philippines, 1980–1981

		Kilos per Capita per Year
1980	March	108.4
	June	110.4
	September	98.2
	December	103.6
1981	March	103.4
	June	115.1

Source: Philippines Ministry of Agriculture 1983.

sonal price patterns occur throughout the developing world. For example, millet prices in Niger rose 80 percent between July and August of 1996 (FAO 1997b).

A detailed study of dietary intake in Mozambique (Rose et al. 1999) vividly illustrates the impact of the hungry season. As shown in Table 6.4,

Table 6.4   The Comparative Nutrient Intakes for the Hungry Season and the Harvest Season for a Sample of Smallholders in Montpuez, Mozambique, 1995–1996

	Harvest	Hungry
	Percentage of requirements	
Calories	91	63
Protein	148	79
Vitamin A	23	88
Niacin	103	64
Calcium	42	42
Iron	92	64

Source: Rose et al. 1999.

average calories per person per day in the village drop from about 2,000 in the harvest season, to about 1,430 during the hungry season. Thirty to forty percent of people surveyed had calorie intake that was insufficient to replace the calories used in normal daily activity. Maize—the source of 60 percent of calories in the average diet during the harvest season—has disappeared from the diets of many during the hungry season; it is replaced by manioc, peanuts, and sorghum—less desirable substitutes that are not eaten as much when maize is available.

One nutritional bright spot for the hungry season diet described in Table 6.4 is the abundance of vitamin A. This comes from the increase in consumption of fruits and vegetables such as pumpkin squash during the hungry season. The increase in consumption of wild fruits and vegetables during the hungry season appears to be a widespread phenomenon. Falconer (1990) reviews the literature and finds a number of studies that stress the importance of wild plants and animals as sources of food during the hungry season in different parts of the developing world. In one Zambian village, wild foods are found to make up 42 percent of the diet during the hungry season, compared to 7 percent during the rest of the year. In rural Bangladesh, people eat an average 1 gram per person per day of food from wild plants for the ten months following the rice harvest; then in the May-June hungry season, this increases to 191 grams per person per day. (See Box 6.2 for descriptions of the hungry season.)

■ Who Is Undernourished?

In which countries is the problem of undernutrition the worst? Tables 6.5, 6.6, and 6.7 show that the answer to this question depends on the way in which the extent of undernutrition is measured.

If we look at calories available per person as a percentage of average

Box 6.2   The Hungry Season in Zambia and Malawi

Data such as those presented in the accompanying text give us some idea of
the quantitative aspects of the hungry season. But a more complete picture
emerges from some vivid descriptions.

A *Washington Post* reporter visiting Zambia during the hungry season
found this (Gillis 2003:A-1):

"When the people by the lake began to starve, they fell back on the
knowledge of their ancestors. They picked poisonous fruits from the bush and
boiled them for three days to eliminate the toxin concocting a barely palatable
dish. But sometimes hungry children would sneak a taste early . . . and the
poison would make them ill. Kebby Kamota, father of 11, could take it no
longer. 'Three days! Three days!' He shouted explaining how long his children would sometimes go without food."

A Peace Corp volunteer (Kluender 2003) in Zambia describes the onset of the
hungry season like this:

"I can tell the change of season by signs rather than months. When there
are mangoes, rain, disease, funerals and kids crying at night, it's the hungry
season."

A CIMMYT report (2003) describes how Agness Pungulani, a single mother
in Malawi, copes:

"During the . . . hungry season, markets were devoid of grain [and] local
traders were selling maize at [two-and-a-half times the normal price]. When
the food stocks disappeared, Pungulani . . . foraged, drank tea from wild
occra leaves in place of evening meals, and pounded banana tree roots into a
crude flour approximating their preferred maize staple. . . . A neighbor . . .
says, "This flour tastes sour, but we eat it because we have no choice." The
hungry season normally arrives during January-February in this part of
Malawi, but lately families have run out of grain as early as September and
must survive until the March harvests."

A *New York Times* reporter describes the joyful end of the hungry season in
Malawi.

"Late one afternoon, during the long melancholia of the hungry months,
there was a burst of joyous delirium in Mkulumimba. Children began shout-
ing the word 'ngumbi,' announcing that winged termites were fluttering
through the fields. These were not the bigger species of the insect, which can
be fried in oil and sold as a delicacy for a good price. Instead, these were the
smaller ones, far more wing than torso, which are eaten right away. Suddenly,
most everyone was giddily chasing about; villagers were catching ngumbi
with their fingers and tossing them onto their tongues, grateful for the unex-
pected gift of food afloat in the air. . . . Most every year, Malawi suffers a
food shortage during the so-called hungry months, December through March.
. . . Families often endure this hungry period on a single meal a day, sometimes nothing more than a foraged handful of greens."

Table 6.5 Countries That Rank High in Undernutrition Based on Dietary Intake and Requirements

Average calories per capita per day as % of average daily requirement, 2001		Percentage of population suffering from undernutrition, 1998–2000	
Country	Percent	Country	Percent
Congo, D. R.	69.8	Congo, D. R.	73
Burundi	72.5	Somalia	71
Tajikistan	73.4	Afghanistan	70
Afghanistan	74.0	Burundi	69
Eritrea	75.7	Tajikistan	64
Somalia	76.1	Eritrea	58
Armenia	83.2	Mozambique	55
Mongolia	83.6	Haiti	50
Zambia	84.5	Angola	50
Cambodia	86.2	Zambia	50
Sierra Leone	86.3	Tanzania	47
Central African Rep.	86.6	Sierra Leone	47
Angola	87.0	Armenia	46
Liberia	87.4	Central African Rep.	44
Mozambique	88.4	Ethiopia	44
Tanzania	89.1	Kenya	44
Madagascar	89.9	Mongolia	42
Kenya	90.4	Rwanda	40
Haiti	90.8	Madagascar	40

Sources: Calories per capita day intake from FAOSTAT food balance sheets. Calories per capita per day requirements calculated from population by age and sex according to the U.S. Census for 2000 and the calorie requirements in Table 3.2. Percentage of population suffering from undernutrition from FAO 2002, *State of the World's Food Insecurity*.

requirements, the worst-off countries are the Democratic Republic of Congo (Kinshasa), Burundi, Eritrea, and Somalia in Africa, and Afghanistan and Tajikistan in Asia. If we look at anthropometric indicators of child nutrition, North Korea and Afghanistan top the list, with Burundi, Eritrea, and Somalia scoring badly as well. If we look at mortality rates for children under five as an indicator of undernutrition, we conclude that Sierra Leone, Angola, and Afghanistan are the worst-off. If we look at the percentage of low-birth-weight babies and children who are underweight, we identify Bangladesh, Haiti, Yemen, and India as the worst. (However, no information on low birth weight is available for Afghanistan, North Korea, and other countries.)

Most of the worst-off countries on these lists are in sub-Saharan Africa. However, one other aspect is worth noting: the lists of low-birth-weight babies and anthropometrically small children have a number of Asian countries near the top. Ramalingaswami, Jonsson, and Rohde (1996) discuss this phenomenon. They suggest the explanation may be a combination of the following:

Table 6.6   Countries That Rank High in Undernutrition Based on Anthropometric Measurements of Children Under Age 5, 2000

Stunted (low height for age)		Underweight (low weight for age)		Wasted (low weight for height)	
Country	Percentage	Country	Percentage	Country	Percentage
Korea, Dem.	59.5	Korea, Dem.	60	Afghanistan	25
Zambia	59	Afghanistan	48	Korea, Dem.	18.7
Burundi	56.8	Bangladesh	47.8	Somalia	17.2
Nepal	54.1	Ethiopia	47.1	Maldives	16.8
Afghanistan	52	Nepal	47.1	Eritrea	16.4
Yemen	51.7	India	47	India	15.5
Ethiopia	51.2	Yemen	46.1	Laos PDR	15.4
Malawi	49	Cambodia	45.9	Cambodia	15.3
Madagascar	48.6	Burundi	45.1	UAE	15.2
Guatemala	46.4	Eritrea	43.7	Mauritius	15
Cambodia	46	Mali	43.3	Sri Lanka	15
India	45.5	Maldives	43.2	Benin	14.3
Nigeria	45.5	Laos PDR	40	Niger	14.1
Congo, D.R.	45.2	Niger	39.6	Madagascar	13.7
Bangladesh	44.8	Pakistan	38.2	Burkina Faso	13.2
Lesotho	44	Myanmar	36	Oman	13
Mauritania	44	Congo, D.R.	34.4	Djibouti	12.9
Tanzania	43.8	Burkina Faso	34.3	Yemen	12.9
Rwanda	42.7	Madagascar	33.1	Nigeria	12.4
Comoros	42.3	Vietnam	33.1	Togo	12.3

Source: UNICEF 2003, Table 2.

- "Girls and women in South Asia are less well regarded and less well cared for than in sub-Saharan Africa." Poor nutrition among pregnant women causes low-birth-weight babies.
- "Differences in standards of hygiene between the two regions [South Asia and sub–Saharan Africa] are very pronounced. . . . This all-round poor hygiene increases the burden of illness, and [causes] significantly higher levels of malnutrition among South Asia's children."
- Quality of childcare is higher in sub-Saharan Africa than in South Asia.

It is interesting to notice that the small size of babies and children in South Asia does not translate into high rates of child mortality. Finally, we should note that the tables describe Afghanistan during the period before the military action that removed the Taliban government in 2002.

Some readers may wonder if we have forgotten to consider undernutrition in the developed world. The incidence of undernutrition in the developed world is generally so close to zero that it does not contribute much to

Table 6.7 Countries That Rank High in Undernutrition According to Infant and Child Health, 2000

Under-5 Child Morality Rates		Low Birth Weights	
Country	Per thousand	Country	% of births
Sierra Leone	180	Bangladesh	30.0
Angola	172	Haiti	28.3
Afghanistan	165	Yemen	25.7
Niger	159	India	25.5
Liberia	157	Chad	23.5
Mali	142	Iraq	23.1
Somalia	133	Sierra Leone	22.0
Guinea-Bissau	132	Pakistan	21.4
Congo, Dem. Rep.	128	Nepal	20.9
Mozambique	126	Guinea-Bissau	19.5
Mauritania	120	Comoros	18.4
Chad	118	Burkina Faso	18.3
Ethiopia	117	Philippines	17.5
Malawi	117	Côte d'Ivoire	17.2
Central African Rep.	115	Sri Lanka	17.0
Burundi	114	Ecuador	16.1
Guinea	112	Burundi	16.0
Zambia	112	Mali	16.0
Nigeria	110	Myanmar	16.0
Burkina Faso	105	Madagascar	15.2

Sources: UNICEF 2003, Table 2.

the worldwide numbers. In the period following the breakup of the former Soviet Union, undernutrition became a problem in some areas. The situation in the United States is described in Box 6.3.

What Kinds of People Are Undernourished?

Of course, hunger knows no boundaries: it afflicts the young, the old, the healthy, the sick, the working, the unemployed. But there are groups of people among whom undernutrition is more common.

Within any given country, malnutrition is likely to be more prevalent in rural areas. The World Bank (*World Development Report 1990*:238) calculated that, among the forty-two countries they classified as low-income in 1988, rural people represented 65 percent of the population. Rural incomes are usually considerably below urban incomes and, because undernutrition is so closely associated with low-income populations, a pretty strong argument can be made that the majority of the world's hungry are rural. Because of this, and because so many policies affecting the price and availability of food to both rural and urban consumers impinge on the rural sector of the economy, we make a heavy emphasis in this book on policies

Box 6.3   Undernutrition in the Developed World

All of our attention here has been on poor countries. What about rich countries such as the United States? Perhaps you have heard claims that thousands of children in this American city or that American state go to bed hungry every night. The source of those claims, and the most in-depth study of hunger in the United States, is a USDA report on Food Security in the United States (Nord, Andrews, and Carlson 2003).

That report concludes that food insecurity afflicts 12.5 percent of people and 18.1 percent of children in the United States (pp. 16–17). But what is food insecurity? The report based its definition on a survey of ten questions (plus an additional eight questions to households with children). Some of the questions are rather subjective, such as: "In the past 12 months, did you worry that your food would run out before you got money to buy more?" Other questions are more concrete, such as: "Did you ever not eat for a whole day because there wasn't enough money for food?"

A household that answered "yes" to more than two of these questions was labeled "food insecure." A household with children could be categorized as "food insecure" if they "couldn't afford balanced meals" and "relied on a few kinds of low cost food." If the household answered "yes" to six or more of the ten questions (eight or more of the eighteen questions asked to households with children), the household was labeled "food insecure with hunger." This more severe form of food insecurity afflicts 3.4 percent of people and 0.8 percent of children in the United States.

Of the households in the "food insecurity with hunger" category, only a tiny number (about 0.1 percent of all households) reported that their children went without eating for a whole day at any time during the year, and only 1 percent reported that adults went without eating for the whole day at any time in the year; 0.2 percent of households said that adults went without eating for at least one day in almost every month.

For poor families in the United States, running out of food with no money to buy more can be a difficult time. But compare the descriptions in this box to the descriptions of the "hungry season" in Box 6.2. By international standards, the undernutition problem in the United States is almost undetectable. The incidence of hunger is low because incomes in the United States—even incomes of the poor—are high by world standards, and because of public programs (such as food stamps) and private efforts (such as church-run food pantries) to help poor families.

affecting the rural sector. The tension that exists between the rural and urban sectors of developing countries is discussed in some detail in Chapter 22. As the world moves into the twenty-first century, developing economies are expected to become increasingly urban, but even then, rural-oriented policies will remain especially significant among those aimed at undernutrition.

Children as a group are by far the most vulnerable to undernutrition, especially at weaning time—that transitional period during which an infant's diet is changed from 100 percent breast milk to 100 percent other foods—a transition that can be abrupt but that, in the third world, often takes place during an eighteen-month time span, say, between six months and two years of age. While infants are being moved from breast milk toward other foods, their requirements for a calorie- and protein-dense diet are still very high, and in cultures where the diet is dominated by grains, providing an appropriate diet for weaning children takes a special effort.

Pregnant women and lactating mothers are the next most vulnerable to undernutrition, and old women may be next in line. During times of extreme food shortages or famines, these groups are almost always the most at risk, but at these times a broader segment of the population, including large numbers of able-bodied men, is likely to be affected also.

We hear occasional reports of food deprivation based on gender. Roger Winter (1988), director of the U.S. Committee for Refugees, writes about the Dinka people in Sudan, who have been plagued both by drought and a scorched-earth strategy the Sudanese army used to subdue the Dinka's rebellious tendencies. Winter reports that many refugee groups consist chiefly of physically weakened young men and boys: "Women and children often are left behind, displaced and without access to international assistance or protection. They are dying in shockingly large numbers. In some areas, virtually all children under 3 are dead. Young girls are rare: In a society beset by war, with an economy based on cattle herding, girls are allowed to starve so that resources can be devoted to their brothers" (p. A-25).

The Punjab in northwest India has the highest ratio of males to females in India. A study of the area (Das Gupta 1988) reported that the youngest daughters in families with many children are often selectively deprived of both medicine and the more nutritious foods in order that their brothers may be better cared for. Although coauthor Foster and colleagues looked, they did not find evidence of this practice during their unpublished 1981 study of Bagbana village.

A bias against girls is by no means universal. WHO data on underweight children breaks down the prevalence by sex of child. In sixty countries, the percentage of boys who are underweight is higher than the percentage of girls who are underweight. In thirty-two countries, more girls are underweight than boys.

When examining the at-risk groups, the emphasis on women and children does not mean that undernutrition never affects adult working men. Although clinical signs of undernutrition are rare in this group, significant numbers appear to suffer an energy depletion that limits work capacities and productivity.

So far, we have examined the number of people suffering from undernutrition, as well as the trends, geographic location, and seasonality of hunger, and the people most vulnerable to it. But undernutrition occurs in individuals on a case-by-case basis. If we can identify the characteristics of a family that predispose them to an occurrence of undernutrition, we may, at the same time, uncover clues as to appropriate policies for reducing its prevalence.

Arnold and his colleagues (1981) examined data collected in 1979 by the National Nutrition Council of the Philippines. Their sample contained 722 families from seven provinces. To be included in the sample, a family had to have at least one preschool child. The purpose of the study was to see if family data could be used to predict the presence of an undernourished child. So the preschool child with the lowest level of nutrition of all a family's preschoolers was chosen as the subject. This child, therefore, became the dependent variable, and what Arnold's group tried to predict was the percentage of standard weight-for-age of this child. See Table 6.8 for some of the main findings of the study. Variables with a positive correlation coefficient have a positive influence on percentage of weight-for-age. That is, the higher the value of the variable, the more likely the subject child is to be well nourished. Some of the relationships are fairly obvious. The more education the father and mother have and the more income the family has, the better nourished the subject child is likely to be.

The importance of weaning age becomes clear when you think about it. The Philippines is a country of rice eaters, and rice is low in both protein and fat. Therefore, the longer a child is breast-fed, the longer is the time it is receiving an appropriately protein-rich, calorie-dense diet.

Table 6.8   Correlation of Socioeconomic Variables with Percentage of Standard Body Weight-for-Age, Philippine Preschoolers (Under Six Years Old), 1979

Socioeconomic Variable	Correlation Coefficient	Number of Families Sampled
Number of years of formal education of the mother	.27	721
Number of years of formal education of the father	.26	716
Income, farming families	.12	213
Income, nonfarming families	.35	499
Age of weaning if subject child is weaned	.34	545
Type of infant feeding	−.37	718
1 = breast alone, 2 = mixed, 3 = bottle alone		
Total number of household members	−.25	722
Birth order of subject child	−.21	722

Source: Arnold et al. 1981.

Note: All variables were significant at the .01 level except income, which was significant at the .07 level.

Variables with a negative correlation coefficient (those at the bottom of Table 6.8) have a negative influence on percentage of weight-for-age. Thus, mothers who bottle-fed their babies almost exclusively were more likely to have undernourished children than those who breast-fed exclusively. Children of mothers who mixed bottle- and breast-feeding tended to be better off than those who were bottle-fed only and worse off than those who were breast-fed only. Children in large families were more likely to be undernourished than children in small families. And within the same family, children born later were more likely to be undernourished than their older siblings. Speculation has it that mothers sometimes give up, if slightly, on the youngest child after they have already borne three or four children (S. Scrimshaw 1978:389; 1984).

Another study has shown that the age of the mother at the time of giving birth may influence nutritional status. Children of mothers who at the time of their children's births were younger than twenty or older than thirty are more likely to be undernourished than are children born of mothers between twenty and thirty (Rustein 1984).

Sometimes special circumstances exacerbate an already unfortunate situation and increase still further the possibility that a child will be undernourished. In 1980, coauthor Foster and colleagues had occasion to visit a number of Filipino families, each of which had at least one third-degree undernourished child. In most cases, in addition to the usual problems of low income, low education of the parents, and a number of children in the household, some special situation or stressor existed that might have significantly contributed to child undernutrition—for example, the mother suffered from tuberculosis and was always tired; the mother liked to gamble and left her one-year-old in the care of her four-year-old; the mother had borne twins and thought they carried a curse; the father was living with another woman; or the father was working in the city and came home only every other Sunday.

PART 2

Causes of Undernutrition

The main causes of undernutrition can be traced to economic, demographic, and health variables. Part 2 is devoted to each of these causes of undernutrition. The concept of food security demonstrates the interrelatedness of these causes, and with this in mind we begin Part 2.

7

Economics: Supply and Demand

To this point, we have focused on the effects, measurement, and prevalence of undernutrition. The next section of the book will describe the factors that influence the occurrence and extent of undernutrition. Economics serves as the organizing framework for this discussion. This chapter is intended to be a very brief introduction to economic principles.

■ An Elementary Example of Supply and Demand

Alfred Marshall, a nineteenth-century British economist, is the father of modern economics. He used a simple example of a boy gathering raspberries to illustrate the concepts of supply and demand. Imagine a boy walking through the woods who spots a patch of raspberry bushes. The boy reaches out and plucks a raspberry and pops it in his mouth. He gets a burst of pleasure: he was hot, thirsty, and hungry; the raspberry refreshes him. As he continues to eat raspberries, two things occur. First, the pleasure from eating additional raspberries subsides; the pleasure he gets from eating the twentieth raspberry is less than the pleasure he got from that first raspberry. This may be because he is no longer as hungry, hot, and thirsty, or because the novelty of eating raspberries has worn off, or because the twentieth raspberry is not as ripe as the first one. Second, the boy discovers it is harder and harder to find raspberries to pick. He has to kneel on the ground, or reach into the brambles to reach additional raspberries.

If we put this experience on a graph it would look like Figure 7.1. The downward-sloping curve shows the pleasure the boy gets from each successive raspberry: he gets a lot of pleasure from the first berry, slightly less additional pleasure from the second, still less from the third, etc. The upward-sloping curve shows the amount of effort needed to obtain each successive berry: the first requires very little effort, the second requires a little more, the third even more, etc.

We can also use the graph in Figure 7.1 to track the boy's reasoning. Should I eat the first raspberry? Yes: the pleasure from that is very high and

Figure 7.1   The Boy in the Berry Patch

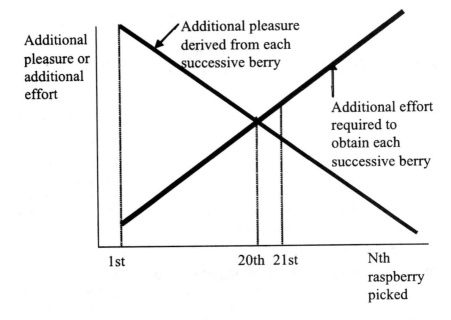

the cost of obtaining it is very low. Likewise, the second, and the third. When he gets to the twentieth berry, the pleasure from that berry has dropped, and the cost of obtaining it has increased, but it is still (just bare-ly) "worth it"—the pleasure derived exceeds the effort needed to obtain it. When he considers the twenty-first berry, he realizes that the berry is no longer worth the effort. In terms of the graph, the intersection of the "addi-tional pleasure" curve and the "additional effort" curve shows the point at which the boy stops.

We can characterize the boy's decision as an "optimal" decision in the following sense. The boy's decision is one that maximizes the boy's "sur-plus pleasure," defined as the pleasure from consuming minus the discom-fort of gathering the berries. This illustrates a fundamental principle of eco-nomics: an optimal decision is one in which the "marginal benefits"—in our example, the additional pleasure gained from eating one more berry—equals the "marginal costs"—the additional effort needed to pick the berries. Note that in the raspberry example, there is no money—the boy does not put a dollar value on his pleasure or on his effort. Yet, there is an implicit comparability: the boy can say, "The pleasure from the berry is worth (or not worth) the additional effort."

■ A Producer's Supply Curve, and a Consumer's Demand Curve

The fundamental concepts of economic behavior are contained in the story of the raspberries. The only difference when it comes to modern economics is that the comparability of pleasure and effort is made explicitly in monetary terms: Figure 7.2 is exactly like Figure 7.1 except that the Y-axis in the figure is now "price" or dollars per unit of the good.

The downward sloping curve is an individual consumer's *demand* curve. It shows how much of a good the person would like to consume at all the different possible levels of price. An alternative interpretation is that the demand curve shows the maximum amount per unit the person is willing to pay for all the different possible levels of consumption. The downward slope of the demand curve means that as the price of a good falls, a consumer would like to consume more of the good. (See Box 7.1 for an example of a downward-sloping demand curve.)

The upward-sloping curve in Figure 7.2 is an individual producer's *supply* curve. It shows how much of a good the person would produce at all the different possible levels of price. Alternatively, it shows the minimum amount per unit that the person would require to produce at each of the different possible levels of production. The upward slope of the supply curve means that as the price of a good increases, a producer is willing to produce more of the good. The concepts of costs of production and the technical relationships between input and output are discussed in Box 7.2.

Figure 7.2 Supply and Demand Curves

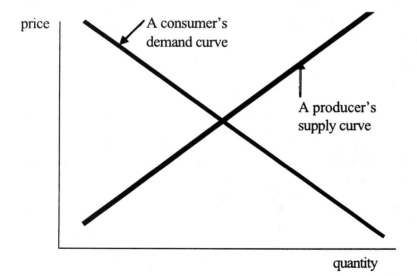

Box 7.1   Demand Curves Slopes Down

The city of London (England) has a problem: too many people driving too
many cars. Economists have a solution: raise the price of driving in London
and people will consume less of that good (driving in London). In February
2003, a congestion fee of £5 (about $8) was imposed on all cars driving in a
zone of central London during every weekday. Cameras record the license
plate numbers of cars entering the zone to ensure that drivers paid the
required fee for that day. The hoped-for result was that automobile traffic
would be reduced by 15 percent by the year 2010. Economists estimated that
the £5 fee would reduce traffic by 12–17 percent. But by early April 2003,
traffic loads appeared to have stabilized at a level 20 percent lower than previous levels. The demand curve for driving in central London was flatter
(economists would say, "the elasticity of demand was higher, in absolute
value") than economists predicted. But the economists were right in the direction of their prediction: if you want people to consume less of a good, raise
the price of the good.

Sources: See Blow, Leicester, and Smith 2003 or Transport for London 2003.

■ Aggregate Supply, Aggregate Demand, and Markets

Of course in real world markets, consumers and producers are not matched
up one by one. A single potato farmer may grow enough potatoes to feed
hundreds of people, and a single consumer may buy different kinds of food
from many different farmers. But the market serves as a place where many
consumers and many farmers can interact in a process that sets an equilibrium price at the point where the *aggregate supply curve* intersects the
aggregate demand curve illustrated in Figure 7.3. Recall that the individual
producer's supply curve shows how much of a good the producer will produce at different price levels. If we add up (aggregate) those quantities for
all producers, we have a picture showing the total quantity that would be
produced at different price levels. Likewise, we add up quantities demanded by individual consumers to obtain the aggregate demand curve.

The point at which the aggregate supply and demand curves intersect
shows the equilibrium price and aggregate quantity. If the price is above
this equilibrium price, producers want to sell a greater quantity than consumers want to buy. Producers who cannot find a buyer for their output will
try to attract buyers by offering a lower price. If the price were to fall below
the equilibrium price, some buyers would be unable to buy the quantity
they wish, and the price will be bid up.

In a complex economy with many consumers, many producers, and
many goods, the prices determined by the interaction of aggregate supply

Box 7.2   Why the Supply Curve Slopes Upward

There is a physical and a cost basis for the relationship between price and the amount that a farmer will try to produce. Let us start with the underlying physical relationship, using as our example the relationship between the amount of seed planted in one field (say a hectare of land) and a crop yield. The raw data we assume are given in Table A and plotted in Figure A. The top curve in Figure A represents the total yield from varying amounts of fertilizer (total physical product or production function). The bottom curve represents the yield added by each successive increment of 10 units of seed (marginal physical product).

Table A: Hypothetical Yield Response to Varying Amounts of Seed

Seed	Yield	Marginal Physical Product
0	0	39
10	39	13
20	52	9
30	61	5
40	66	0
50	66	-2
60	64	

Figure A

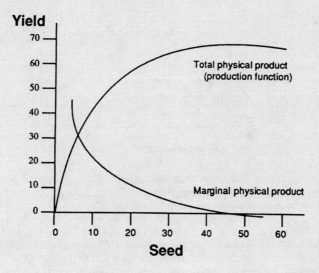

(continues)

Continued

What we have in Figure A is a graphic representation of the fact that, as we increase the amount of an input used, holding other inputs constant, we experience diminishing returns to successive inputs (thus the downward-sloping marginal physical product curve—which is often called diminishing marginal returns). The functional relationships we are talking about here are based on observations that have been made in the real world.

Now let us combine the variable inputs commonly used to increase production on our hypothetical one hectare of land. As we increase production we not only add more seed, but more fertilizer, more labor, and maybe other inputs such as irrigation water and pesticides. These things cost money. As we increase production, we could, at various amounts produced, add up the costs of the things we are using to increase production and plot these sums to get a cost curve.

The cost curve would say very much the same thing that Figure A says, except that it would measure costs, instead of seed, along the horizontal input. (The relation between cost and production is based on the underlying physical relationships between inputs and production.) We diagram our cost curve in Figure B. Because the fixed cost of land is not included in our set of costs, we identify the costs in this diagram as variable costs.

Figure B

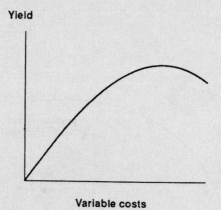

Yield

Variable costs

Notice in Figure B that, although not specifically diagrammed, as yield increases there are diminishing marginal returns to costs, just as there were diminishing marginal returns to seed in Figure A.

It is a convention of economics to draw cost curves with the cost on the vertical axis and the yield on the horizontal axis. So let us redraw Figure B in the conventional way, namely as shown in Figure C. (To see what happens to the cost curve when this is done, you might want to trace Figure B and then flip it over and look at it from the back side so as to get Figure C.)

(continues)

Continued

Figure C

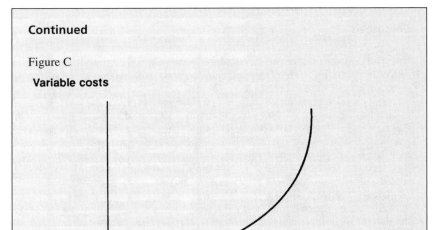

Variable costs

Yield

With Figure C, instead of thinking about what happens to yield as we increase costs by one unit, we can think about what happens to costs as we increase yield by one unit. If you examine Figure C you will see that we produce under conditions of increasing marginal cost. For each additional unit of yield from our hectare of land, we have to spend somewhat more on our bundle of variable costs. These increasing marginal costs are diagrammed in Figure D.

Figure D

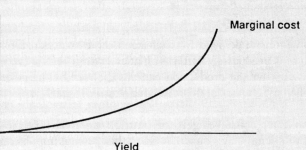

**Marginal cost
(vertical scale is
expanded from
the scale in
Figure c)**

Marginal cost

Yield

(continues)

Continued

Thus we see that we produce under diminishing marginal returns, which results in producing with increasing marginal costs. The two are based on the same underlying physical relationship.

For an individual producer, the marginal cost curve (Figure D) is the price schedule at which he is willing to produce various amounts of goods for the market. He is willing to produce up to the point where the price equals his marginal cost of production. If he is producing at this point and we want to motivate him to produce more, barring a shift in technology or a reduction in the costs of some of his inputs, we will have to pay him more. This is represented in Figure E as shifting production from A to B, which is motivated by an increase in price from P1 to P2.

Adding up the marginal cost curves (individuals' supply curves) for all the individual producers yields the supply curve for the industry. Increasing the price of the product will motivate the industry to produce more.

Figure E

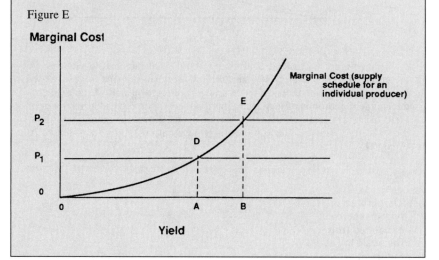

and aggregate demand for each good serve to organize or direct consumption and production patterns. Under certain restrictive assumptions, the consumption and production patterns dictated by the price mechanism will be the best choices in the following sense.

• Each consumer gets the most pleasure possible out of the money he has to spend. The consumer does this by making sure he gets the same amount of pleasure from the last dollar he spends on each good. To see what this means, suppose it were not the case; instead, suppose that the last dollar spent on bananas provided the consumer with very little pleasure,

Figure 7.3   Aggregate Supply and Demand

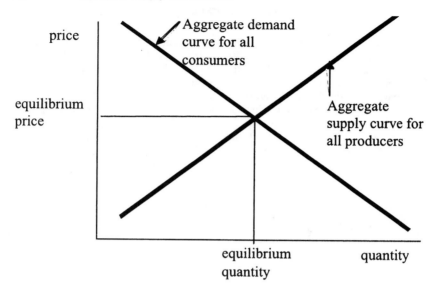

compared to the last dollar spent on tomatoes. In this case, the consumer would be happier if he took some of the money spent on bananas and bought tomatoes with that money.

• Each producer produces at the point that gives the highest profits (revenue minus cost). The producer does this by producing every unit for which the price received exceeds the additional cost of production, and by refusing to produce any additional units.

This description of how a competitive market equilibrium, in which each producer and consumer acts in his or her own self-interest, results in an allocation of goods that is (in the sense described above) optimal for the group as a whole is at the heart of Adam Smith's image of an "invisible hand" guiding economic activity. (See Box 7.3.) This concept will be discussed more fully in Chapter 16, where criticisms of the "economics approach" to policy analysis will be explored.

■ Combining Goods Together into Groups

In many economic discussions, and frequently in this book, we will refer to commodities that are not actually single goods. We have some idea of what it means to talk about the price of a tomato, or the price of a banana, or the price of a bushel of corn or a pound of chicken wings. But when we talk about the price of "food" or the quantity of "food," that is an abstract con-

---

Box 7.3   Adam Smith's Invisible Hand

"[E]very individual . . . neither intends to promote the public interest, nor knows how much he is promoting it. . . . [B]y directing that industry in such a manner as its produce may be of the greatest value, he intends only his own gain, and he is in this, as in many other cases, led by an invisible hand to promote an end which was no part of his intention. Nor is it always the worse for the society that it was no part of it. By pursuing his own interest he frequently promotes that of the society more effectually than when he really intends to promote it. I have never known much good done by those who affected to trade for the public good. It is an affectation, indeed, not very common among merchants, and very few words need be employed in dissuading them from it."

Source: Adam Smith, *Wealth of Nations,* Book IV. Online at: http://socserv2.socsci. mcmaster.ca/~econ/ugcm/3ll3/smith/wealth/index.html

---

cept. In the rest of this chapter, we will talk about "aggregate supply" and "aggregate demand" as shorthand terms meaning aggregate supply and demand of food.

■ How Demand Changes over Time

One important aspect of our study of world food problems is to understand how supply and demand for food have changed in the past and how they might be expected to change in the future. In terms of the previous section: What causes aggregate demand and supply curves to move around? In this section we examine factors that shift the aggregate demand for food.

Recall that aggregate demand for food shows the total quantity of food demanded at every level of price. The total quantity of food demanded at any given price might increase for any of the following reasons: (1) the number of the people in the economy increases, (2) people in the economy have more money to spend on all goods, so part of the additional income is spent on food, (3) people's tastes change so that the person gets more pleasure out of food compared to other nonfood goods. (Economics students will recognize that we have failed to mention a fourth factor: [4] prices of other nonfood items increase, so that the pleasure per dollar of additional expenditure on those nonfood goods declines.)

Population Growth Shifts the Aggregate Demand Curve

It is obvious that aggregate demand for food depends on how many individual consumer demand curves we are aggregating. This is the usual departure point for discussions of the world hunger problem: Can food supplies keep up with population growth? Or how many mouths are there to feed? This will be the focus of Chapter 9 and population policy will be discussed in Chapter 19. For the present, let us simply note that in the supply-demand context, an increase in population causes an outward shift in the aggregate demand curve for food. At any particular price level, the aggregate quantity demanded is higher because there are more people contributing to the aggregate demand. Holding all other factors constant (and in particular assuming that the aggregate supply curve stays in the same place), the effect of the outward shift in aggregate demand is to increase the price, and the higher price induces farmers to produce more food, so that aggregate equilibrium quantity increases.

Changes in Income or Income Distribution
Shift the Aggregate Demand Curve

It is important to emphasize that aggregate demand for food is not the same thing as "quantity of food that will provide every individual a healthy diet," nor is there any implicit promise that the equilibrium price will guarantee that the average individual (or all individuals, or even most individuals) will have sufficient food. Aggregate supply and demand can describe famine conditions or conditions of great plenty.

An individual's demand curve for food shows how much food he or she would like to buy at every price level, *given his or her income*. A person with a low income will have a demand curve that reflects low quantities. For most goods (so-called normal goods), if the person gets more income to spend, his or her demand curve will shift up and to the right as shown in Figure 7.4: at every price, the person will demand a higher quantity.

How big will the shift be? Economists use the concept of "income elasticity of demand" to measure this. This concept and some measures of the income elasticity of demand will be discussed in more detail later in this chapter. There we will show that the size of the shift is different for a poor person than for a rich person. If a poor person's income increases by 10 percent, the person will spend a lot of the increase on food and the person's demand curve for food will shift a relatively large amount. If a rich person's income increases by 10 percent, the person will spend little of the increase on food and the person's demand curve for food will shift a small amount. This fact has implications for how the aggregate demand for food changes with changes in income distribution.

If everyone's income grows, each person's demand for food will shift out and aggregate demand will also shift out. If average income stays the same, but income is redistributed from a rich person to a poor person, the aggregate demand curve for food will also shift out, since the poor person's

Figure 7.4   Outward Shift in Demand

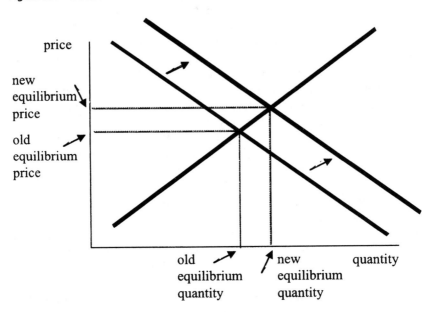

demand for food will shift out by a large amount, while the rich person's demand for food shifts back (in the opposite direction of the arrow in Figure 7.4) but by a smaller amount.

Changes in Tastes and Preferences
Can Shift the Aggregate Demand Curve

A final factor that may shift the aggregate demand curve for food is worth mentioning, even though it may seem obvious: if people's tastes and preferences change over time, that can have an effect on the aggregate demand for food. To see how this works at the level of the individual, we can return to the boy and the raspberries and imagine that the same boy revisits the same raspberry patch the following summer, except that this year he is wearing braces on his teeth. As he begins to eat the raspberries, he discovers that the tiny seeds get stuck in his braces in an annoying way. The pleasure he derives from eating the berries is less. In economics terminology, his individual demand curve has shifted down and to the left.

A "change in tastes and preferences" is not the same thing as a "change in quantity of food a person wants to buy." As the price of food changes, the quantity of food a person wants to buy will change as the person moves along his (not moving) demand curve. As a person's income changes, the quantity of food the person wants to buy will change as his/her demand curve shifts as described above. A change in tastes and preferences causes a change in the quantity of food a person wants to buy even as prices and income remain constant. For example, a person who decides to lose weight by eating less food will have a shift in demand.

In the aggregate, some trends in general behavior may cause a detectable shift in aggregate demand for food in developed countries: an increasing concern with obesity and overeating, increasing interest in diets low in carbohydrates, an increasing interest in food produced "organically," and/or a shift toward a more vegetarian diet.

■ How Supply Changes over Time

We next look at two factors that may cause shifts in the aggregate supply of food over time: availability (or price) of resources used to produce food, and technological change.

Changes in Availability of Resources Used to Produce Food.

If the resources used to produce food become more readily available—if the price of those resources falls—then at any level of output price, farmers will be willing to produce more. In the berry patch analogy, this is equivalent to an increase in the density of berries on the bush, or a decrease in the density of the thorns. Because it is less costly to produce an additional unit, more units are produced. An increase in production at every price level means an outward shift in supply, such as that illustrated in Figure 7.5.

Some simple examples illustrate this. If a farmer obtains more land, then at every price level, he will produce more output; his individual supply curve will shift out. If the farmer has more children able to work in the field, the farm's supply curve will shift out. If somebody gives the farmer some fertilizer to use on his land, the supply curve will shift out. If a dry creek begins to run with water so that the farmer can irrigate, the supply curve will shift out. If the general weather pattern changes to be more conducive to agricultural production, the supply curve shifts out. If the soil on the farm is eroded, or soil nutrients deplete, the supply curve shifts back (in the opposite direction of the arrows in Figure 7.5.) All of these—land, labor, fertilizer, water, weather, soil—are examples of productive resources; changing their availability shifts the supply curve.

When productive resources are bought and sold on a market, changes in general availability are reflected in the level of price for the resources. If fertilizer becomes more plentiful, the fertilizer price drops, and the supply of agricultural output shifts out. Or (as we will see later in the book) a government program to reduce fertilizer price (or to reduce the price of any other productive resource) has the same effect: it reduces farmers' production costs and causes an outward shift in the supply of agricultural output.

Figure 7.5   Outward Shift in the Supply Curve

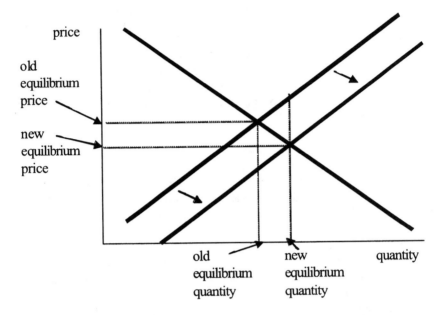

A technological improvement is some kind of new knowledge that allows farmers to produce more output with the same resources. Often the new knowledge is embodied in some piece of equipment (e.g., the invention of the plow) or other input (a new variety of seed). But the concept is broad enough to encompass improvements in the ability to predict weather patterns, or a better understanding of agronomic processes. A technological improvement is similar to a reduction in the price of a productive resource: both reduce the cost to the farmer of producing an additional unit of output, and both shift the supply curve out.

■ Using the Concept of Elasticity
to Quantify Economic Changes

So far in this chapter we have focused mainly on the direction of changes: as price goes up consumers reduce the quantity of food demanded and producers increase the quantity of food supplied; as income goes up, consumers increase the quantity of food demanded. But by how much? If the price of food increases by 3 percent, how much will quantities supplied and demanded change? If a person's income increases by 12 percent, how much will he or she increase the quantity of food purchased?

Economists answer these questions using a concept called "elasticity."

An elasticity measures the percentage change in quantity supplied or demanded in response to a one-percentage-point change in price or income. Here we will limit our attention to three types of elasticity. *Income elasticity of demand* measures the extent to which a demand curve shifts out in response to an increase in income. *Price elasticity of demand* measures the steepness of the demand curve—how much does quantity demanded fall as price increases (or how much does quantity demanded rise as price decreases) as we move along a demand curve? *Price elasticity of supply* measures the steepness of the supply curve—how does quantity supplied change in response to a change in price as we move along a supply curve?

Income Elasticity of Demand

In simplest terms, income elasticity of demand is the percentage change in the consumption of something, such as rice, when a 1 percent change occurs in income. You can easily see that this elasticity will change depending on your income level. If a poverty-stricken Indian villager suffered a 1 percent decrease in income, he might decrease his consumption of rice by half a percent or so. But a wealthy stockbroker who suffered a 1 percent decrease in income might not change her rice consumption at all. (She might spend less on recreational travel, for instance. But this is getting ahead of our story.)

Let us look at some general ways in which food consumption changes as income rises or falls. Table 7.1 provides an illustration, for a third world country, of how consumption of calories and protein increases as income increases or decreases. (In Table 7.1, expenditure subgroup is used as a proxy for income category.) The table, by the way, provides yet another illustration of the relationship between low income and undernutrition.

In Figure 7.6, more general than Table 7.1, we see differences in food consumption, converted to an equivalent amount of cereal grains, as income changed in a number of countries between 1966 and 1982. The curve is a best-fit trend line for the data. Notice how the rate of increase in consumption falls off as income increases. What is happening is that the proportion of the household budget spent on food decreases as income increases. The first person to write about this was Ernst Engel, and the phenomenon has become known as Engel's law.

In Figure 7.7 we can see, in some detail, changes in food consumption patterns associated with changes in income for a low-income region of East Java, Indonesia. Only the families in the top half of the income groupings (the right-hand half of Figure 7.7a) were receiving at least the 1,900 calories cited in the footnote to Table 7.1 as the minimum appropriate for Indonesians. Figure 7.7b provides a second illustration of Engel's law: As income rises, the percentage of income spent for food declines from 75 for the lowest-income families in the sample population to 60 for the highest-

Table 7.1   **Calorie and Protein Intake Estimated from the Fifth National Socioeconomic Survey (Susenas V), All Indonesia, 1976**

Expenditure Subgroup (Rupiahs per Capita per Month)	Percentage of Total Population	Calories per Capita per Day	Grams Protein per Capita
Less than 2,000	15.3 ⎱ 39.1	1,387	22.2
2,000–2,999	23.8 ⎰	1,870	32.3
3,000–3,999	19.5	2,034	40.2
4,000–4,999	13.6	2,084	47.0
5.000–5,999	8.8	2,288	52.7
6,000–7,999	9.4	2,533	60.9
8,000–9,999	4.2	2,794	69.7
10,000–14,999	3.8	3,066	79.1
Over 15,000	1.6	3,284	93.3
Total	100		
Average		2,064	43.3

Source: Hutabarat 1990, as quoted in Dixon 1982:6.
Note: Dixon (1982:4) reports that minimum nutritional requirements for Indonesia are 1,900 calories and 39.2 grams of protein per day, based on the 1973 FAO/WHO recommendations and the distribution by age and body weight of Indonesians. Groups below that amount can therefore be considered undernourished. Note that, because of wastage in marketing and preparation, the amount available for consumption must be greater than the actual calorie or protein intake. For Indonesia, the minimal daily requirements of food available are 2,100 calories and 45.9 grams of protein. In 1976 the exchange rate for rupiahs were U.S. $1 = Rp 145.

income families. Figure 7.7c shows how the food expenditure mix changes as income increases. As income grows, the East Javanese spend a smaller proportion of their food budget on starchy staples—cassava, rice, maize, and wheat flour—and a larger proportion on other items, especially animal products. This phenomenon is called Bennett's law, which states that the *starchy staple ratio* (the ratio of starchy foods such as cereals and root crops to other foods in the diet) falls as income increases. Figure 7.7d shows how the energy derived from various food sources shifts as income rises. The lowest-income people in the sample derive half their food energy from cassava (see Box 7.4); but as income rises, they quickly substitute other foods, especially rice, for cassava.

Commodities such as cassava, which people consume less of as their incomes rise, are known by the ignominious name of *inferior goods.* In Figure 7.8, we see that, for the world as a whole, diet changes follow Bennett's law. Carbohydrates make up about 70–75 percent of the dietary calories of the lowest-income countries and only 45–50 percent of the dietary calories of the highest-income countries. For the world as a whole, then, the cereals and root crops are inferior goods. Contrast this income

Figure 7.6   Food Consumption and Income, Selected Countries, 1966–1982

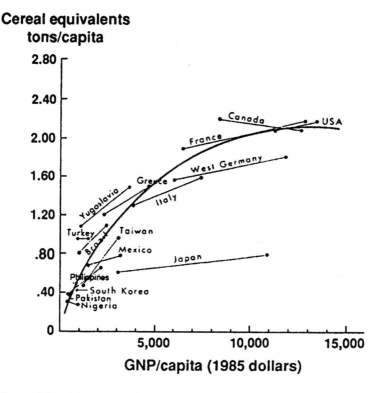

**Cereal equivalents
tons/capita**

Source: Adapted from Rask 1986.

consumption response to the change in consumption of fats and sugars as income increases.

The figures shown here certainly do not define the diet for every individual in each of the income categories shown. They do, however, identify clear tendencies toward changes in consumption patterns with changes in income.

Quantifying income elasticities.   As we said earlier, income elasticity of demand is the percentage change in the consumption of something, such as rice, when there is a 1 percent change in income.

For very small changes in income—for instance, when the percentage change in income is 1 percent or less—we can express income elasticity of demand algebraically as:

Figure 7.7   Relationships Between Income Level and Nutritional Status, East Java, 1977–1978

a. Energy (Kcal)

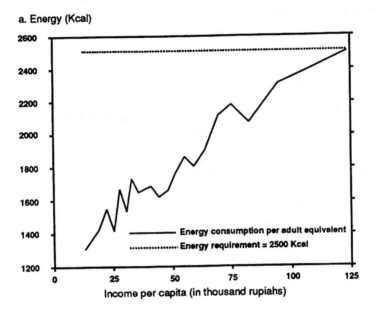

b. Food expenditures (percentage of income)

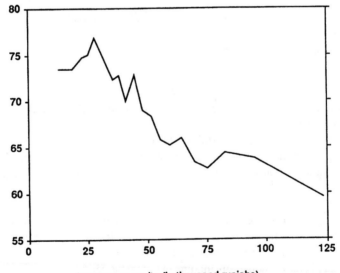

Income per capita (in thousand rupiahs)

(continues)

Figure 7.7   Continued

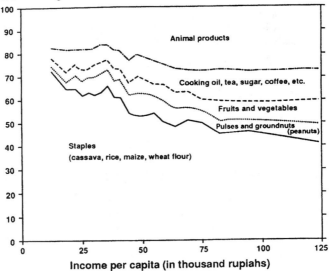

c. Percentage of food budget

Income per capita (in thousand rupiahs)

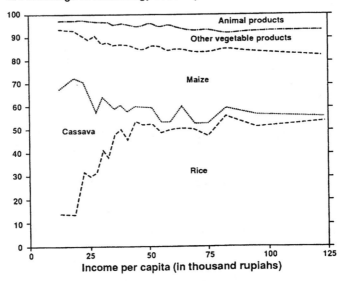

d. Percentage of total energy consumption

Income per capita (in thousand rupiahs)

Source: Ho 1984.

Note: Income is shown in thousands of Rupiahs. An income of Rs. 125,000 in 1977/78 was worth something over $200. The study region included Madura and the nearby regency of Sidorajo.

Box 7.4 Cassava

Cassava is a common food source in the tropics, especially among low-income people. It is a member of the spurge family (genus *Manihot*) and, in Africa, is usually called manioc. The fleshy rootstock is high in the starch known to English speakers as tapioca.

One source (Indonesia Oleh Direktorat Gizi Department Kesehatan R. I. 1979:19) gives the major nutritional constituents for 100 grams of dried cassava as: calories, 338; protein, 1.5 g; fat, 0.7 g; and carbohydrate, 81.3 g. There is some feeling among nutritionists that the protein in cassava is largely unavailable. If this is the case, consuming cassava is very close to consuming straight starch.

In the tropics cassava is so easy to grow it has been called "the Lazy Man's Crop." If you want some, just cut a foot or so of stalk from a live plant and stick it in the ground where it can get plenty of sunshine and some rain. Wait six to nine months and dig up the rootstock. The tuberous roots will keep only a week or so out of the ground, but if you are in no hurry do not dig it up; it will usually store for a year or so in the ground. Thus it can be used as insurance against famine during periods of food scarcity.

It is unfortunate that cassava leaves are seldom eaten, for they are high in vitamin A.

To some people, a full-grown cassava plant resembles a miniature papaya tree, while to others it looks more like an overgrown marijuana plant.

$$E = \frac{\% \text{ change in consumption}}{\% \text{ change in income}} = \frac{\dfrac{QD_2 - QD_1}{QD_1}}{\dfrac{Income_2 - Income_1}{Income_1}}$$

where: E = Elasticity of demand with respect to income
QD_1 = Quantity demanded at old income level ($Income_1$)
QD_2 = Quantity demanded at new income level ($Income_2$)

In the real world of constantly changing incomes and prices, trying to estimate demand elasticities is a lot more difficult than the above equation suggests. We leave descriptions of how this is done to others (e.g., Deaton and Muellbauer 1980; Huang 1985; Johnson, Hassan, and Green 1984). For purposes of this discussion we accept elasticity estimates done by others and concentrate on their meaning and implications for policy planners.

T. J. Ho (1984) calculated income elasticity for the East Javanese consumers whose food consumption patterns were outlined in Figure 7.7. She found the income elasticity of expenditure on food to be 0.58. That is, for this community, a 1 percent increase in income will produce a 0.58 percent increase in spending for food.

Figure 7.8   Percentage of Calories Derived from Fats, Carbohydrates, and Proteins by Annual GNP per capita, 2001

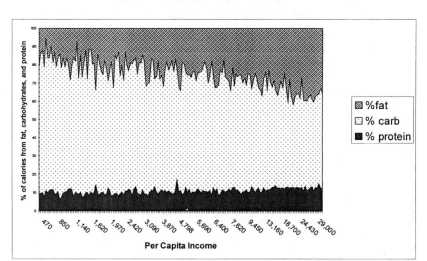

For purposes of illustration, let us hypothesize that this community spends half its income on food and, to make the computations simple, let us assume that its income is $100. A 1 percent increase in income raises income to $101. If food spending increases by 0.58 percent, these people will spend 29 cents more on food, for a total of $50.29. The remaining 71 cents of increased income will be spent on nonfood items, bringing the total for that category (housing, clothing, paying off debts, etc.) to $50.71. We can deduce, therefore, that the income elasticity of demand for nonfood items in this community is 1.42.

Had this community increased its spending on food by exactly the same percentage (and in this case exactly the same dollar amount) as its spending on nonfood items, that would indicate that the income elasticity of demand for both food and nonfood items is exactly one (1.0).

In a 1992 article, Bouis and Haddad review the literature and report a wide range of calorie-income elasticities, from 0.01 in Nicaragua to 1.18 in India. They argue that the wide range is attributable in large part to the different methods that different studies use to collect data on calories and the different conceptual measures they have of "income." They conclude that if appropriate measures are used, elasticity estimates fall in the 0.08–0.14 range.

Ho (1984) estimates the income elasticity of demand for calories to be 0.28 and for protein to be 0.52. These elasticities condense some of the information in Figure 7.7d. Review this graph and notice again how these people are substituting rice for cassava as their incomes increase. To a lesser extent, they are substituting animal products and other vegetable products for cassava at the same time. Calories from cassava are cheaper than calories from rice, other vegetables, or meat. Therefore, as they increase their spending on food, they buy fewer calories per rupiah and more of other food properties such as protein content and flavor. That is what the income elasticity figures (low for calories and high for protein) are telling us.

If you find this hard to grasp, here is another way of looking at those elasticity figures for calories versus protein. A 1 percent increase in income yields only a 0.28 percent increase in consumption of calories but a more generous 0.52 percent increase in protein consumption. That is, as income changes, these people change their consumption of protein more (in percentages) than they change their consumption of calories. While you could easily have come to this conclusion without the aid of the elasticity figures, what you get from the elasticity calculations is how much the people of East Java change their consumption of these two nutrients when income changes. That is the beauty—and the importance—of elasticity. It quantifies things.

Of course, people do not go to the market and buy nutrients like calories and protein. They buy food. So let us look at some income elasticity figures for particular commodities and see how these elasticities change with income. A detailed table of income elasticities in various countries for a variety of food groups and nutrients can be found at the USDA website (www.ers.usda.gov/data/internationalfooddemand).

How Income elasticity changes as income changes. Table 7.2 shows some income elasticities for three income groups in rural Brazil. Notice that, except for cassava flour, the income elasticity figures are positive. That is, for most foods, consumption increases as income increases. Cassava flour, with a negative income elasticity, is an inferior good.

Notice also that the absolute value (value without regard to sign) of the numbers in this table tends to decrease from low- to high-income consumers. That is, food consumption among low-income consumers is considerably more responsive to changes in income than it is among high-income consumers. This phenomenon is found among all third world populations.

When the low-income consumer in the Brazilian sample receives a 1 percent increase in income, he or she tends to increase rice consumption by about 2 percent. But the high-income consumer tends to change his or her consumption of rice by less than 0.2 percent when income changes by 1 percent. We call the low-income family's consumption response own-price *elastic.* That is, a 1 percent change in income yields a greater than 1 percent change in consumption. On the other hand, we call the high-income fami-

Table 7.2   Income Elasticities for Calorie Intake, Selected Foods, by Income Group, Rural Brazil, 1974–1975

	Income Group		
	Lowest 30 Percent	Middle 50 Percent	Highest 20 Percent
Cassava flour	−3.50	−1.59	−.356
Rice	1.99	.172	.173
Milk	2.27	.147	.172
Eggs	1.93	.630	.114
Mean per capita calorie intake	1,963	2,432	2,771

Source: Gray 1982:26.

Note: The 1974–1975 National Household Expenditure Survey (ENDEF) of the Brazilian Geographical and Statistical Institute was used as the data base from which to calculate these income elasticities.

ly's consumption response own-price *inelastic*. A 1 percent change in its income produces a less than 1 percent change in consumption. If a family changed its consumption of rice by exactly 1 percent when its income changed by 1 percent, we would say it had an income elasticity of demand for rice of one—neither elastic nor inelastic.

Remember that the elasticity figures show percentage change in consumption with a 1 percent change in income. The income elasticity of demand for rice in rural Brazil is about the same as the income elasticity of demand for eggs. But because rice makes up 15 percent of the total calories consumed among this income group, and eggs only 0.5 percent, a 1 percent change in income results in a far greater change in actual consumption of rice than of eggs (see Table 7.3). The nutritional significance of an elasticity, therefore, depends not only on the magnitude of the elasticity but on the magnitude of consumption of the goods under consideration.

Price Elasticity of Demand

How food consumption changes with price. As Figures 7.2 and 7.3 show, quantity demanded normally increases in response to a price decrease. But by how much? The consumption response to a decline in the price of a food item can be complex. Let us think about what might happen to consumption among the poorest 30 percent, in terms of income, in Brazil if the price of rice were to fall substantially.

A fall in the price of rice would likely result in the consumption of more rice. But it might well be that not all the increased purchasing power that results from a fall in the price of rice will be spent on rice. Some of it

Table 7.3   Changes in Calorie Consumption Resulting from a 1 Percent Increase in Income, Selected Foods, Lowest 30 Percent of Consumers by Income, Rural Brazil, 1974–1975

	Kilo-Calories	Percentage of Total Kilocalories Consumed	Income Elasticity	Change in Kilocalories Consumed Resulting from a 1 Percent Increase in Income
Cassava flour	440	22.4	−3.50	−15.4
Rice	296	15.1	1.99	5.9
Milk	41	2.1	2.27	.9
Eggs	7	.5	1.93	.1
Other	1,152	59.9		
Total kilocalorie intake	1,963		.46	1,940
Total change in entire diet				9

Source: Calculated from Gray 1982:20, 26.

might be spent on purchasing more of other foods, such as eggs, and some of it might be spent on purchasing nonfood items, such as entertainment.

This percentage change in rice consumption as a result of a 1 percent change in the price of rice is its *own-price elasticity*. The percentage changes in the consumption of a variety of other things, from eggs to entertainment, resulting from a 1 percent change in the price of rice (a fall in price, in this case) are the *cross-price elasticities* of demand.

Cross-price elasticities tend to be small. The cross-commodity price impact of a change in the price of rice, for instance, may be spread across a multitude of goods and services. Data on cross-price elasticities are harder to come by and may be less reliable than income and own-price elasticities. Furthermore, much sound analysis of the nutritional impact of policy alternatives can be done with what we know about income and own-price elasticities. Therefore, as mentioned earlier, in this book we will not deal much with cross-price elasticities.

Quantifying own-price elasticities.   Remember that price elasticity of demand is the percentage change in consumption of something, like rice, when a 1 percent change occurs in its own price.

For very small changes in price (for instance, when the percentage change in income is 1 percent or less) we can algebraically express elasticity of demand with respect to price as:

$$E = \frac{\substack{\% \text{ change} \\ \text{in consumption} \\ \hline \% \text{ change} \\ \text{in price}}}{} = \frac{\dfrac{QD_2 - QD_1}{QD_1}}{\dfrac{Price_2 - Price_1}{Price_1}}$$

where: E = Elasticity of demand with respect to price
QD_1 = Quantity demanded at old price
QD_2 = Quantity demanded at new price

As with income elasticity of demand, estimating these elasticities is a lot more difficult than the above equation suggests. So again we leave descriptions of how this is done to others. A comprehensive set of demand elasticities in various countries for a variety of food groups and nutrients can be found at the USDA website.

Table 7.4 shows a set of income and price elasticities for major food groups in Indonesia. These figures are for the complete spectrum of incomes, not broken down by income groups. Notice that for Indonesian society as a whole, all the income elasticities are positive and all the price elasticities are negative. This is exactly what the theory predicts: income elasticities are positive, meaning that an increase in income causes an outward shift in demand as in Figure 7.4; price elasticities are negative, meaning demand curves are downward-sloping.

Elasticities quantify consumers' behavior in the face of changing purchasing power. If income increases 1 percent, you can expect most consumption responses to be positive. But if price increases 1 percent, you can expect the usual consumption response to be negative. It is so common for price elasticities to be negative that the minus sign is often omitted. We will use the minus sign when quoting specific price elasticities to remind you of the inverse relationship between change in price and change in consumption.

Elasticity figures show you the relative importance consumers attach to the various foods in their diets. Items considered essential or necessary tend

Table 7.4 Income and Price Elasticities for Selected Foods, Indonesia

	Income Elasticity	Own-Price Elasticity
Corn and cassava	.3	−.26
Spices	.3	−.25
Rice	.7	−.63
Coconut	1.1	−.88
Tea and coffee	1.1	−.90
Vegetables and fruits	1.2	−.97
Prepared food	1.2	−1.01
Fish	1.3	−1.04
Sugar	1.4	−1.15
Drinks	2.1	−1.71
Livestock and livestock products	2.2	−1.73

Source: Boediono 1978:362.

to have elasticities below 1.0. Think of it this way: when income falls by 1 percent, consumption of necessities falls by less than 1 percent. Or if the price of a necessity rises by 1 percent, consumption falls by less than 1 percent. From Table 7.4, it appears that, by and large, Indonesians regard corn and cassava, spices, and rice as necessities.

Conversely, items considered luxuries tend to have elasticities above 1.0. If income falls by 1 percent, the consumption of luxuries falls by more than 1 percent as people cut back on luxuries and concentrate what income is left on necessities. If the price of a luxury rises by 1 percent, people are more likely to cut back substantially on consumption of that luxury than if the price of a necessity rises by 1 percent. Table 7.4 shows that Indonesians generally regard livestock and livestock products as luxuries. This is commonly the case in third world countries.

How price elasticities change as income changes.   Per Pinstrup-Andersen and colleagues (1976; Pinstrup-Andersen and Caicedo 1978) were the first to show that one could estimate price (and income) elasticities by income groups as well as by the community as a whole. They divided their Cali, Colombia, sample population into five income groups, and estimated elasticities for each income group as well as for their entire sample. Some of the elasticities calculated in their groundbreaking study are shown in Table 7.5.

Notice how responsiveness to change in price generally diminishes as

Table 7.5   **Estimated Direct Price Elasticity of Demand by Income Group, Cali, Colombia, 1969–1970**

	Low Income			High Income		
	I	II	III	IV	V	Average
Cassava	−.23	−.28	−.25	−.00	−.00	−.19
Potatoes	−.41	−.42	−.31	−.00	−.00	−.26
Rice	−.43	−.40	−.40	−.26	−.18	−.35
Maize	−.63	−.55	−.44	−.00	−.00	−.44
Bread/pastry	−.65	−.56	−.32	−.24	−.00	−.31
Beans	−.82	−.78	−.64	−.45	−.25	−.60
Peas	−1.13	−1.13	−.76	−.59	−.52	−.70
Eggs	−1.34	−1.23	−1.26	−.75	−.35	−.92
Oranges	−1.39	−.96	−.79	−.64	−.29	−.69
Milk	−1.79	−1.62	−1.12	−.64	−.20	−.77
Pork	−1.89	−1.61	−1.12	−.82	−.70	−1.01
Daily calorie intake as percentage of requirement	89	99	117	132	1,718	119

Source: Pinstrup-Andersen et al. 1976:137–138.

you move from low-income to high-income consumers. From this table it appears that high-income consumers in Cali could not care less about small changes in the price of cassava, potatoes, maize, or bread. And even with regard to pork, which the average consumer considers just over the edge into the luxury category, high-income consumers have a demand elasticity with respect to price of less than one (a 1 percent change in the price of pork will generate a less than 1 percent change in pork consumption among these consumers). In contrast, low-income consumers are fairly responsive to changes in food prices. They consider cassava, rice, potatoes, bread, and beans necessities, but they regard animal products and fresh fruit as luxuries.

Since this pioneering study, a number of other studies have been done that relate food price elasticities to income. Alderman (1986) provides a useful survey of those studies.

Price Elasticity of Supply

The final elasticity we will look at is the supply elasticity, which measures the percentage change in output produced in response to a 1 percent change in price of the output. This can be approximated by:

$$E = \frac{\substack{\text{\% change} \\ \text{in quantity produced}}}{\substack{\text{\% change} \\ \text{in price}}} = \frac{\dfrac{QS_2 - QS_1}{QS_1}}{\dfrac{Price_2 - Price_1}{Price_1}}$$

where: E = Elasticity of supply with respect to price
QS_1 = Quantity produced at old price
QS_2 = Quantity produced at new price

Estimates of supply elasticities find that supply is also "inelastic": a 1 percent increase in price will induce less than a 1 percent increase in quantity supplied. Lopez (1980), for example estimates a supply elasticity of 0.01 for crops and a supply elasticity of 0.472 for animal products. Table 7.6 shows some short-run supply elasticities for several farm products in African countries. (The "short run," in this case, refers to the fact that these elasticities measure the response of farmers when the quantity of land they are using and the quantities of other fixed inputs such as tube wells are not allowed to vary.)

Although the evidence is not conclusive, it appears that agricultural supply elasticities are somewhat higher in the developed world than in the developing world (Askari and Cummings 1976; Herdt 1970:518–519), indicating that farmers in developing countries are somewhat less responsive to changes in prices than are farmers in the developed world. If this is

Table 7.6   Short-Run Supply Elasticities, Selected Crops, African Countries

	Elasticity
Wheat	.31
Maize	.23
Sorghum	.10
Groundnuts	.24
Cotton	.23
Tobacco	.48
Cocoa	.15
Coffee	.14
Rubber	.14

Source: World Bank 1986:68; data are derived from Askari & Cummings 1976 and Scandizzo & Bruce 1980.

the case, it is most likely explained by three characteristics of farmers in developing countries: (1) they are less involved in the market economy—they sell a smaller percentage of their production and therefore are less impressed by swings in market prices; (2) they use lower quantities of purchased inputs relative to output sold and are therefore less able to adjust their production to variations in market prices; (3) they are more risk-averse than farmers in the developed world—they do not like spending large amounts on purchased inputs when a chance exists that because of low prices, the investment may not pay off. Nevertheless, hundreds of estimates of supply response to price show a positive relationship between price and production (supply curves do slope up).

Similar results are obtained for long-run aggregate supply elasticities. ("Long run" elasticities are evaluated allowing all inputs, including land and major capital items, to vary in quantity when the output price changes.) Because all inputs are allowed to vary, long-run supply elasticities are generally higher than short-run supply elasticities. In the developing world, the aggregate supply elasticity of agricultural output with respect to price appears to range between 0.3 and 0.9. Among higher-income developing countries the range is 0.6 to 0.9, and among the poorest developing countries the range is 0.3 to 0.5 (Chhibber 1988).

■ Economics and the Study of Undernutrition

The factors mentioned above as influencing the demand and supply for food, are the fundamental factors that influence the extent of undernutrition. We will discuss these factors in Chapters 9–14. All of these factors influence the extent of undernutrition by affecting the price of food. In addition, the level and distribution of income influences the extent of undernutrition by affecting the ability of individuals to afford adequate food.

We should reemphasize that an individual's demand curve for food reflects how much food the person would like to buy at various price levels given the amount of money the person has to spend. A person with low income may go hungry, or be severely undernourished, while buying the quantity of food specified on his/her demand curve at the prevailing price. This causes some people to view economics as a heartless discipline that has no sympathy for human suffering. But the concepts of supply and demand are not intended to be prescriptions for the world's problems; rather, they are a model for understanding the complex ways in which the world works. Chapter 8 will show how economic concepts can help us understand undernutrition from the standpoint of the individual.

8

The Concept of Food Security

> The world has ample food. The growth of global food production has been
> faster than the unprecedented population growth of the past forty years.
> . . . Yet many poor countries and hundreds of millions of poor people do
> not share in this abundance. They suffer from a lack of food security,
> caused mainly by a lack of purchasing power.
> —Reutlinger et al. 1986:1

In the early 1970s, rising fertilizer prices, spurred by the Organization of
Petroleum Exporting Countries oil cartel, and a couple of years of lacklus-
ter grain harvests that included a bad crop year in the Soviet Union, combined with gradually increasing demand to draw down worldwide grain
reserves and send the price of grain skyrocketing. The spike in food prices
during the early 1970s is illustrated in Figure 6.2 (on p. 78).

In 1974, the shock of finding that "the global grain bin was nearly
empty" (Gilmore and Huddleston 1983:31) channeled food-policy thinking
in the direction of the security of national and international grain reserves.
The phrase "food security" entered the literature, and food security was discussed as a problem of grain-importing nations (e.g., Chisholm and Tyers
1982).

But, as the worldwide food shortage seemed to evaporate in the
1980s, while the numbers of hungry remained high, the thinking on food
security shifted from concern over national food supplies to concern over
hungry people. Reutlinger and his colleagues (1986:1) captured this shift
toward a concern for people when, in 1986, they defined food security as
"access by all people at all times to enough food for an active, healthy
life."

By focusing on people, food security thinkers sometimes shift the main
emphasis concerning the world hunger problem away from food production
and toward the purchasing power of those families at risk for undernutrition. We do not say that food production is no longer considered important
in the hunger problem; it is. Food shortages result in high prices for food,
which in turn make it difficult for the poor to purchase adequate supplies. A
broader recognition now exists of the hunger problem: that food produc-

123

tion, income of the poor, and a mix of other variables all influence the incidence of undernutrition.

■ The Food Security Equation

Anderson and Roumasset (1985) have developed a series of inequalities for conceptualizing the risk of food insecurity on a national scale. By adapting these inequalities to the household level, we can better understand the concept of food security as well as what delivers the risk of food insecurity to a household.

In its simplest form, the food security equation compares the value of the food production deficit in a household with the income and liquid assets that household has available to purchase food. Almost any household, even that of a landless worker, can raise *some* food at home, if nothing more than a tomato plant near the back door, so we can assume that any household at risk for food insecurity has a food production deficit that must be made up with food purchases. In simplest form, therefore, we can develop the food security equation as follows:

$$\text{Value of food production deficit in a household (HH)} \leq \text{Income and liquid assets available to purchase food}$$

The food production deficit in a household is that food needed, over and above any home production, in order to provide all household members at all times with enough food for an active, healthy life. The value of that deficit is simply the minimum cost of purchasing such a supply of food. For a similar approach to food security see Box 8.1.

Families make decisions on how to allocate their expenditures among such competing needs as food, housing, clothing, medical care, and entertainment. The right-hand side of the equation says that, for food security, the income and liquid assets (including savings) available in the household's food budget must be at least enough to purchase enough food to cover the food production deficit.

A household becomes more food-secure when the right-hand side of the equation is bigger relative to the left. It becomes less food-secure when the left-hand side of the equation is bigger relative to the right. The risk of food insecurity is the probability that the left-hand side of the equation will be bigger than the right.

We said above that, by focusing on people, food security thinkers tended to shift the emphasis on the world hunger problem away from food production and toward the purchasing power of those families at risk for undernutrition. But the beauty of an equation is that it forces you to look at

---

Box 8.1 Amartya Sen

The 1998 Nobel Prize in economics was awarded to Indian economist Amartya Sen, who has written extensively on the economics of hunger. Sen's organizing framework is similar to the exposition of food security as presented in this chapter. Sen uses the term "entitlements" to refer to an individual's ability to acquire food. "Since food . . . [is] not distributed freely, people's consumption depends on their 'entitlements', that is, on the . . . goods over which they can establish ownership through production and trade, using their own means. Some people own the food they themselves grow, while others buy [food] in the market on the basis of incomes earned" (Sen 1990).

Sen points out that hunger can exist even when there are not food shortages in the aggregate. In this framework, hunger can be seen as an "entitlement failure"—the failure of a person to assert an entitlement right to a quantity of food large enough to provide adequate nutrition. Production, income, and price all work together in defining a person's entitlements; and entitlements depend on social, political, and cultural systems in which the person lives.

---

the balance between variables. In the food security equation, we concern ourselves not only with the right-hand side, the income and liquid assets available in the family's food purchase budget, but equally with the left-hand side, the value of the household's food production deficit. This left-hand side of the equation can be factored into two components, the food purchase requirement and the price of food, for the value of the food production deficit is the product of these two variables. So the equation can be rewritten as follows:

$$\text{Food purchase requirement} \times \text{Price of food} \leq \text{Income and liquid assets available to purchase food}$$

Now we can demonstrate how the price of food affects food security. If the price goes up, the left-hand side gets bigger, and we see a greater risk of food insecurity. If the price goes down, the risk of food insecurity is reduced.

The food purchase requirement in our equation can be shown as the difference between two factors: household food consumption requirement and household food production. The greater the household's food production the less the food purchase requirement; the smaller the household's food consumption requirement the smaller the food purchase requirement. We can rewrite the equation again, using HH as shorthand for households:

$$\left\{ \begin{array}{c} \text{HH food} \\ \text{consumption} \\ \text{requirement} \end{array} - \begin{array}{c} \text{HH food} \\ \text{production} \end{array} \right\} \times \begin{array}{c} \text{Price of} \\ \text{food} \end{array} \leq \begin{array}{c} \text{Income and liquid} \\ \text{assets available} \\ \text{to purchase food} \end{array}$$

For any given family, to the extent that we can adopt policies to assure the left-hand side of the above equation is smaller than the right-hand side, we will reduce the risk of food insecurity. Therefore, it makes sense to examine each variable in the equation separately and to discuss what sorts of things influence it.

Household Food Consumption Requirement

The household food consumption requirement is affected by the number of people in the household and, as was pointed out earlier, by their age, sex, and working status. (Other things being equal, a family with few children will have an easier time feeding itself than a family with many children—a situation sometimes overlooked.) Because, as we discussed earlier, good health reduces the need for food, good health reduces the household food consumption requirement. Childbearing increases the food needs of the mother during pregnancy and lactation and thus increases the consumption requirement.

Household Food Production

The poorest people in the world are generally landless, and the relationship between household production and food security is mainly relevant to families with land. Nevertheless, many families have no rights to farmland on which to grow small amounts of food around their houses or to keep a few productive scavenging animals such as chickens, ducks, a pig, a goat, or a cow.

The level of food production in a farming household is influenced by a complex set of variables including the amount and quality of land available and the education of the farm manager and his workers. The quantity and quality of technology and capital available is important; how this technology and capital are used is also important and is usually heavily influenced by a multitude of government incentives and disincentives that can include tariffs, export taxes, price controls, and subsidies of purchased inputs. Agricultural research and education have a powerful influence on quantity produced.

The level of food production of households taken together influences the next variable in the equation—the price of food.

The Price of Food

The price of food is influenced by the quantity produced, as discussed above. But all that is on the supply side. The price of food is also influenced by the demand side: the size of the population as well as the per capita income and the tastes and preferences of consumers. Governments often attempt to influence the price of food with tariffs, export taxes, price controls, and subsidies of purchased inputs.

Income and Liquid Assets Available to Purchase Food

The income and liquid assets position of a household is the result of complex factors, among them the education of its members, its capital position, its land position, its employment opportunities, attitudes toward work, the cost of transportation to and from work, and health.

9

It Is Not Food Versus Population

Land, unlike people, . . . does not breed.
—Heilbroner 1953:82 (paraphrasing Malthus)

◼ Thomas Malthus

The debate over food versus people started with an argument between the young reverend Thomas Robert Malthus and his father. The elder Malthus was enthusiastic about a recently published book that promised a future world devoid of "disease, anguish, melancholy, or resentment" (Godwin 1793). Young Thomas was not impressed. In fact, he was so skeptical about such a utopian future that he wrote down his objections. The father was so struck with Thomas's words that he encouraged his son to publish them (Heilbroner 1953:69–70). First issued anonymously in 1798 as *An Essay on the Principle of Population as It Affects the Future Improvement of Society*, Malthus's "essay" was never short and by its sixth edition, still claiming to be an essay, covered some 600 pages of detailed argument. For Malthus in his own words, see Box 9.1.

The Malthusian thesis postulated that the reproductive capacity of humans must put continual pressure on the "means of subsistence." Human numbers, he said, could increase by "geometric" progression: 2, 4, 8, 16, 32, 64, 128, 256 (we now call this progression *exponential*). Malthus did not see how subsistence could increase any faster than an "arithmetic" progression: 1, 2, 3, 4, 5, 6, 7, 8, 9 (we now call this progression *linear*). Unlike people, land does not breed, and Malthus thought that the potential for human numbers to increase exponentially must therefore put continuous pressure on our food supply.

Malthus enumerated a long list of checks to population growth, including war, "sickly seasons, epidemics, pestilence, and plague." Humans themselves, Malthus thought, would be unable to check their own population growth because the only way he knew how to limit family size was through, as he put it, "moral restraint." (The technology of contraception was next to nonexistent at the time.) And in Malthus's view, given the "passion between the sexes," moral restraint was not strong enough to effective-

129

> **Box 9.1   Excerpts from "An Essay on the Principle of Population" by Thomas Malthus, 1798**
>
> "It has been said that the great question is now at issue, whether man shall henceforth start forwards with accelerated velocity towards illimitable, and hitherto unconceived improvement, or be condemned to a perpetual oscillation between happiness and misery, and after every effort remain still at an immeasurable distance from the wished-for goal. . . ."
>
> "I think I may fairly make two postulata. First, That food is necessary to the existence of man. Secondly, That the passion between the sexes is necessary and will remain nearly in its present state. . . ."
>
> "Assuming then my postulata as granted, I say, that the power of population is indefinitely greater than the power in the earth to produce subsistence for man. Population, when unchecked, increases in a geometrical ratio. Subsistence increases only in an arithmetical ratio. A slight acquaintance with numbers will shew the immensity of the first power in comparison of the second. . . ."
>
> "By that law of our nature which makes food necessary to the life of man, the effects of these two unequal powers must be kept equal. . . ."
>
> "This implies a strong and constantly operating check on population from the difficulty of subsistence. This difficulty must fall somewhere and must necessarily be severely felt by a large portion of mankind. . . ."
>
> "Taking the population of the world at any number, a thousand millions, for instance, the human species would increase in the ratio of—1, 2, 4, 8, 16, 32, 64, 128, 256, 512, etc. and subsistence as—1, 2, 3, 4, 5, 6, 7, 8, 9, 10, etc. In two centuries and a quarter, the population would be to the means of subsistence as 512 to 10: in three centuries as 4,096 to 13, and in two thousand years the difference would be almost incalculable, though the produce in that time would have increased to an immense extent. . . ."
>
> "No limits whatever are placed to the productions of the earth; they may increase for ever and be greater than any assignable quantity. Yet still the power of population being a power of a superior order, the increase of the human species can only be kept commensurate to the increase of the means of subsistence by the constant operation of the strong law of necessity acting as a check upon the greater power. . . ."
>
> *Source:* The full text of this excerpt can be found online at: http://socserv2.socsci. mcmaster.ca/~econ/ugcm/3ll3/malthus/popu.txt.

ly limit human fertility. Therefore, lurking in the shadows, always ready to impose the ultimate check on population growth, would have to be famine. "Famine stalks in the rear, and with one mighty blow, levels the population with the food of the world" (Heilbroner 1953:83).

There was plausibility to the Malthusian argument. It was, in fact, a precursor to the now widely accepted ecological principle that any population will expand until it fills the ecological niche available to it. What

Malthus did not foresee was that there would eventually be other checks to human population growth besides war, pestilence, and famine; that changing attitudes about family size, a kind of "small is beautiful" philosophy, could combine with a new technology in the form of effective and simple contraception to limit population growth. Nor did he foresee the enormous increases in agricultural production that would accompany the application of science to farming.

Important as Malthus's book was for the thesis it espoused, it was more important as a stimulation to thinking among people who read it. Charles Darwin, for instance, reports that he happened to read Malthus "for amusement," yet this reading inspired the theory of natural selection and survival of the fittest that would dominate his *On the Origin of Species* (Bettany 1890; Herbert 1971).

Others were not amused. As one biographer put it, "Malthus was not ignored. For thirty years it rained refutations" (James Bonner, as quoted in Heilbroner 1953:76). In the storm of protest that followed the publication of his essay, Malthus was compared to Satan and denounced as an "immoral, revolutionary, hard-hearted, and cruel atheist" (Bettany 1890:ix). But the strongest refutation of the seeming inevitability of a perpetual tendency toward famine that Malthus postulated lies in what has happened since he wrote his essay.

Since 1800 the population of the world has, in fact, grown exponentially—or nearly so (Figure 9.1). On the other hand, the growth of world population seems destined to stop eventually through a process demographers call the demographic transition.

■ The Demographic Transition

The world appears to be going through a pattern of growth known as the *demographic transition*. Originally described by Frank Notestein (his definition is found in Box 9.2), the literature contains a number of ways of defining the term. We adopt and paraphrase from a conceptualization by Carl Haub (1987:19) of the Population Reference Bureau in Washington, D.C.

The theory of demographic transition offers a general model for the gradual evolution of a population's birth and death rates from the preindustrial to the modern pattern, which results in an S-shaped curve of population growth through time. According to the theory, population growth goes through four stages, illustrated in Figure 9.2:

Stage I. Preindustrial stage: Birth rates are high and fertility uncontrolled, with the birth rate exceeding the death rate and generally within the range of 25 to 45 per thousand. Periodic famines, plagues, and wars cause brief periods of population loss. Population grows, but slowly.

Figure 9.1   Growth of Human Population

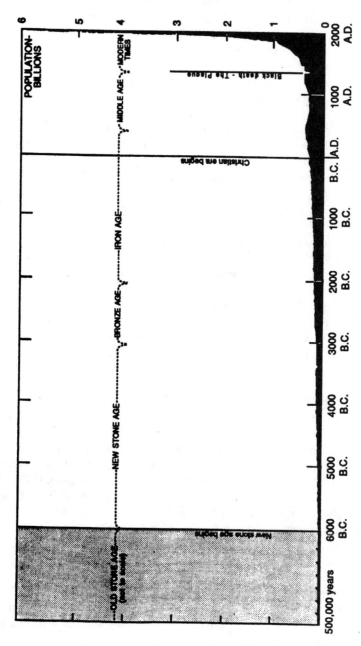

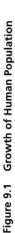

Source: The 0.002 percent estimate, Frejka 1973:15; other material taken from the Population Reference Bureau.

Note: It took many thousands of years of man's existence on earth for the population to reach a billion, around the year 1830. Up until about 1700 the human population had grown very slowly; the average rate was probably less than 0.002 percent per year. Then the growth rate began to gradually increase. In the early 1970s it rose above 2 percent, over 1,000 times the rate of growth of the ancients. In 1998 the world's population growth rate was down to 1.35 percent. Current projections are that world population growth should approach zero around the year 2100.

Box 9.2   Terms Commonly Used by Demographers

Age cohort, or cohort: All the people in a population within a given age range (Each bar in a population pyramid represents a particular age cohort.)

Annual growth rate, or growth rate: Crude birth rate minus crude death rate divided by 10, which expresses the rate as a percentage

Child dependency ratio: The ratio of the dependent children to working-age adults

Crude birth rate, or birth rate: The number of births per year per thousand individuals in the population

Crude death rate, or death rate: The number of deaths per year per thousand individuals in the population

Demographic transition: A pattern of population growth experienced by Western industrialized democracies and involving an S-shaped curve of total population change through time. Frank Notestein (1945) identified three stages in the transition: (1) High growth potential: birth and death rates are high, life expectancy is short, and population growth is slow; (2) transitional growth: birth rates remain high but death rates are falling; population growth rates increase, sometimes to the point that there is said to be a population explosion; (3) incipient decline: the birth rate follows the death rate downward; population continues to grow until birth rate reaches the death rate.

Dependency ratio: The ratio of dependent to working-age adults—those from 15 to 65 (percentage of the population dependent divided by the percentage of working age)

Dependent adults: (Usually) those people who are 65 or over

Dependent children: (Usually) those people who are under 15 years old

Dependent population: Dependent children and dependent adults

Doubling time: The number of years it takes the population to double, growing at the present annual growth rate, compounded. (You can figure out how long it will take a population to double, if it grows at a constant annual rate compounded, by dividing the number 70 by the annual, percentage, growth rate.)

(continues)

Continued

Gross reproductive rate (GRR): The number of female children a newborn female will have during her lifetime if current levels of fertility by age of female continue through time

Infant mortality rate: the number of babies who die during their first year of life per 1,000 babies born

Life expectancy at birth, or life expectancy: The average expected age of death of newborns who follow a given age-specific mortality schedule

Net reproductive rate (NRR): The expected number of daughters per newborn female, after subjecting those newborn females to a given set of mortality rates. (NRR is lower than GRR because some of the newborn females will die before completing their reproductive years.)

Population momentum: The tendency for population growth to continue beyond the time that replacement-level fertility has been achieved; that is, even after the net reproduction rate has reached one. The momentum of a population in any given year is measured as a ratio of the ultimate stationary population to the population of that year, given the assumption that fertility remains at replacement level. Using this definition, the World Development Report 1989 provides population momentum figures for 129 countries and an example of how the calculation is done (World Bank 1989: 214-215).

Population pyramid: A graph of the population distribution according to age and sex. Two basic kinds of pyramids are used: The first type, a numerical pyramid (such as Figure 11.1), plots numbers of people in each age and sex group; the second, a relative pyramid (such as Figure 11.2), plots the percentage distribution of people according to age and sex. The major difference between the two kinds is that the numerical pyramid increases in area as the population grows, while the relative pyramid always maintains a constant area (you can think of it as 100 percent). Thus, the two kinds of pyramids may appear to exhibit different dynamic characteristics.

Total fertility rate, or fertility rate: The total number of births a female has during her lifetime

Figure 9.2   The Theory of Demographic Transition

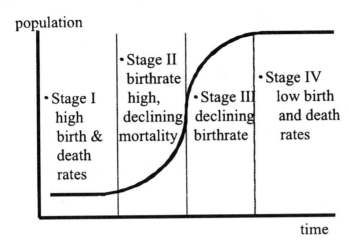

Stage II. Mortality decline before fertility decline: With better public health services and more-reliable food and water supplies, death rates fall and life expectancy increases. If no accompanying decrease in the birth rate occurs, the population growth rate rises and population grows rapidly.

Stage III. Fertility decline: At some point, usually as the country urbanizes and industrializes, the birth rate decreases in response to desires to limit family size. Population continues to grow rapidly for a while. But eventually birth rates approach death rates, and population growth slows. The growth rate may even fall to zero or below.

Stage IV. Modern stage: By this point both the birth rate and death rate are low, around twelve per thousand. After the birth rate falls as low as the death rate, population size stabilizes if the total fertility rate remains at two children per woman. If the total fertility rate creeps up slightly from two, population size increases slowly, although family size remains small.

There is abundant evidence to support the validity of the theory of demographic transition. First, we can find developed countries in which all four stages of demographic transition have occurred. The experience of Sweden, for example is shown in Figure 9.3. In the decades before 1805, Sweden was in the last phase of Stage I, with birth rates and death rates approximately equal, but high. Stage II in Sweden covered the seventy years between 1805 and 1875, as death rates began to fall, but birth rates stayed high. Stage III in Sweden covered the one-hundred-year period between 1875 and 1975, as birth rates declined faster than death rates. Sweden is now in Stage IV, with birth and death rates approximately equal,

Figure 9.3   Birth and Death Rates, Sweden, 1751–1984

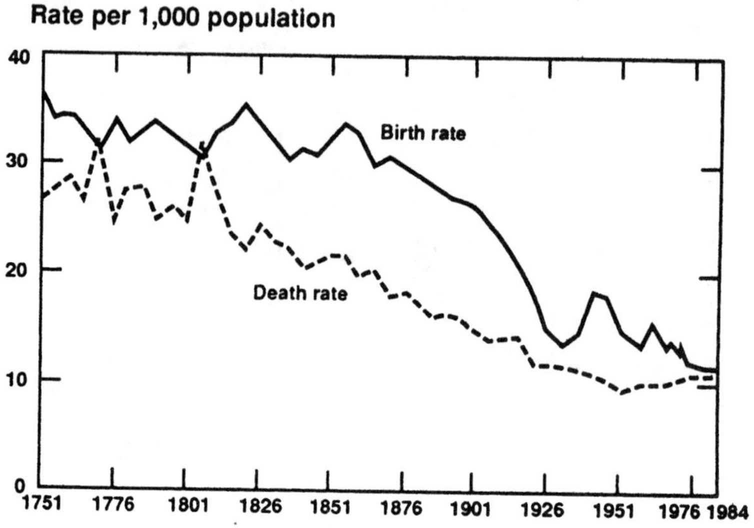

Rate per 1,000 population

Source: Adapted from Haub 1987:20.

but low. (In fact, currently the birth rate in Sweden is slightly below the death rate.)

A second source of evidence supporting the theory of demographic transition is a comparison of population growth rates in developed countries to those in developing countries. For example, in the period 1995–2000, the population of Africa (where many of the poorest countries of the world are) grew at a rate of 2.35 percent per year; the population of Asia (where there are many developing countries) grew at a rate of 1.41 percent per year; and the population of Europe grew at a rate of only 0.02 percent per year. In what are today's developed countries, the demographic transition is essentially finished (look at recent birth [fertility] and death [mortality] rates in the industrial market economies in the *World Development Report* table on health [World Bank 1997:198–199]). But in developing countries, the process of demographic transition is still under way. Compare the demographic transition as shown in Figure 9.3 (with Sweden as representative of the developed world) and Figure 9.4 (with Mexico as representative of the developing world). The death rate decline in Sweden began shortly after 1800 and took approximately 150 years to fall from 30 to 10. The more dramatic death rate decline in Mexico did not begin until about 1915 and took only 40 years to fall to 10 per thousand. Birth rates in Mexico remained above 40 per thousand until the early 1970s, when they began a rapid decline. Consequently, by the early 1970s

Figure 9.4   Birth and Death Rates, Mexico, 1895/99–1908/95

Rate per 1,000 population

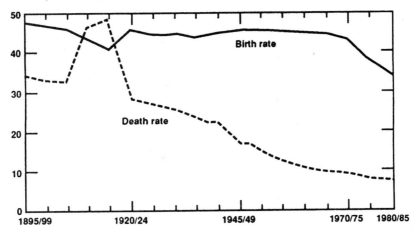

Source: Adapted from Haub 1987:20.

Mexico's population growth rate was above 3 percent, yielding a doubling time of fewer than 23 years.

Figure 9.5 makes this point a little more generally: population growth is higher in less developed countries. The countries with high population growth rates are bunched at the left of the figure in low per capita incomes. The rich countries generally have lower rates of population growth. This has two implications. First, economic growth, or improved economic prosperity, can be a powerful policy mechanism for reducing population growth. This will be discussed in more detail in Chapter 19. Second, since population is growing fastest among groups of people who have low incomes, the growth in demand for food may lag behind population growth. When we get to future projections in Chapter 24, we will assume that a 50 percent increase in population translates into a 50 percent increase in demand for food; in reality this may overstate the impact on demand.

A final piece of evidence supporting the theory of demographic transition is shown in Figure 9.6. For the world as a whole, the growth of population is slowing down, after peaking in the late 1980s. At that point in time, the world as a whole moved from Stage II to Stage III. Note that the rates of growth are still positive—world population continues to grow; but the *rate* of growth is slowing over time. In addition, the U.S. Census predicts that the rates of growth in population will continue to decline for the next fifty years. (The sharp dip in population growth rates in the late 1950s and

Figure 9.5   Population Grows Faster in Countries with Lower per Capita Income: Evidence from 165 Countries, 2001

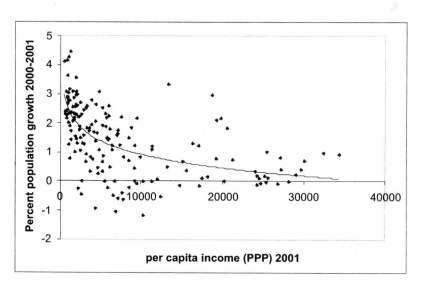

Source: World Bank *World Development Indicators,* 2003.

early 1960s corresponds with the Great Leap Forward Famine in China, discussed in Chapter 2.)

Lester Brown and Hal Kane point out a less happy road to population stabilization. Criticizing the optimistic view of demographic transition, they say:

> As we approach the end of the twentieth century, a gap has emerged in the [demographic transition] analysis. The theorists did not say what happens when second stage population growth rates of 3 percent per year begin to overwhelm local life-support systems, making it impossible to sustain the economic and social gains that are counted on to reduce births. Unfortunately, trends that lead to ecological deterioration and economic decline are also self-reinforcing: Once populations expand to the point where their demands begin to exceed the sustainable yields of local forests, grasslands, croplands, or aquifers, they begin directly or indirectly to consume the resource base itself. . . . This . . . reduces food production and incomes, triggering a downward spiral in a process we describe as the demographic trap. All countries will complete the demographic transition, reaching population stability with low death and birth rates, or will get caught in the demographic trap, which eventually will also lead to demographic stability—but with high birth rates and high death rates. (Brown and Kane 1994:55–56)

Figure 9.6   Annual Growth Rate of World Population, Historical and Projected, 1950–2050

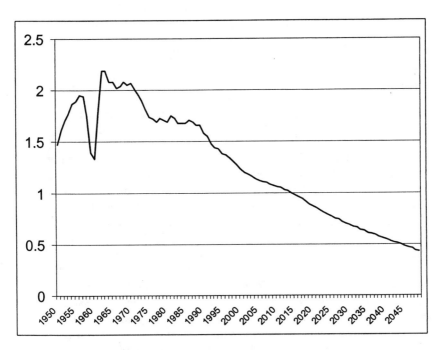

Source: U.S. Census Bureau website.

If the world's population growth does, in fact, stop as projected, humans will have succeeded in controlling their own numbers without war, pestilence, and famine—something Malthus did not expect.

■ Projections of Future World Population
As we consider the future prospects for world food supply and demand, we think first of population. How many mouths will there be to feed? The U.S. Census Bureau, basing its statistics on the growth rates shown in Figure 9.6, projects that by the year 2050, world population will be about 9.08 billion, 50 percent higher than the current (2003) population of 6.34 billion (see Table 9.1).

The UN has also made population projections into the future. The UN projections are based on assumptions about how life expectancy will change in the future, and about how fertility rates will change. See UN Population Division (2002a) for a description of these assumptions.

Table 9.1   Population in the Year 2050: Four Projections

Projection	Population Size in 2050 (millions)	Percentage Increase from 2000	Average Annual Rate of Growth (%)
UN Low	7,409	22.04	0.40
UN Medium	8,919	46.92	0.77
U.S. Census Bureau	9,084	49.44	0.81
UN High	10,633	75.16	1.13

Source: United Nations Population Division 2002b; U.S. Census Bureau website

Life expectancy at birth is assumed to increase as average nutrition continues to improve and as average incomes continue to rise. The improvements are assumed to be greatest in countries where life expectancy is the lowest, and therefore where potential for improvement is the greatest.

These assumptions mean that life expectancies are projected to increase substantially in some parts of the world. Babies born in Africa in 2050 are expected to live sixteen years longer than babies of their grandparents' generation born in 2000 (UN Population Division 2002b). This may sound like quite a dramatic increase. But life expectancy has increased by substantial amounts in other areas: Life expectancy in Saudi Arabia increased from 53.9 years in the early 1970s to 70.9 years in the late 1990s; in Indonesia, the increase over the same period was 15.7 years, from 49.2 to 64.5; in South America as a whole, the increase was from 60.5 to 69 over the same period (UN Population Division 2002b). The UN's assumption is, therefore, within the range of historical experience.

It is more difficult to make reasonable assumptions about future levels of fertility. As a result of this difficulty, the UN presents three possible scenarios, or *variants*. The *medium variant* assumes that fertility in each declines (from its current level of about three children born to an average woman of childbearing age) until it reaches a level of 1.85 children per woman. (This is below the "replacement level"—the number of children each woman would give birth to, on average, to ensure that two children survived to puberty. Even if the fertility rate fell to the replacement level, population would continue to grow because of increases in life expectancy.) In the *high variant,* fertility is assumed to be 0.5 percent above the medium variant. In the *low variant,* fertility is assumed to be 0.5 percent below the medium variant.

Again, to put these projections in historical context, let us examine recent experience. For the world as a whole, fertility rates dropped from 4.5 in 1970–1975 to 2.8 in 1995–2000. In Asia, where economic growth has been exceptionally strong in the last twenty years, fertility rates dropped from 5.1 in the early 1970s to 2.7 in the late 1990s. In Europe, fertility was at the replacement rate of 2.1 in the early 1970s; by the late 1990s, the number dropped to 1.4 (UN Population Division 2002b). Thus, the UN's low variant assumption is that fertility worldwide will drop to levels currently observed in Europe.

Based on these assumptions, the UN's three population projections are shown in Table 9.1. The medium variant is quite close to the U.S. Census Bureau's prediction. How good are the projections? Table 9.2 shows UN projections of world population in 2000 made at different points in time. Several things are notable:

- For obvious reasons, near-term projections are more accurate than long-term projections.
- However, the projection made in the early 1960s was remarkably close to the actual population that existed in 2000; the 1963 projection was off by only 3 or 4 percent.
- All of the projections (except the last one) overestimated the actual population. It is generally true that projections of future population have gotten lower over time. For example, Table 9.1 in the second edition of this book reported the 1996 projections of the population in year 2050; the U.S. Census projection was 9,350 million and the UN medium variant was 9,850 million. Six or seven years later, those projections have been revised downward.

Table 9.2   Past Projections of World Population in the Year 2000: How Good Were Those Projections?

Projection made in year	Projected population in 2000 (billions)
1957	6.28
1963	6.13
1968	6.49
1973	6.25
1980	6.12
1984	6.12
1988	6.25
1990	6.26
1992	6.23
1994	6.16
1996	6.09
1998	6.06
Actual 2000	6.07

Source: National Research Council 2000.

A report published in the journal *Nature* (Lutz, Sanderson, and Sherbov 2001) criticized the UN methods of projections and made a set of projections to the year 2100. The median projection of that report tracked closely with the UN medium variant through 2050. The Lutz et al. median projection calls for world population peaking at about 9 billion during the decade of the 2060s and then declining.

The specter of AIDS hangs over any discussion of future population. The projections shown in Table 9.1 include estimates of increased mortality as a result of AIDS. The UN estimates that at the end of 2002 about 40 million people were infected with the virus (human immunodeficiency virus or HIV) that causes AIDS. The problem is especially severe in parts of sub-Saharan Africa (see Table 9.3). Although the world hopes that medical science can make progress on AIDS treatment, it is still the prognosis that many of these 40 million people will die from AIDS during the next five to twenty years. In 2002, an estimated 3 million people died of AIDS worldwide. To put this number in perspective, recall that over 50 million people died in 1995 from all causes. If all HIV-positive people died within five years, that would increase the number of deaths during the period by about 10 percent or less. One review of the literature concludes:

> At the world level, AIDS is unlikely to suppress population size or growth rates. However, the impact of AIDS may be felt by some individual countries. For example, the U.S. Bureau of the Census predicts that in some countries populations in 2020 will be considerably smaller as a result of the AIDS pandemic—45 percent smaller in Uganda, 35 percent in Rwanda, and 30 percent in Malawi. (Lynn Brown 1997)

Table 9.3   Percentage of Adult Populations (Ages 15–45) Infected with the HIV Virus, 2001

Country	% infected by HIV
Botswana	39.4
Lesotho	33.5
Zimbabwe	33.5
Swaziland	33.3
Namibia	24.4
Zambia	21.1
South Africa	19.9
Malawi	15.2
Kenya	15.0
Cent. Afr. Rep.	12.8
Cameroon	12.2
Mozambique	11.7
Rwanda	11.4
Burundi	11.4
Sub-Saharan Africa	8.9

Source: UNAIDS/WHO Reference Group for Estimates, Modelling, and Projections 2002.

■ Current Trends in per Capita Food Production

Not only did Malthus not expect humans to willfully control their own population size, he did not expect our food supply to keep up with a dramatic, exponential growth in our population. The last half of the twentieth century experienced the most rapid growth of population in the entire history of the world, yet during this period of breakneck population growth, food production grew even faster; so per capita food production gradually increased.

The factors contributing to growth in food production will be discussed in Chapters 12–14. Here we simply note the facts: food production has continued to grow faster than population. As Table 9.4 shows, worldwide food production per capita has increased steadily over the past thirty-five years, growing about 5 percent per decade. Food production per capita in the developing world has grown much more rapidly. In the developed world, food supply grew faster than population from the early 1960s until the late 1980s. Since 1990, food production has continued to grow, but at a slower pace than population, so production per capita has declined. The situation in sub-Saharan Africa is an exception to the worldwide trend: food output per capita has declined steadily over the forty-year period. By 2001 food production per capita was about 15 percent lower than it was in 1961.

A World Bank study (Mundlak, Larson, and Crego 1996) concludes that worldwide food supply is growing faster than food demand: "Has supply lagged demand? If that were so, agricultural prices would have risen. They didn't." They find that median prices to farmers dropped by 0.61 percent during the 1967–1992 period, and that 71 percent of world production from 1967 to 1992 came from countries in which (inflation-adjusted) farm prices fell. This study finds that median growth rate in agricultural production was 2.25 percent per year. (*Median growth rate* means that one-half of

Table 9.4   Index of Food Production per Capita for Selected Areas and Years (Index of Production, 1989–1990 = 100[a])

Year	Sub-Saharan Africa	Developing Countries	Developed countries	World
1961	115.6	75.4	77.3	83.9
1971	117.5	79.9	89	89.9
1981	102.1	87.2	97.2	94.7
1991	99.3	103.6	98.3	100.6
2001	99	125.7	95.4	109.3

Source: FAO STAT
Note: a. See Box 14.5 for a description

the world's food production takes place in countries with agricultural growth rates of less than 2.25 percent.) The study confirms that in most countries, per capita agricultural production grew—food became more plentiful.

FAO data on nutrient availability per capita also shows steady improvement. As Figure 9.7 shows, since 1961 worldwide calories per capita have increased over 20 percent, from 2,235 calories per person per day to 2,712 calories per person per day. Similarly, protein availability has increased about 17 percent to 72.4 grams per person per day. These levels of nutrients are sufficient for an adequate diet for the average person. One interpretation of this states that *if the world's food supply were evenly divided among the people of the world, there would be enough food for everybody.*

So an important question in any discussion of the incidence and perma-

Figure 9.7   Growth in Calories per Capita per Day, Worldwide, 1961–2001

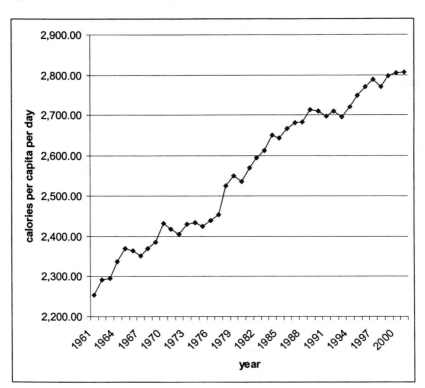

Source: FAOSTAT.

nence of world hunger is how the world's food supplies are allocated among the people of the world. In the next chapter, we look at purchasing power—and its components, income and food prices—as the immediate problem explaining why certain people in the world are unable to afford adequate nutrition.

10

Income Distribution and Undernutrition

> "Get off this estate!"
> "What for?"
> "Because it's mine."
> "Where did you get it?"
> "From my father."
> "Where did he get it?"
> "From his father."
> "And where did he get it?"
> "He fought for it."
> "Well, I'll fight you for it!"
> —Carl Sandburg 1936:75

Income is central to the problem of undernutrition. A family is hungry because the family is poor. In this chapter we look at two closely related issues. First we look at the distribution of income in the world. What countries are poor? How poor are they? How is income distributed within countries? How are these things changing over time? Second, we look at how changes in income affect the aggregate demand for food.

■ Who Are the Poor?

The World Bank (*World Development Report* 1996) lists thirteen countries with per capita income of less than $200 and fifty countries with per capita income of less than $500. It is hard for most of us to imagine how a person could feed herself on a little over $2.00 per day. And people have needs besides food.

Who are the poorest of the poor? They live in the third world. They are landless or nearly so. If they do have a bit of land, typically they earn more than half their livelihood working for others. Whether they live packed tightly into city slums or sprinkled across the countryside, they are poorly educated, often illiterate, and commonly superstitious. When employed, they accept the most menial of jobs. Some are subsistence fishermen. Some live in relative isolation in upland farming areas. Often they are squatters, neither owning nor renting the land on which they put up their huts. Their food larder is usually almost empty.

Their households are often fragmented, with one or more members away trying to find work so they can send money home. They may be in debt—to wealthier relatives, to friends, to employers, or to the local money-lenders. The household head is often young, not yet having found good employment, but already burdened with the responsibility of raising children. (For a good essay on the poor of a particular region, see Carner 1984.)

■ Comparing Average Incomes in Different Countries

In an international economy, prices are influenced by consumption in all countries. The affordability of food for poor people in one country is influenced by the consumption patterns of affluent people in other countries. As we look at the distribution of income in the world, we note that average per capita incomes are very different from one country to another (see Tables 10.1 and 10.2). To pick the most dramatic example, in 2001, per capita income in Democratic Republic of Congo was $80 per year, while per capita income in Switzerland was $38,330. The average person in Switzerland earned about five hundred times the amount earned by the average person in Mozambique (World Bank 2003).

Incomes, as the term is used here, refers to the gross national product (GNP) or the closely related concept gross domestic product (GDP) or gross national income (GNI), which measure the total value of goods and services produced in the economy. The richest ten countries in the world have less than 10 percent of the world's population but produce over 60 percent of the world's goods. The poorest fifty-six countries support more than 50 percent of the world's population but produce less than 5 percent of the world's goods.

An Alternative Way of Comparing Incomes in Different Countries: Purchasing Power Parity

Some economists have expressed doubt about whether the usual method of comparing GNP per capita in different countries gives an accurate view of the quality of life in those countries. The usual method—as reflected in the numbers in the previous section—translates the value of goods and services in a country from the local currency to U.S. dollars by using the market exchange rate. In effect, this measure translates local currency into dollars by considering how many units of the local currency it would take to buy a dollar on the foreign exchange market.

An alternative method translates local currency into a dollar equivalent by comparing the purchasing power of the local currency to the pur-

Table 10.1   Income and Population of 18 Largest Economies in the World, 2001

	2001 GNP ($ billions)	Percentage of World Total	2001 Population (millions)	Percentage of World Total Population
United States	9,781	31.1	285	4.6
Japan	4,523	14.4	127	2.1
Germany	1,940	6.2	82	1.3
United Kingdom	1,477	4.7	59	1.0
France	1,381	4.4	59	1.0
China	1,191	3.8	1,272	20.8
Italy	1,130	3.6	58	0.9
Canada	682	2.2	31	0.5
Spain	588	1.9	41	0.7
Mexico	550	1.8	99	1.6
Brazil	529	1.7	172	2.8
India	477	1.5	1,092	17.8
Korea, Rep.	448	1.4	47	0.8
Netherlands	390	1.2	16	0.3
Australia	386	1.2	19	0.3
Switzerland	277	0.9	7	0.1
Argentina	261	0.8	37	0.6
Russian Federation	259	0.8	145	2.4
Sub-total	26,270	83.7	3,648	59.5
World total	31,400	100	6,130	100

Source: World Bank, *World Development Indicators 2003.*
Note: These are the 18 countries that have the largest GNI of all countries. The countries with the highest per capita income would be a different list and would show a greater intensity of income concentration.

chasing power of the dollar. In effect, this measure translates how much it would cost in the local currency spent in the local market to buy the same quantity of goods that could be purchased in the United States with one dollar. Using this conversion method, the richest country (the United States by this measure, rather than Switzerland) has a per capita income sixty times larger than the per capita income of the poorest country (Malawi by this measure, rather than the Democratic Republic of Congo). (See Table 10.2.) Compare this factor of sixty to what we reported above—that the average income in the richest country was five hundred times that of the poorest country—based on exchange rate comparisons of GNP per capita.

It is difficult for readers who grew up and live in the United States or other developed countries to wrap their minds around a number that says the average income per person in a country is $80 a year, or $270 per year. Box 10.1 describes the life of a poor person who lives in Malawi.

Table 10.2   2001 GNP per Capita for Selected Countries, Using Exchange Rate Comparison and Purchasing Power Parity Comparison

	GNP per capita ($)	
Country	Exchange rate comparison	Purchasing power parity comparison
D.R. Congo	80	630
Burundi	100	680
Ethiopia	100	800
Malawi	160	560
Tanzania	270	570
Mali	290	770
India	460	2,820
China	890	3,950
Brazil	3,070	7,070
Germany	23,560	25,240
United States	34,280	34,280
Japan	35,610	25,550
Norway	35,690	29,340
Switzerland	38,330	30,970

Source: World Bank, *World Development Indicators, 2003.*

Box 10.1   Life in Rural Malawi

The figures cited in the text tell us that Malawi is one of the poorest countries in the world; average income per capita (PPP method) is less than $2 a day. But what does this really mean? How can a person live on $2 a day? It is difficult—perhaps impossible—to convey the depth of poverty experienced by people in rural Malawi. Reporter Barry Bearak (2003), writing for the *New York Times Sunday Magazine*, visited the Malawian countryside and describes the life of Adilesi Faisoni, a grandmother in the village of Mkulumimba.

A photograph accompanying the article shows her "worldly goods": a cup, three bowls, a cooking pot, some hearth stones and stirring sticks, a cleaning rag. That's it. No electricity, no furniture, nothing. She owns a single set of clothes. Her grandchildren wear used T-shirts from the United States with pictures of Power Rangers and Teenage Mutant Ninja Turtles. The clothes are ragged and worn. Her house is a 9-foot by 12-foot mud hut. She lives here with her daughter and ten grandchildren. How do they all fit? "We squeeze like worms."

Her diet is almost exclusively *nsima*, a thick porridge made from maize meal. During the hungry months, she may only eat a single bowl each day. "There is no way to get used to hunger," she tells the reporter. "All the time something is moving in your stomach. You feel the emptiness. You feel your intestines moving. They are too empty and they are searching for something to fill up on."

Last year, the maize meal ran out, and her family had to eat pumpkin leaves and wild vegetables. Her husband starved to death. "There was nothing to do but beg, and you were begging from others who needed to beg."

Does Income per Capita Measure What Is Important?

Some readers may at this point be a little skeptical about exactly what these average per capita numbers mean. And there are some legitimate concerns. In the following sections we will take up the issue of income distribution. Related to that, other indicators of quality of life, or depth of poverty, in different countries have been developed.

The World Bank tabulates data on the number of people in each country who live in extreme poverty measured by incomes of less than $1 or less than $2 per day. To make these comparable over time, the "$1" poverty line is adjusted for inflation. For the numbers shown in Table 10.3, the $1 standard refers to 1993 dollars; adjusted for inflation, it is equivalent to $1.08 in the year 2000. The United Nations Development Progam (UNDP) compiles an index (the "human development index" or HDI) of indicators of quality of life. This index includes per capita income, but also includes measures of health and education.

Table 10.3 allows us to compare income per capita with these other indicators. Several points emerge:

- The very high-income countries also have high HDIs and no people living on less than $1 per day.
- The countries with low HDIs and high poverty rates also have very low incomes per capita.
- Some countries (compare South Africa to Indonesia) can have similar HDIs even though they have very different incomes.
- Some countries (compare Uzbekistan to Lesotho) can have very different HDIs and poverty rates even though they have the same income per capita.

Despite the fact that income per capita rankings differ from HDI rankings or poverty rate rankings, income per capita is an important indicator of

Table 10.3   Alternative Measures of Quality of Life for Selected Countries, 2001

Country	Income per Capita ($ per year)	Human Development Index	% of population living on < $1/day
Norway	29,620	.944	0
United States	34,320	.937	0
South Africa	11,290	.684	< 2
Indonesia	2,940	.682	7.2
Uzbekistan	2,460	.729	19.1
Lesotho	2,420	.510	43.1
Niger	890	.292	.614
Sierra Leone	470	.275	57

Source: UNDP 2003

quality of life in a country. Figure 10.1 shows that average per capita income is negatively correlated with shorter lives, poverty, and undernutrition.

■ Measuring Income Distribution Within a Country

Another legitimate criticism of average per capita income as an indicator of quality of life is that it is an average. Some people in the country have incomes above average and some have incomes below the average. Next we look at measures of how income is distributed within a country.

Pareto's Law

For a typical town, when you rank family or individual incomes from low to high and graph them, the result is suggestive of a J. The J-shape is especially pronounced if you graph just the richest people in the town (Figure 10.2).

In the late 1800s the Italian mathematician-economist-sociologist Vilfredo Pareto examined income distribution among the rich and moderately rich in a number of countries and found the J-shaped distribution pattern among them to be remarkably consistent. Furthermore, he was able to fit this pattern to a mathematical formulation that soon became known as Pareto's law. Pareto's law had its problems, and, as it turned out, one of the main benefits of Pareto's work on income distribution was to stimulate others to think about alternative methods of measuring it. (For a concise discussion of Pareto's work on distribution, see Steindl 1987.)

The Lorenz Curve

In 1905, the U.S. statistician Max Lorenz proposed a method of comparing distributions of income and wealth through a cumulative income or wealth curve, the Lorenz curve, an example of which is shown as the dashed line in Figure 10.3. The vertical axis, OC, represents percentage of total income for the group under analysis. The horizontal axis, OE, represents the percentage of individuals (or families) in the group.

To conceptualize how a Lorenz curve is constructed, imagine a group of 100 individuals, each with a different income. Bake a cake that represents the total income of the group. Cut the entire cake into blocks, each block being a length proportional to one individual's income, and distribute the cake accordingly. Now arrange all the individuals in a line according to cake size, with the person having the shortest piece of cake first and the person with the longest piece last. Starting with the person with the shortest piece of cake, have the line pass by a point at which each individual stacks her piece of cake on top of the previous piece until all the pieces are placed in a column. Then the column will represent all the income of the group.

As every tenth person places cake on the column, measure the height

Figure 10.1 Income Matters

Poor people are better off in high income countries

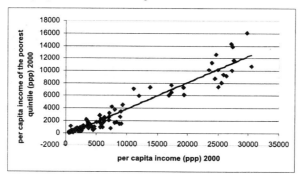

People live longer in high income countries

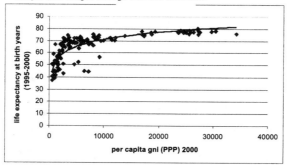

Fewer people are undernourished in high-income countries

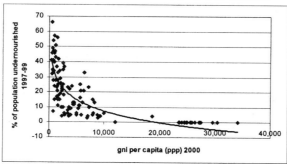

of the column at that time and calculate what percentage of total income is represented so far. On the Lorenz diagram, plot the percentage of total income accounted for so far against the percentage of population accounted for at that time until every person has walked by. Connect the points with a smooth line and you have a Lorenz curve (Cowell 1977:23).

Figure 10.2   Stylized Representation of Income Distribution Among the Rich in a Typical Community

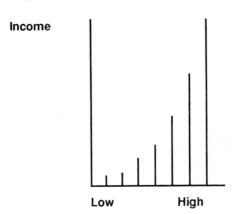

Note: Each vertical bar represents the total income of one individual or family. A line traced across the top of the bars resembles a "J."

Figure 10.3   A Lorenz Curve

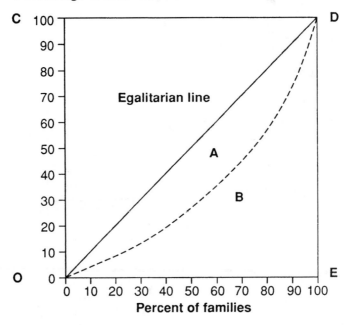

Source: Adapted from Kakwani 1987:244.

The straight diagonal line, OD, in Figure 10.3 is called the *egalitarian line*. If everyone in the group under analysis had exactly the same income, the Lorenz curve would correspond to the egalitarian line. If all the income accrued to one individual, the Lorenz curve would be the right angle represented by OED in Figure 10.3. The more the Lorenz curve bends away from the egalitarian line, the greater the inequality of income.

Figure 10.4a shows a Lorenz curve for the distribution of land owned in a Bagbana village, India, during 1968 and 1981. More than 30 percent of the families in this village own no land, which is why both Lorenz curves in Figure 10.4 track the zero line of land owned for more than a third of the way across the horizontal axis. Notice that inequality in land distribution in this village increased during the thirteen years from 1968 to 1981.

Figure 10.4b shows the Lorenz curve for farm income in this same village over the same period; more people have farm income than own land (many are landless farm workers). During the thirteen years under consideration, the inequality of farm income decreased.

In Table 10.4 some raw data from the Philippines is presented, from which several Lorenz curves could be constructed. To fix the concept in your mind you might try constructing a Lorenz curve for Philippine families for 1983.

The Gini Coefficient

The search for a better method of measuring income and wealth distribution did not end with Lorenz. In 1912 the Italian economist Corrado Gini proposed yet another measure of inequality, the Gini ratio, often called the Gini coefficient (Dagum 1987). Gini used the Lorenz curve as the basis of his ratio. He simply compared the area of the triangle OED (see Figure 10.3) with the area of the lens-shaped piece taken out of that triangle by the Lorenz curve. Labeling the lens-shaped part A and the remainder of the triangle B, the Gini ratio is:

$$\frac{A}{A+B}$$

If one individual in the group has all the income, the Gini ratio becomes one. If the size of A approaches zero, the Gini ratio approaches zero. The range of the Gini is thus from zero to one. Often the ratio above is multiplied by 100 and the Gini is reported on a scale of 0 to 100. At the bottom of Table 10.4 are Gini ratios for the income distribution data shown in that table.

Although popular, the Gini coefficient is open to criticism (Paglin 1974). It shows nothing about the location of the concentration of income inequality among high- versus low-income groups. The shape of the Lorenz curve could conceivably change (with the poor better off and the middle class worse off, for instance) without any change in the Gini. Furthermore,

Figure 10.4   Lorenz Curves for Farm Land and Farm Income, Bagbana Village, India, 1968 and 1981

a. Cumulative land

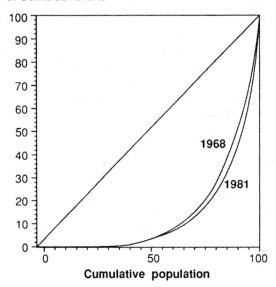

b. Cumulative farm income

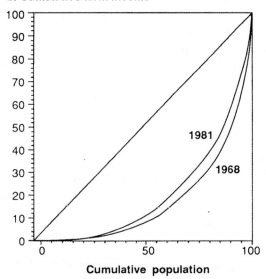

Source: Field surveys by Phillips Foster and his assistants. Lorenz curves by Paul Fishstein.

Table 10.4   Distribution of Total Family Income by Decile and Gini Coefficient, Philippines, 1978–1983

Ranking of Families	Percentage					
	1978	1979	1980	1981	1982	1983
First tenth	0.9	0.8	0.8	0.8	1.0	1.0
Second tenth	2.1	2.0	1.9	1.9	2.0	1.9
Third tenth	3.2	3.1	2.9	2.8	3.2	3.2
Fourth tenth	4.1	4.1	3.9	3.8	3.6	3.7
Fifth tenth	5.3	5.4	5.3	5.1	5.0	5.0
Sixth tenth	6.7	6.7	7.0	6.7	6.4	6.5
Seventh tenth	8.6	8.6	8.9	8.6	8.1	8.3
Eighth tenth	11.4	11.3	11.9	11.6	11.2	11.3
Ninth tenth	16.3	16.0	15.4	16.7	16.1	16.1
Last tenth	41.1	42.0	42.0	42.0	43.4	43.0
Gini coefficient	0.521	0.525	0.527	0.534	0.535	0.533

Source: Philippines National Economic Development Authority 1983:157.

neither the Lorenz curve nor the Gini take account of expected variation in income as people age.

Imagine a group consisting of working adults with ages distributed evenly from twenty to fifty years and with everyone in his twenties paid the same, everyone in her thirties paid the same, but more than those in their twenties, and everyone in his forties paid the same, but more than those in their thirties. In this case, the Gini would be greater than zero, although you might feel the income distribution was equitable.

Now imagine another group with the same income by age, but in which young and old ages predominate, with few in the middle group. The Gini would be higher than before, indicating greater inequality, but you might not think the ratio fairly contrasted the two groups.

Relative Income Share

Lorenz curves and Gini ratios make for useful comparisons and appear frequently in the literature of income and wealth distribution, but they are hard for the layman to understand and time-consuming to explain to politicians. Increasingly, the easy-to-understand relative income share is being used to describe income inequalities. With relative income share, you array the incomes in the population from lowest to highest and divide the population into equal-sized groups, just as you did on the Lorenz curve. Then you calculate the percentage of the total income in each group. And that is it; you have relative income share.

Given time series data, as in Table 10.4, you can track what is happening to any one income category that you may be interested in, such as the poorest, who are the most susceptible to undernutrition.

Relative income share is equally convenient for making comparisons among countries. A good source of such comparisons can be found in the World Bank's annual *World Development Report* table on income distribution (e.g., World Bank, *World Development Report 1996*:196–197).

Income Distributions in Different
Countries and Changes Over Time

Information on income distribution is collected and published by the World Bank and by the United Nations Development Programme. Some of this is presented in Table 10.5. The countries represented in the table account for over 70 percent of the world's population and 80 percent of the total world income. We can see from the table that there is quite a wide variation in the degrees of income equality. Of the countries reported in the table, the most equal distribution, as reflected by the lowest Gini coefficient, is in Japan (Gini = 24.9); the most unequal distribution is in Brazil (Gini = 60.7). The poorest 20 percent of the population controls 10.6 percent of the income in Japan, but only 2.2 percent in Brazil. The richest 20 percent of the population controls 35.7 percent of the income in Japan, but 64.1 percent of the income in Brazil.

Over the last thirty years, there appears to be a trend toward greater inequality of income in many countries. The increase in inequality has been especially pronounced in formerly socialist (Soviet-bloc) countries since the end of the Cold War and the breakup of the Soviet Union. For example, the Gini coefficient in Poland went from 25.5 in 1991 to 33 in 1993; in Bulgaria the increase was from 24 in 1991 to 34 in 1993. Table 10.6 illustrates changes in the Gini coefficient over time for a sample of countries. The increase for China probably represents reforms in the general economic system. However, the increases in inequality were not limited to countries that were replacing a socialist system with a more market-oriented economy. In both the United States and the United Kingdom, inequality increased gradually but substantially over a period going back to the late 1960s. From 1968 to 1991, the Gini coefficients increased from 33 to 38 in the United States, and from 24 to 32 in the United Kingdom. This trend does not appear in every country. For example, Japan and India show little change. Italy showed a substantial increase in equality, with the Gini coefficient dropping from about 40 in the mid-1970s to about 32 in the early 1990s. The World Bank website on income distribution, http://www.worldbank.org/poverty/inequal/index.htm, provides an excellent overview of the literature and data on income distribution.

Table 10.5 Income Distribution in Selected Countries

Country	Year	% of the country's income earned by				Gini coefficient	Country's GNI as % of world total	Population as % of world total
		Poorest 10%	Poorest 20%	Richest 20%	Richest 10%			
U.S.	1997	1.8	5.2	46.4	30.5	40.8	21.8	4.7
China	1998	2.4	5.9	46.6	30.4	40.3	11.4	20.9
Japan	1993	4.8	10.6	35.7	21.7	24.9	7.1	2.1
India	1997	3.5	8.1	46.1	33.5	37.8	6.5	16.8
Germany	1998	2.0	5.7	44.7	28.0	38.2	4.6	1.3
Italy	1998	1.9	6.0	42.6	27.4	36.0	3.2	0.9
U.K.	1995	2.1	6.1	43.2	27.5	36.0	3.2	1.0
France	1995	2.8	7.2	40.2	25.1	32.7	3.2	1.0
Brazil	1998	0.7	2.2	64.1	48.0	60.7	2.8	2.8
Russia	2000	1.8	4.9	51.3	36.0	45.6	2.3	2.4
Canada	1997	2.7	7.3	39.3	23.9	31.5	1.9	0.5
Mexico	1998	1.2	3.4	57.6	41.6	51.9	1.9	1.6
Spain	1990	2.8	7.5	40.3	25.2	32.5	1.8	0.7
S. Korea	1998	2.9	7.9	37.5	22.5	31.6	1.6	0.8
Indonesia	2000	3.6	8.4	43.3	28.5	30.3	1.4	3.5
Australia	1994	2.0	5.9	41.3	25.4	35.2	1.1	0.3
S. Africa	1995	0.7	2.0	66.5	46.9	59.3	1.1	0.7
Pakistan	1998–99	3.7	8.8	42.3	28.3	33.0	0.6	2.4
Bangladesh	2000	3.9	9.0	41.3	26.7	31.8	0.5	2.3
Nigeria	1996–97	1.6	4.4	55.7	40.8	50.6	0.2	1.9
Viet Nam	1998	3.6	8.0	44.5	29.9	36.1	0.4	1.3
Philippines	2000	2.2	5.4	52.3	36.3	46.1	0.7	1.3
Turkey	2000	2.3	6.1	46.7	30.7	40.0	0.9	1.1

Source: Human Development Report, 2003, tables 5, 12, and 13, http://www.undp.org/hdr2003/indicator/index_indicators.html

Table 10.6   Changes in Gini Coefficients Over Time for Selected Countries

	U.S.	U.K.	Taiwan	Japan	Italy	India	China
1968	33.50	24.10	28.90	34.90		31.86	
1969	33.64	24.90		35.70		31.47	
1970	34.06	25.10	29.42	35.50		30.38	
1971	34.30	25.70		36.90			
1972	34.46	26.00	29.02	33.40		31.85	
1973	34.42	25.10	33.60	32.50		29.17	
1974	34.16	24.20	28.09	33.60	41.00		
1975	34.42	23.30	31.20	34.40	39.00		
1976	34.42	23.20	28.40	33.90	35.00		
1977	34.98	22.90	28.00	33.70	36.30	32.14	
1978	35.02	23.10	28.43	32.90	35.98		
1979	35.06	24.40	27.70	33.90	37.19		
1980	35.20	24.90	27.96	33.40	34.29		
1981	35.62	25.40	28.15	34.30	33.12		
1982	36.48	25.20	28.51	34.80	32.02		
1983	36.70	25.70	28.45		32.87	31.49	27.20
1984	36.90	25.80	28.81		33.15		25.70
1985	37.26	27.10	29.20	35.90			31.40
1986	37.56	27.80	29.29		33.58	32.22	33.30
1987	37.56	29.30	29.65		35.58	31.82	34.30
1988	37.76	30.80	30.02			31.15	34.90
1989	38.16	31.20	30.41	37.60	32.74	30.46	36.00
1990	37.80	32.30	30.11	35.00		29.69	34.60
1991	37.94	32.40	30.49		32.19	32.53	36.20

Source: Deininger & Squire 1996.

■ Factors Influencing Income Distribution

Because unequal distribution of income contributes to third world undernutrition, we need to examine the causes of unequal income distribution so that we can, later, consider policies that might reduce undernutrition through changes in income distribution. The causes are many and complex and not fully understood.

Traditional Thinking: Heredity and Environment

Traditional thinking on the causes of differences in income concentrated on heredity and environment; we can develop a list of the leading schools of thought on this subject. Condensing each school in a purposely oversimplified sentence provides an efficient way of leafing through the diversity of opinions. Each school of thought (the list here is excerpted from Chu 1982:18–19) purports to offer at least a partial clue as to that basic income distribution question: Why is A's income greater than B's?

"Because A is smarter," says the *ability school.*

"Because A chose to work harder and/or chose to take more risks, and he was rewarded for this behavior," says the *individual choice school.*

"Because A went to a high-quality, expensive college and got a good education, and she is being rewarded for the educational investment in her," says the *human capital school.*

"Because A came from a well-to-do, supportive family. As a result, he was raised better, learned the habits and attitudes necessary for success, and thus can get and hold a better job," says the *family background school.*

"Because A works in the primary labor market, characterized by large firms and/or labor unions, while B works in the secondary labor market, characterized by small firms and without the protection of labor unions," says the *segmented labor market school.*

"Because A inherited a large fortune from his parents," says the *wealth inheritance school.*

"Because A is a white male and B is a black female," says the *discrimination school.*

"Because A is in her prime years of earnings and B is either substantially younger or older," says the *life cycle school.*

"Because A is lucky," says the *stochastic school.*

Each of these schools of thought could be the subject of considerable discussion as to causes and interrelationships with the other schools. Take the first one, for instance, the "ability school." Ability is constrained by both heredity and environment. But we have learned much in this century about how the developmental potential of an individual can be influenced by a mother's behavior during pregnancy. Poor eating habits, smoking, drug abuse, alcohol abuse, and other activity during a woman's pregnancy can limit the potential of her offspring. Is this part of the "family background school"?

Intelligence tests conducted on over 386,000 Dutch men as they were inducted into the military were correlated with their family size and birth order (whether they were born first, second, etc.). Belmont and Marolla (1973) found a high level of statistical significance when they correlated intelligence with family size and birth order. With the exception that an only child tended to be less intelligent than children in a family with two or three children total, there was a remarkable tendency for intelligence to decrease as family size and/or birth order increased.

In a study in the United States, Blake (1989) found that family size is a major influence on verbal and educational attainment, both of which tend to decrease as family size increases. Do parents, to some extent, determine family size? And if so, is family size a variable that issues from the "individual choice school"?

We have been examining some of the traditional ways of thinking about the causes of inequality of income distribution, schools of thought based largely on heredity and environment or their interaction. Recent research has caused us to study the impact of other variables, such as technology adoption, education, and fertility control, on income distribution.

Technology Adoption

The Kuznets Curve. In his 1954 presidential address to the American Economic Association, Harvard economist Simon Kuznets (1955) hypothesized that during the early phases of development, third world countries might experience increasing income inequalities before "leveling forces become strong enough to first stabilize and then reduce income inequalities." His idea that the path of income inequality through time in the third world would trace the shape of an inverted U became known as the Kuznets curve. Subsequent studies have lent support to Kuznets's hypothesis (Adelman and Morris 1973; Ahluwalia 1976b; Chenery, Robinson, and Syrquin 1986).

Using cross-sectional data of a sample of sixty countries, including forty third world countries, fourteen developed countries, and six socialist countries, Ahluwalia estimated relative income shares as per capita income changed. The result of one of his multiple regressions, which estimates percentage income share for the lowest 40 percent of the population from income variables, is shown in Figure 10.5. In this diagram the income share of the lowest 40 percent of the population declines from around 17 percent at around $150 per capita to about 12 percent at around $400 per capita, and then is back up to around 17 percent when income increases to $3,000. The U shape in Figure 10.5 is not inverted because the diagram tracks a measure of income equality instead of inequality, as in the original statement of the Kuznets curve.

It seems reasonable to postulate that the poor may benefit less from development than the rich. As development takes place, those in the more advanced sector of the economy are likely to be the first to take advantage of it. Therefore, they reap the first gains. After all, when the new productive techniques come along they often require new knowledge and substantial amounts of capital. The railroads and canals and electric companies, which were originally privately owned, are a case in point. It was difficult for the poor even to imagine "making a killing" in these areas.

Modernization could conceivably make the poor worse off. As Ahluwalia (1976b:330–331) puts it: "An aggressively expanding technologically advanced, modern sector, competing against the traditional sector for markets and resources (and benefiting in this competition from an entrenched position in the institutional and political context) may well generate both a relative and absolute decline in incomes of the poor." He concludes from his research, however, that though the initial stages of development are likely to make the poor worse off relative to the rich, these same initial stages are not necessarily inclined to making the poor worse off in absolute terms.

Figure 10.5   Estimated Relationship Between Income Share and per Capita GNP, 60 Countries, Various Years Prior to 1975

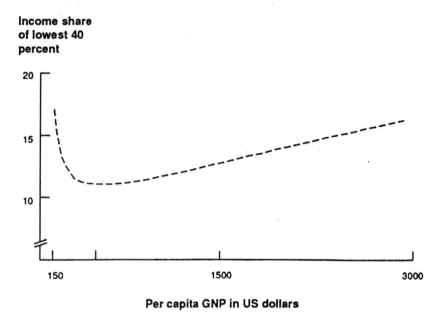

Source: Adapted from Ahluwalia 1976a:133.

An Empirical Analysis of Factors influencing Income Distribution

Ahluwalia's study, which estimated a type of Kuznets curve of income distribution (shown in Figure 10.5), also produced evidence of how some variables besides per capita income affect income distribution. Table 10.7 shows the results of two of his multiple regressions on sixty countries, mentioned above. In these regressions, the variables in the left-hand column are hypothesized to have an impact on the relative income shares.

The numbers in the middle column (equation one) show how the variables in the left-hand column influence percentage income share among the top 20 percent of the population. The numbers in the right-hand column (equation two) show how the variables in the left-hand column influence percentage income share among the bottom 40 percent of the population.

The variables on GNP per capita and GDP growth rate are included to account for the Kuznets curve. The variable at the bottom of the table, "dummy for socialist countries," is included to account for the fact that, by and large, socialist countries have a more equal income distribution than nonsocialist countries. The remaining variables in the equation are included

Table 10.7   Cross-Country Regressions Explaining Income Shares

	Dependent Variable: Percentage Income Shares			
	Top 20 Percent		Lowest 40 Percent	
Explanatory Variables	Direction of Influence of Variable	Equation One	Direction of Influence of Variable	Equation Two
Constant	−	9.07 (0.27)[a]	+	77.93 (4.11)
Log per capita GNP	+	50.35 (2.13)	−	47.28 (3.50)
(Log per capita GNP)	−	8.16 (1.98)	+	7.65 (3.35)
Growth rate of GDP	−	0.11 (0.32)	+	0.11 (0.55)
Literacy rate	−	0.09 (2.21)	+	0.06 (2.56)
Secondary school enrollment	−	0.14 (2.48)	+	0.02 (0.74)
Growth rate of population	+	3.59 (4.29)	−	1.19 (2.56)
Share of agriculture in GDP	−	0.25 (2.23)	+	0.04 (0.65)
Share of urban population	−	0.10 (1.68)	+	0.06 (1.79)
Dummy for socialist countries	−	9.41 (3.27)	+	8.57 (5.35)
R^2		.76		.69
F		22.31		6.21
SEE		4.6		2.6

Source: Ahluwalia 1976a:131.
Note: Note that on each explanatory variable the signs switch between the top 20 percent and the bottom 40 percent of the population.
   a. Values in parentheses are T ratios. For this sample, a T value of 1.68 indicates significance at the 10 percent level for a two-tailed test.

to see how they influence relative income share when the influence of the Kuznets curve and socialism are accounted for.

    The signs on the numbers are of particular interest to us in examining the regression because they tell us the direction of influence that the related variable has on percentage income share when the other variables are at their average value. (Because the units of measurement of each of the variables influence the size of the regression coefficients—the numbers not in parentheses—and because we do not have these units of measurement, the size of the numbers is not of particular interest to us here. The size of the numbers in parentheses is important because they are the results of a test of significance—the bigger the number, the more likely its variable is to be of significant influence.)

First look at signs for the "dummy for socialist countries." In equation one, the sign for this variable is negative, meaning that socialism tends to lower the percentage income share of the top 20 percent of the population. In equation two, the sign is positive. That is, socialism tends to raise the relative income share of the lowest 40 percent of the population.

Now examine the signs for the other variables. Increasing the literacy rate, the rate of secondary school enrollment, the share of agriculture in the GDP, and the share of urban population appear to increase the relative income share of the poor and to reduce the relative income share of the rich.

The share of agriculture in the GDP variable is not significant for the poor (T = 0.65), so we will not consider this variable important. As the percentage of the urban population increases, relative income share of the poor increases. This seems reasonable, because urban people generally enjoy higher incomes than rural people, and as rural people move to the city in search of better jobs the total income distribution may become more equal. However, because of problems of crowding, pollution, crime, and so on associated with growth in third world cities, it is hard to argue for urbanization as a means to reduce income inequality.

Literacy rate and secondary school enrollment are good indices of overall education among the poor in third world countries. The wealthy see to it that their children get an education somehow or other; the illiterates and those without even a secondary education are usually the poor. Increasing the rate of literacy and secondary education makes the poor potentially more productive and gives them better access to employment and better-paying jobs, thus reducing income inequality.

The influence of population growth rate on relative income share is harder to understand. It is the only one of the variables considered here for which increasing its value makes the poor worse off relative to the rich. The relationship between income and population is dicussed more fully in Chapters 9 and 19.

■ An Illustration of Why Income Distribution Matters

In the world as a whole, low-income people tend to underconsume food while high-income people tend to overconsume it. In an influential monograph published in 1976, Reutlinger and Selowsky attempted to quantify this under- and overconsumption. Figure 10.6 is representative of their work on this subject.

For purposes of developing the data from which Figure 10.6 was drawn, Reutlinger and Selowsky assumed that income elasticity of demand

**Figure 10.6   Calorie Consumption by Income Groups, Latin America, 1965
(with Calorie–Income Elasticity Equal 5o 0.15)**

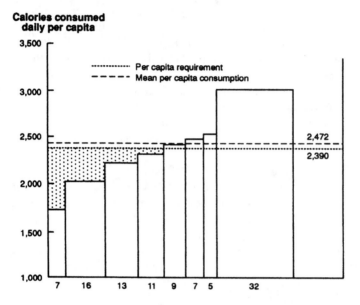

**Percentage share of total population by income group,
lowest income on left and highest on right**

Source: Adapted from Reutlinger & Selowsky 1976:20.

Note: If an income elasticity of 0.15 seems low to you, remember that income elasticities decline as income rises. The income elasticities we have quoted so far are mostly for very low income. For example, Ho's estimate was 0.58 for the East Javanese sample. The income elasticity estimates shown for calories in Table 7.2 were for rural Brazil, which, by and large, is poorer than urban Brazil, where such elasticity estimates run lower. Remember also that income elasticities for particular foods shown (as in the case of Tables 7.2 and 7.3) tend to run higher than income elasticities for calories as a whole. The median calorie elasticity for low-income families (consuming 1,750–2,000 calories per capita per day) among 19 estimates examined by Alderman (1984:37) was 0.405.

for calories was 0.15. Subsequent estimates based on data from seventeen developing countries put the income elasticity of demand for calories at 0.15 or 0.16 (Reutlinger et al. 1986:64), suggesting that this original assumption was reasonable. As noted in Chapter 7, Bouis and Haddad (1992) conclude, after an extensive review of existing literature, that a number in the range of 0.08–0.14 is a reasonable estimate.

Figure 10.6 plots calorie consumption by income groups in Latin America, given 0.15 as the estimate for overall income elasticity of demand for calories. The dashed horizontal line cutting across the vertical bars represents FAO-recommended per capita daily calorie consumption for adult equivalents. The dotted horizontal line close by represents average daily adult equivalent calorie consumption. With a little imagination you can see two stepped triangles in this figure: one (the shaded triangle) represents the total calorie deficit among low-income people, while the other triangle (the boxes above the dotted line) represents overconsumption among the rich. We refer to these as the *Reutlinger triangles.*

Figure 10.6 is a visualization of the nutritional impact of differential purchasing power among third world income groups. As the rich and the poor both bid for food in the marketplace, the poor simply do not have as much clout as the rich. The rich bid food away from the poor.

As per capita income increases, people, especially the rich, eat more livestock and livestock products. Over the past century the worldwide demand for livestock and livestock products has increased to the point that the world livestock herd, which in the 1800s was largely a scavenging herd (cows ate grass; chickens, pigs, and ducks ate table scraps), is now eating substantial amounts of grain. In 1983 and 1984 about one-third of the world's grain production was fed to livestock (Reutlinger et al. 1986:24). As the rich consume meat, milk, eggs, and other livestock products, they are, to some extent, bidding grain away from the poor. To recapitulate: income distribution is important in nutrition for two reasons: (1) the greater the distance between the rich and the poor, the greater is the capacity and the tendency of the rich to bid food away from the poor; and (2) the greater the concentration of income in the hands of a wealthy few, the greater is their tendency (because of their high incomes) to purchase and consume livestock products. The more the wealthy consume livestock products, the more dependent the livestock herd becomes on grain as it switches from scavenging and eating grass. The more the price of grain is bid up to satisfy the wealthy's demand for animal products, the harder it is for the poor to buy the grain they need for minimal nutrition.

The Redistribution-Incentive Paradox

Programs that transfer purchasing power from the rich to the poor will reduce the size of both of the Reutlinger triangles, thus improving nutrition (the upward-sloping line that is the hypotenuse of the right triangles will become more horizontal). By eliminating all differences in income, the Reutlinger triangles could also be eliminated, and food would, presumably, be fairly evenly distributed across the population.

Two major and vastly different countries—China and the Soviet Union—have experimented with programs that greatly reduced differences in income. As they succeeded, they reduced differences in food consumption, but at the same time they experienced difficulties with food production.

Before their respective socialist revolutions, both countries enjoyed healthy agricultural economies. In 1917, the year of the Russian Revolution, the world's leading agricultural geographers (Finch and Baker 1917:13) wrote that "the Russian Empire leads the world in both acreage and production of wheat. . . . Nearly one-fifth of the average harvest is exported." China's socialist revolution was completed after World War II. Before that war, China accounted for 93 percent of the world's soybean exports.

Both Russia and China went from being major food exporters before their socialist revolutions to major food importers afterwards. And during the 1980s both countries tried to reintroduce market-oriented incentives, in part to bolster their flagging agricultural productivity.

There appear to be nutritional gains from reducing the size of the Reutlinger triangles through redistributing income, yet income redistribution, carried to extremes, appears to introduce incentive problems that could conceivably lead to low levels of food consumption for all. It seems, then, if your goal is to improve nutrition for all, there is not much point in debating the relative merits of laissez-faire, free-enterprise capitalism (which can produce large Reutlinger triangles) versus extreme socialism (which appears to lead to problems in agricultural productivity), for both of these extremes may lead to widespread hunger problems. In reducing undernutrition, then, the appropriate debate with reference to income redistribution should center on how much and by what methods to do it. That is, to what extent should the rich be taxed, and how should the money going into the tax till be spent?

Does Income Equality Promote Growth?

A study in the late 1970s answered this question with a tentative yes. Ahluwalia, Carter, and Chenery (1979) examined twelve countries for which they had data on growth and income shares for a ten-year period. They found that the countries most successful in reducing income inequality were also the countries with the highest rates of growth in per capita incomes.

Recently a more comprehensive study by the World Bank (Deininger and Squire 1997) failed to make a strong correlation between growth and income inequality. Of the eighty-eight countries whose per capita GDP grew for a decade, income inequality improved slightly in about half the cases and worsened slightly in the other half. However, the study found that the distribution of *wealth* (as measured by land ownership) does strongly affect growth. Countries having great inequality of wealth grow more slowly than countries with less inequality. For example, fifteen developing countries have a Gini coefficient (for land distribution) higher than 70. Of these fifteen countries, only two showed growth rates higher than 2.5 percent per year during the period 1960–1992.

Global Redistribution:
Do Incomes Grow Faster in Poor Countries?

No matter how large the income disparities that exist within a country, they are dwarfed by the differences in income between rich and poor countries. How can such enormous differences exist between countries? One obvious answer to this question is that much more investment in productive capital occurs in rich countries; people in those countries are more productive because they have more and better capital, better equipment in their work-places, better roads and communications, and better education. Many economists believe that as time passes, income per capita in poor countries will catch up with income in rich countries; in other words, incomes per capita will *converge*. Investors will discover that investing in poor countries with low levels of capital has a higher payoff than investing in rich countries where there are high levels of capital; this investment will increase the capital stock in poor countries and therefore increase production per person in those countries.

In Table 10.8, we see mixed evidence about whether this *convergence theory* is correct. Over the last decade, income per capita grew faster in middle-income countries (2.4 percent per year) than in high-income countries (1.7 percent). But low-income countries lag behind (1.2 percent per year growth). Among developing countries, the South Asian numbers reflect strong growth in India (4.1 percent annual growth during the 1990s) and the East Asian numbers reflect strong growth in China (9.2 percent growth during the 1990s). Two areas show negative growth. Sub-Saharan Africa's low-income growth is persistent over a quarter century, though

Table 10.8 Annual Growth Rate of per Capita Income (PPP), 1975–2000 and 1990–2000

Region	Growth rate 1975–2000	Growth rate 1990–2000
Developing countries in:		
East Asia & Pacific	5.9	5.7
Latin America & Caribbean	0.7	1.7
South Asia	2.4	3.3
Sub-Saharan Africa	−0.9	−0.3
Eastern block and former Soviet Union	Not available	−2.4
Low-income countries	1.5	1.2
Middle-income countries	1.8	2.4
High-income countries	2.1	1.7

Source: UNDP, *Human Development Report 2003*.

during the last decade the news is slightly less bad. The large negative growth rates observed in parts of the former Soviet bloc reflect the fact that during the 1985–1995 period, these economies underwent severe problems adjusting to a new economic system. If we eliminate both groups of countries—China and India with their high positive growth rates and the former Soviet-bloc countries with their high negative growth rates—we find that middle- and low-income countries had an annual rate of growth in per capita income of –0.44 percent over the last decade. This is substantially below the positive growth rates of 1.7 percent per year in the high-income countries. Maddison (1995) finds stronger evidence for convergence by looking at income growth over a long period (1820 to the present).

Changes in the World Distribution of Income and How It Has Changed over Time

So far we have talked about two sources of income disparity: income disparity within countries that appears to be growing in many countries over the past decades, and income disparity between countries that may be declining. What does this mean to the overall distribution of income in the world?

A description of the world distribution of income is found in Box 10.2. Notice that most incomes in the United States are at the top end of the world distribution. For example, if a college student spends $30,000 a year on tuition, room, and board, that student spends more than the annual incomes of 95 percent of the world's population. A single person at the poverty line in the United States earns more than about 80 percent of the world's population. See Box 10.3 for a more detailed picture of poverty in the United States.

A paper by Sala-i-Martin (2002) estimated the world distribution of income and how it changed over time. He concluded that income is becoming more equally distributed over time. He estimated Gini coefficients that fell from about .66 in the 1970s to .65 in the 1980s to .63 in the 1990s. This has translated into a reduction in poverty worldwide (measured by the percentage of people living on incomes of less than $2 per day, adjusted for inflation). Sala-i-Martin found that this poverty rate declined from 40 percent in 1970 to less than 20 percent by the late 1990s. China's poverty rate fell from about 75 percent in 1970 to 20 percent in 1998. The reduction in poverty was found in every geographical area, except for Africa, where poverty rates increased from 53 percent in 1970 to 64 percent in 1998.

Box 10.2   World Distribution of Income: Who Is Rich?

Who is rich? Would you say that all people in the top half of the income distribution are rich? Or do you have to be in the top quarter, or the top 10 percent or the top 5 percent? Or would you say that only the richest 1 percent of the population are "the rich"? This is a subjective judgment, and well-intentioned, well-informed people can come to different conclusions. Once you have decided how you would define "rich," use the table below to find out how much a rich person earns (according to your definition). We predict you will be surprised.

Using data such as that shown in Tables 10.2 and 10.5, we constructed an estimated world distribution of income. For each country, we calculate the average income in each quintile, and then assume that everybody in that quintile earns the average income of his/her group. Using this simplification, we then calculate how many people earn less than $1,000, how many less than $2,000, etc. In the table below, we show the world distribution of income in 2001 using the PPP comparison.

As described in the text, this method of comparing incomes attempts to adjust for different costs of living, so that a person making $5,000 in one country has approximately the same standard of living as a person making $5,000 in another country. The countries used for our exercise account for 86 percent of the world's population and 96 percent of the world's income in 1995. Therefore, the countries omitted are relatively poor countries, and our estimate of the distribution may be biased in the upward direction—perhaps people are not as rich as we make them out to be.

So . . . are you one of the rich?

World Distribution of Income 2001

This proportion of the world's population (in percentages)	Earns less than this income per person (in U.S. dollars)
50	2,801
65	4,632
75	7,189
80	9,516
85	13,324
90	19,963
95	33,714
98	56,037
99	76,434
99.5	100,334

Box 10.3   Poverty in the United States

Box 10.2 suggested that a person at the poverty line in the United States would have higher income than 80 percent of the people in the world. How does the life a poor person in the United States compare to the life of Malawian Adilesi Faisoni described in Box 10.1?

A single person is categorized as "poor" in the United States if his income is below $9,359 a year; for a family of four, a family income below $18,392 makes you poor.

In the United States:

95.4 percent of poor households have air conditioning.

99.5 percent of poor households have a refrigerator

97.5 percent of poor households have a color television; 54.8 percent have more than one color TV; 26 percent of poor households have a large-screen TV; 62.9 percent have cable or a satellite dish.

11

Other Factors Influencing
Demand for Food

Chapter 9 presented some projections about the size of the world's population—it could grow by over 50 percent over the next fifty years. Does this mean that if food supply grows by 50 percent we will have enough extra food to feed those extra mouths? To answer that question we must first examine the factors that influence food consumption per person. In Chapter 10, we discussed how demand for food increases as income increases, and we examined some trends in per capita income levels and the distribution of income. In this chapter, we ask the question: What factors influence the amount of food and the types of food consumed per capita?

■ Population Characteristics and Demand for Food

How does average demand for food change as a result of characteristics of the population? We saw in Chapter 3 that nutrient requirements depend on age, sex, pregnancy and breast-feeding status, and physical activity level.

Age Structure

The age composition of a population (*age structure*) is one of the most important features of that population. It is a reflection of the underlying demographic conditions of the preceding decades and at the same time is an important determinant of future demographic patterns.

Population pyramids. The most convenient way to visualize the age structure of a population is through a graph of population distribution according to age and sex, called a *population pyramid.* Conventionally, population pyramids represent age cohorts by five- or ten-year intervals, and place males on the left of a vertical line and females on the right, with the youngest cohort at the bottom. The graphic representation of the age cohorts can be either the actual numbers or the percentage distribution. Figure 11.1 shows a numerical population pyramid for the industrialized nations versus the third world in the year 1985, with projections to 2025. The horizontal lines across both sets of pyramids mark the dividing lines

Figure 11.1   Population Pyramids for Less and More Developed Countries, 1985 and Projections to 2025

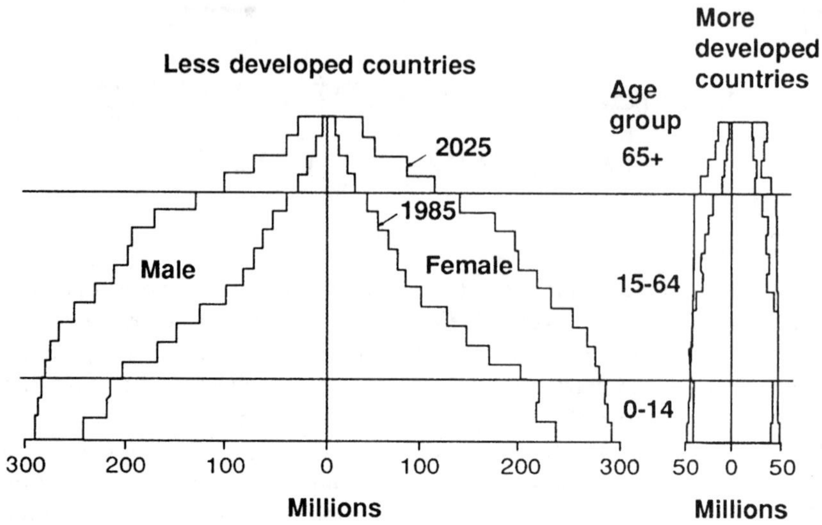

Source: Adapted from Merrick et al. 1986:19.

that are commonly, but arbitrarily, placed to separate the dependent age categories (in this case, below fifteen years or above sixty-five years) from the working-age population. Such numerical population pyramids do a nice job of making visible the differences in actual population size, third world versus developed world, and they can also show demographic features such as the higher survival rate of older women (notice the difference between the numbers of men and women in the oldest cohort for the 2025 projection for the developed world). But to make comparisons from one country to another, or from one time period to another within a country, pyramids showing percentage distribution (relative pyramids) are usually more helpful.

Figure 11.2 shows relative pyramids for two developed countries (the United States and West Germany) and one third world country (Morocco). The total area in each pyramid is exactly the same and represents 100 percent of the population of each country. The relative size of the youngest age cohort (zero to five) is reflective of the magnitude of the birth rate in the previous five years in each country. In 1972, the birth rate in Morocco was 45 per thousand; in the United States it was 16; and in West Germany, 10.

Demographic patterns in the recent past can often be read directly from current population pyramids. For instance, during World War II and imme-

Figure 11.2   Age Structure in Morocco, United States, and West Germany, 1985

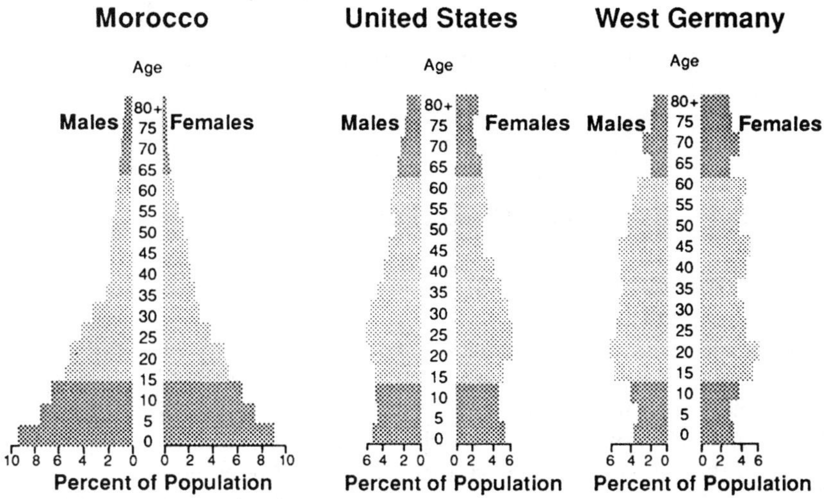

Source: Adapted from Haub 1987:21.

diately afterward, birth rates in Germany decline. In 1985, the year of the pyramid shown in Figure 11.2, people born between 1945 and 1950 were between thirty-five and forty years old. They are shown in the cohort 35. Notice the narrowness of Germany's pyramid during that year. By contrast, the United States experienced a fifteen-year baby boom starting immediately after World War II, which shows as a bulge in the 1985 pyramid extending from cohorts 25 through 35.

Age structure is of interest to demographers because, as we have noted above, it provides clues about past and future demographic patterns. It is important to policymakers because of its impact on two things we will discuss next: (1) momentum in population growth and (2) dependency ratios.

Momentum in population growth. Over a long period, a population would just reproduce itself if individual couples produced exactly the right number of children to replace themselves, allowing for some children to die before they arrived at childbearing age. In most populations this number comes to just over two children (that is, about 2.1) per couple (or per woman). In this discussion, we assume that 2.1 children, on the average, will handle replacement. If a population has remained constant for a couple of generations and then its fertility rate rises higher than 2.1, it will grow. (We are assuming no net immigration or emigration and no improvements in healthcare that raise average life expectancy.) If, on the other hand, its fertility rate falls below 2.1, it will shrink. For that reason, a fertility rate of 2.1 is considered the replacement level (Merrick et al. 1986:6).

You might expect that when the fertility rate of a rapidly growing population falls to 2.1, births and deaths would be in balance, and population growth would stop. This is not the case, at least not immediately. The reason is demographic momentum. A population that has had high fertility in the years before reaching replacement-level fertility will have a much younger age structure than a population with low fertility before crossing the replacement threshold. Consider the three countries in Figure 11.2. West Germany has a fertility rate of 1.4. It has already stopped growing, with a population growth rate of minus 0.2 percent. Notice that a substantial proportion of its population is over thirty-five. The United States has a fertility rate of 1.9 and rate of natural increase of 0.7 percent. (Immigration is now causing the United States to grow faster than that.) It also has a more youthful population than West Germany. But an enormous proportion of the population of Morocco, which in 1982 had a fertility rate of 6.9, is below thirty-five years of age. Morocco's rate of natural increase was 3.2 in 1982. It fell to about 2.6 in 1989. Now suppose that Morocco's fertility rate should suddenly fall to 2.1. Would its population growth stop immediately? No, because of the large numbers of young people in the childbearing years relative to the older years. Would it stop soon? No, because of the large number of people below fifteen who will be moving into the childbearing years.

As noted above, the rate of natural increase of population in the United States is 0.7 percent even though its fertility rate is 1.9, just below replacement level. This is caused by momentum. To reinforce your understanding of momentum in population growth, study Figure 11.3. On a worldwide basis, population momentum means that "even if there were a sudden reduction of fertility to the level strictly needed to replace the population, the world population would still increase by more than 2 billion" by the year 2050 (FAO, WFS Background Paper no. 4, 1996a).

Dependency ratios. When the age structure of a population is known, the dependency ratios can be easily calculated. The dependency ratio is usually defined as the ratio of dependents to working-age adults. As mentioned before, working-age adults are generally identified as those from fifteen to sixty-five. But dependents are commonly split into groups by age, and two more ratios are then defined: The adult dependency ratio is the percentage of the population sixty-five and over divided by the percentage of the population between fifteen and sixty-five; the child dependency ratio is the percentage of the population below fifteen divided by the percentage of the population between fifteen and sixty-five.

In a rapidly growing population, the burden of dependent children per

Figure 11.3   A Demonstration of Momentum in Population Growth

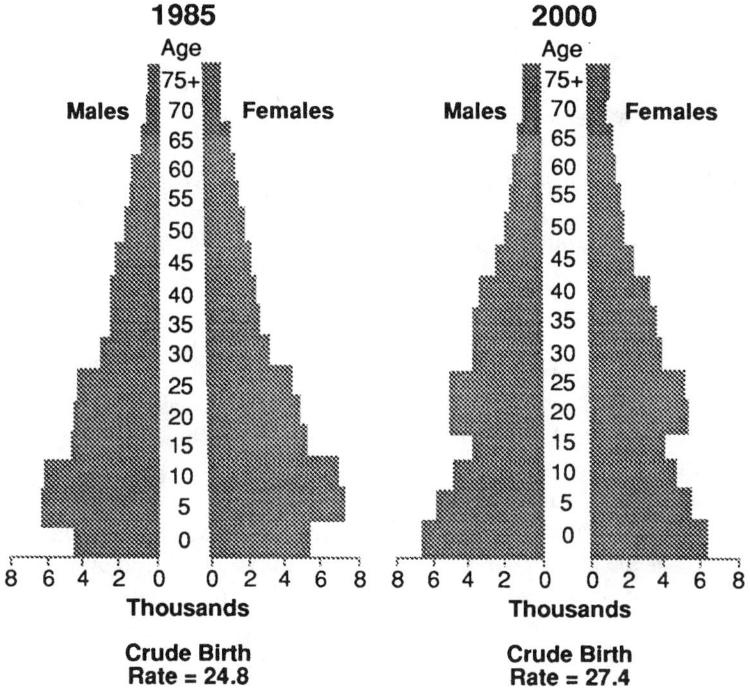

1985

Age

Males   75+   Females
         70
         65
         60
         55
         50
         45
         40
         35
         30
         25
         20
         15
         10
          5
          0

8 6 4 2 0   0 2 4 6 8

Thousands

**Crude Birth
Rate = 24.8**

2000

Age

Males   75+   Females
         70
         65
         60
         55
         50
         45
         40
         35
         30
         25
         20
         15
         10
          5
          0

8 6 4 2 0   0 2 4 6 8

Thousands

**Crude Birth
Rate = 27.4**

Source: Adapted from Haub 1987:14.

Note: The pyramids here demonstrate the effect of age structure on population change. In 1985 this population had a noticeable bulge in the age groups 5–9 and 10–14, the result of a recent baby boom. In this population about half of all the childbearing takes place in the twenties. When the bulge groups reach their twenties, the number of births will rise disproportionately. In this example the total fertility rate is held constant at 3.1, as is mortality. In 1985 the crude birth rate was 24.8 per 1,000 but by the year 2000 it will have increased to 27.4, as a result of the bulge groups reaching childbearing years. The growth rate will have increased from 1.65 in 1985 to 1.84 in the year 2000.

adult is far greater than in a slowly growing population or one with zero population growth. Compare again the population pyramids in Figure 11.2, this time with regard to the child dependency ratio. In West Germany, which in 1985 had essentially zero population growth, 15 percent of the population was below fifteen years of age, and 70 percent was in the age group fifteen through sixty-four. The child dependency ratio was thus 0.21; that is, 0.21 children per working adult. Another way of looking at these data is to say that some 4.7 adults were available, on the average, to raise and educate each child.

In Morocco, whose population was growing at just over 3 percent at the time the pyramid was drawn, 42 percent of the people were children and 54 percent were in the working-age group (fifteen to sixty-four). That produces a child dependency ratio of 0.77. In Morocco, then, there were only 1.3 adults available, on the average, to raise and educate each child. (Raw data for calculating dependency ratios were furnished by the Population Reference Bureau.)

The age structure of population in the future. What kind of age structure will we see in the future? The theory of demographic transition described in Chapter 9 predicts that as living conditions improve, life expectancy will increase, followed by declining fertility rates. This implies that in the future there will be a smaller percentage of children and a larger percentage of adults. Future population pyramids will be narrower.

If there are proportionately more adults than children, the need for food will grow faster than the population. The simple example in Table 11.1 illustrates this point. Although population increases by 50 percent, calorie requirements increase by 54 percent because the future population is 66 percent adult rather than the present 60 percent. This effect can also be seen in comparisons of current energy requirements in different geographical areas. Because of the high proportion of children in Africa's population compared to the United States and Canada, average calorie requirements in Africa are 2,150 calories compared to 2,400 in North America (FAO, WFS Background Paper No. 4, 1996b). The projections of the impact of changing age structure on per capita calorie requirements are shown in Table 11.2. In Africa, where the age structure is projected to change the most, per capita calorie requirements are expected to increase by 7 percent (to 2,300 calories per person per day) over the next fifty years. In Asia and Latin America, the increase is 2 percent. In the developed world, no change is projected (except for a slight decline in requirements in Europe, attributable to an increase in percentage of elderly people in the population).

Table 11.1   An Example Demonstrating How Changing Age Structure of a Population Can Affect Food Requirements

	Present	Future
Number of children (requiring 1,800 calories per capita per day)	4 million	5 million
Number of adults (requiring 2,700 calories per capita per day)	6 million	10 million
Total population	10 million	15 million
Total calorie requirements	23,400 million	36,000 million
Calories per capita per day	2,340	2,400

Table 11.2   Estimated Effects of Demographic Factors in Average Calorie Requirement per Capita per Day (percentage increase or decrease from 1995)

	Africa	Asia	Europe	Latin America and the Caribbean	North America	Oceania
Age structure	+7	+2	−1	+2	no change	no change
Change in percentage of pregnant women	no change	−1	no change	no change	no change	no change
Change in level of physical activity	−3	−4	−1	−2	−1	−1
Change in average height	+2	+2	no change	+2	no change	+1

Source: FAO, WFS Background Paper No. 4.

■ Other Demographic Characteristics and Food Requirements

Average per capita food requirements in a population also depend on other characteristics of the people. In this section, we discuss likely impacts on per capita food requirements over the next fifty years from three factors: (1) the number of pregnant women in the population; (2) the average amount of physical activity in the population; (3) the average height of people.

Pregnancy.   Pregnant and breast-feeding women require higher caloric intake. Two opposing trends exist here. As the base of the population pyramid contracts, we see an increase in the ratio of women of childbearing age to total population. On the other hand, the drop in fertility rates means that each woman of childbearing age is becoming pregnant fewer times during her lifetime. As Table 11.2 shows, the FAO estimates no net effect on average per capita food requirements, except for a 1 percent decline in Asia.

Physical activity.   Anyone who has ever exercised in an attempt to control her weight knows that physical activity burns calories. On a worldwide scale, what is likely to affect average per capita calorie requirements is not "average visits to the gym," but the average physical activity of adults on the job. Farming (especially in developing countries) requires more physical activity than many city jobs. Therefore, as urban populations grow faster than rural populations in the future, we should expect to see a decline in the average activity level. As Table 11.2 shows, the FAO projects that this change will cause a reduction in per capita food requirements of from 1 to 4 percent.

Height. Good nutrition during infancy and childhood can cause a person to become a taller adult. But taller adults need more calories to maintain their bodily functions. The FAO projections are based on an underlying assumption that food supplies will continue to grow faster than food demand; thus the incidence of undernutrition will decline, and there will be less stunting. Table 11.2 shows that this is expected to add 2 percent to energy requirements in developing countries, and to have no substantial effect in the developing world.

Compared to the changes in population characteristics described above, growth of per capita income is likely to have a much bigger effect on food demand. As we saw in Table 10.8 during the 1980s and 1990s, per capita income grew at an annual rate of 1.5–2.1 percent, depending on the country grouping. If income per capita grows at a rate of between 1 and 3 percent per year, at the end of fifty years, average income will be higher by between 64 percent and 338 percent, as shown in Table 11.3. As discussed in Chapter 7, estimates show that the income elasticity for food is between 0.1 and 0.3. This means that a 1 percent increase in a person's income will increase the quantity of food demanded by the person by from 0.1 to 0.3 percent. If we apply this to the growth in income projected in Table 11.3, we obtain growth in per capita food demand of between 6.4 percent (if income grows by 64 percent and income elasticity is 0.1) and 101 percent (if income grows by 338 percent and income elasticity is 0.3).

The most likely scenario is at the low end of this range, for two reasons. First, although average growth of per capita incomes in the 2–3 percent range have been observed over a decade, it may be hard to sustain this high of a level for fifty years. Second, income elasticities decline as income increases; therefore the 0.1 elasticity is probably more realistic than the 0.3 elasticity.

So a good guess about how food demand per capita will grow over the next fifty years is that it will grow by 5–20 percent. Is this a reasonable guess based on historical experience? Growth of this magnitude would mean that (assuming constant prices) the worldwide average intake of calories per capita might grow from the current 2,806 per day to a level between 2,946 (equivalent to the current average diet in China) and 3,508

Table 11.3   The Power of Compound Growth

If income per capita grows at an annual rate of:	Then income after 50 years will be higher by a factor of:
1%	1.64 (about one-and-a-half times current income)
2%	2.69 (over twice current income)
3%	4.38 (over four times current income)

calories per day (approximately equivalent to the current average diet in Hungary). For an additional comparison, between the early 1960s and the early 2000s, worldwide consumption of calories per person grew about 24 percent.

Growth in Population and Growth in Food per Capita—A Multiplicative Effect

Notice that growth in per capita food consumption magnifies the impact of growing population. Imagine a country in which a thousand people consume 2,500 calories per day—total food consumption in the country is 2.5 million calories per day. Now suppose the population grows to two thousand, and per capita calories grows to 3,000; now total food consumption in the country is 6 million calories per day. The population has grown by 100 percent (from one to two thousand), but food consumption has grown by 140 percent (from 2.5 to 6 million). Not only are there more mouths to feed, but each mouth is eating more. The practical effect of this is illustrated in Table 11.4. If population grows by 50 percent over the next fifty years, and if per capita food demand grows by between 5 and 20 percent, total food demand will grow by between 57.5 and 80 percent.

■ Dietary Diversification and Demand for Food

As average incomes go up, people do not simply eat more food; they eat different kinds of food. In particular, they eat more meat and animal products, and they consume fewer calories from cereals. To illustrate this, consider the diets of various countries and country groups shown in Table 11.5.

In the mid-1990s, average calories consumed per day worldwide were about 2,700, with about 400 (15 percent) coming from animal products and about 2,300 from plant sources. According to FAO estimates, it took about 4,800 *plant-derived calories* to produce these 2,700 calories. Thus, it took about 2,500 plant-derived calories to produce the 400 calories from animal

Table 11.4   Growth in per Capita Food Consumption Magnifies the Effect of Population Growth

If population grows by 50% over the next 45 years, and if per capita food demand grows by ___%	then total food demand will grow by ___%
5	57.5
10	65
15	72.5
20	80

products—a ratio about about 6:1. (See Box 11.1 for a discussion of estimates of the number of plant-derived calories needed to produce a human-consumed calorie from various animal products.)

In 1995, people in developing countries consumed about 12.5 percent of their 2,570 calories as animal products. Suppose this percentage rises to 15 percent (approximately the world average today) by the year 2050. Even

Table 11.5   Calories (per Capita per Day) from Cereals and Animal Products in Various Countries and Country Groups, 1995

	Nigeria	India	China	Brazil	U.S.	All Developing Countries	All Developed Countries
Income/capita ($)	260	340	620	3,640	26,980	4,771	24,930
Calories from animal products	79	170	506	543	989	315	861
Calories from cereals	1,057	1,483	1,578	889	847	1,435	1,018
Total calories	2,508	2,388	2,741	2,834	3,603	2,570	3,192

Source: FAOSTAT Statistical Database, 1998.

Box 11.1   Plant-Derived Calories Needed to Produce a Calorie from Animal Products

In a background paper for the 1996 World Food Summit, FAO (1996a) published estimates that it takes:

- 11 plant-derived calories to produce 1 calorie of beef or mutton
- 4 plant-derived calories to produce 1 calorie of pork or poultry
- 8 plant-derived calories to produce 1 calorie of milk
- 4 plant-derived calories to produce 1 calorie of eggs

Time Magazine (Usher 1996) cited a conversion rate of 16:1 for cattle.

Fitzhugh (1998) argues that these numbers are too high. Animals can eat grass, crop residues, waste, and by-products that are not part of the human diet. He estimates that the correct conversion rate is 2.3–3.4 plant calories for each calorie of animal products.

If we convert the figures on the world's food balance sheet from kilograms to calories, we find that the ratio of calories used in animal feed to calories of animal products eaten by humans is about 2.3–2.5 to 1. Although we will use the higher FAO estimates in our projections and discussions in the text, it should be noted that this may overstate the impact of dietary diversification.

if caloric intake remained constant at 2,570, this shift to animal products would mean that each person would need 8.7 percent more plant-derived calories. The calculation is as follows: The current diet is 315 calories from animal sources, and 2,255 from plant sources; if 6.25 plant-derived calories are needed to produce one animal product calorie, this means the current diet requires 4,224 plant-derived calories; if calories from animal products rise to 15 percent of 2,570 (385 calories), the future diet would require 4,591 plant-derived calories. This is an 8.7 percent increase in plant-derived calories. To put it somewhat differently: if diets in developing countries were slightly more diversified (15 percent animal products instead of the current 12.5 percent)—even with no increase in calories per capita—the effect on food demand would be the same as an 8.7 percent increase in population.

Consider a different scenario—suppose that by the year 2050, people in developing countries have incorporated meat into their diets to such an extent that their diets resemble diets in developed countries today. In this case, the future developing country diet would be 27 percent animal product calories (693 out of 2,570). Converting this to plant-derived calories, and adding the 1,877 calories consumed directly from plant sources, yields about 6,200 plant-derived calories—a 47 percent increase from the present diet.

■ Total Impact of Demographic Changes on Food Demand: Alternative Scenarios

The same multiplicative effect described above between population growth and growth in consumption per capita applies more generally to all the effects described in this chapter. To review, using examples:

- If population grows by 50 percent, and population characteristics cause food demand to grow by 5 percent per capita, total demand grows by more than 50 percent—demand will be (1 + .50) x (1 + .05) = 1.575, or 57.5 percent above current levels.
- If population grows by 50 percent, and if changes in population characteristics give food demand a 5 percent boost, and if (in addition) income increases demand per capita by 15 percent, total demand grows by 81 percent. (The computation is [1 + .50] x [1 + .05] x [1 + .15] – 1).
- If diversification of diets has an additional impact on effective (or plant-equivalent) demand of 10 percent, the total growth in demand is 99 percent.

In these examples, the numbers were chosen to be "in the reasonable range." They are by no means intended as an exact projection.

We can learn two important lessons from the above. First, notice the impact of taking changes in demographic characteristics into account. Population grows by 50 percent (in the example); but total food demand grows by 99 percent—nearly double the growth in population. Even though none of the demographic effects is large in and of itself—5 percent growth in demand per capita because of population characteristics, 15 percent growth because of income growth, 10 percent growth because of diet diversification—the cumulative effect is large. Second, notice the frequent use of the word "if" in the above example. In making projections about the future, this word has to be used a lot. It is useful to construct alternative scenarios to see how much variation results. Table 11.6 shows a number of scenarios about possible growth in demand for food.

In constructing scenarios, we must be internally consistent. We should not assume that incomes per capita will be stagnant and that a large amount of dietary diversification will take place simultaneously; dietary diversification is a result of growth in incomes. The scenario laid out in the example above—and much of the discussion in this chapter—is based on a fundamentally optimistic outlook. Prosperity is assumed to increase; food supplies are assumed to keep pace with demand. As a result, life expectancy increases and fertility declines; the age structure of the population changes toward fewer children and more adults; average per capita income increases, and with it demand for food; increased prosperity also encourages increased consumption of meat relative to plant sources of calories. The scenario is optimistic—but it is also consistent.

The requirement of internal consistency carries with it a certain element of self-correction of projections. For example, if we adopt more pessimistic assumptions—prosperity declines and food supply fails to keep pace with demand—we see several implications. First, population may

Table 11.6   Various Scenarios About Growth in Demand for Food to the Year
2050, Expressed as Percentage Increases

Scenario	Effect of Population Growth	Effect of Population Characteristics	Effect of Increasing Income	Effect of Dietary Diversification	Total Impact
A	50	5	15	10	99
B	65	5	15	10	119
C	90	5	15	10	152
D	40	5	15	10	86
E	65	0	15	10	109
F	65	0	5	10	91
G	65	0	20	10	118
H	80	0	5	5	98
I	40	0	20	20	101

grow more rapidly than anticipated—the decline in fertility rates is dependent (according to the theory of demographic transition) on the increase in life expectancy attributable to prosperity. However, the change in age structure or in average height of the population will not be as large as projected above (and may move food demand in the opposite direction). Similarly, lower growth in incomes will result in a smaller increase in calories per capita and less dietary diversification. Thus, although population growth is larger (under this pessimistic scenario), other factors are less important. Scenario H in Table 11.6 demonstrates this: income growth is lower, therefore growth in calories per capita and dietary diversification are smaller, but population growth is larger; the result is that demand approximately doubles—the same as we see in scenario A. Scenario I demonstrates a more optimistic scenario: income growth and dietary diversification are greater, but population growth is slower; the result is that demand approximately doubles. This demonstrates the *self-correcting* mechanism at work.

12

Agricultural Land and Water

The last few chapters help us analyze questions such as: How much food is enough? How many people will need to be fed? How much food will the average person eat? How does the average level and the distribution of income in the world influence the answers to these questions? Next, we turn to the supply side. Will there be enough food? How can we increase the supply of food to make food more affordable? Prices of food are not etched in stone and handed down from on high. They are determined in the market day-by-day and week-by-week through the interplay of supply-and-demand forces. When the supply of food increases, prices drop, food becomes more affordable, and hunger decreases. In this chapter we begin an examination of the factors that determine food supply.

■ The Basic Equation of Food Supply

The typical way to analyze the food supply is to focus on crops, and to split up output according to the following simple equation.

$$\text{Total output} = \frac{\text{Output}}{\text{Acre}} \times \text{Number of Acres}$$

Typically "output per acre" is referred to by the shorthand term "yield." Of course, one might think that this equation ignores the possibility of getting food from animal products. But, as described in Chapter 11, animal food products require animal feed, and animal feed comes from crops. And only 16 percent of calories worldwide come from meat products. About 50 percent comes from cereal crops (rice, wheat, maize, etc.). Therefore we will discuss food production primarily from the perspective of crop production.

The equation obviously splits into two factors: land area and yield. In our discussion in Chapters 12 to 14, we will explore four principal influences on current and future agricultural output:

- Quantity of available agricultural resources—land and water
- Quality of agricultural resources
- Intensity of input use on the land
- Technological change

This chapter deals with the first of these influences. Chapter 13 deals with the interrelationship of agricultural production and environmental quality. Chapter 14 deals with input use and technological change.

■ Available Land

Of course, one way to increase food production is to increase the amount of land devoted to agricultural production. Data in Table 12.1 show that agricultural land has increased slowly but steadily. Worldwide, total land in agriculture increased 2.8 percent during the 1960s, 2.3 percent during the 1970s, 3.7 percent during the 1980s, and 2.1 percent during the 1990s.

The growth in total agricultural land masks some changes of land use within agriculture. As Figure 12.1 shows, total arable land ("arable land" is land on which crops are grown) grew at nearly exactly the same rate as total agricultural land until the late 1980s; since then arable land has stayed about constant, while total agricultural land has continued to grow. This growth in total agricultural land reflects the growth in land used as permanent pasture, and is consistent with the addition of meat and dairy products to the average diet, described in Chapter 11.

But can the rate of increase in agricultural land use continue into the future? An FAO report estimates that there are 2.57 billion hectares of "rainfed land with crop potential" in developing countries, excluding China

**Table 12.1   Worldwide Agricultural Land Use, 1961–2001
(in thousands of hectares)**

	Agricultural Area	Arable Land	Permanent Pasture
1961	4,504,580	1,278,834	3,147,858
1966	4,564,049	1,295,275	3,186,922
1971	4,632,629	1,318,312	3,227,576
1976	4,686,492	1,332,794	3,261,190
1981	4,739,950	1,345,094	3,297,564
1986	4,849,234	1,386,415	3,359,216
1991	4,917,373	1,389,412	3,413,256
1996	4,994,401	1,394,987	3,474,548
2001	5,021,734	1,401,667	3,489,834

Source: FAOSTAT Statistics Database 2003.

(Alexandratos 1995:162–163). Of this 2.57 billion, about .75–.85 billion are currently used. At first blush, this would appear to be very good news. But much of this potential land (67 percent) is hilly, or has poor soil or drainage. As Table 12.2 shows, the potential for increased production on good-quality land is considerably more limited. Nevertheless, there does

Figure 12.1   Indices of Worldwide Land Use in Agriculture, 1961–2001 (1984–1986 = 100)

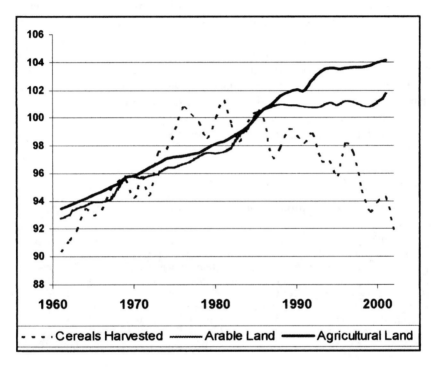

Source: FAOSTAT.

Table 12.2   Land Use and Availability in Developing Countries (in millions of hectares and excluding China), 1996

	Good Soil/Terrain	Poor Soil or Terrain	Total
Currently used for crops	547	213	760
Land with crop potential	848	1,722	2,570
Use as % of potential	64%	12%	30%

Source: Derived from FAO, World Food Summit, Background Paper No. 1, 1997.

appear to be potential to bring new land under cultivation; the area of this potential agricultural land is perhaps 30 percent of the current area. The potential differs significantly from region to region. In South Asia, the Near East, and North Africa, there is little potential for expansion. In Brazil and the Republic of the Congo (and surrounding African countries), there are large tracts of land that could be brought under agricultural production. (See Grigg 1993, chapter 6, for additional discussion.) Box 12.1 describes a large area of currently unused land in Brazil.

The last paragraph seems to imply that it is possible to increase the amount of land under cultivation significantly, perhaps by 30 percent or more. However, this calculation requires an additional assumption: that no land currently under cultivation is lost to agriculture. There are three reasons to be concerned that land currently used for agricultural production might not be usable for agriculture in the future. First, as population grows, and urban areas expand, some farmland is paved over. The impact of suburban sprawl is obvious in parts of the United States. However, worldwide urban areas and other human settlements take up only 3 percent of the land mass. Therefore even significant urbanization will have a small quantitative

---

Box 12.1   Expanding Agricultural Land in the Brazilian Cerrado

One place that there is substantial opportunity for adding land to agricultural use is in the Brazilian savannah. About one-quarter of the area of Brazil (200 million hectares) is in an ecological system known as the *cerrado*. The cerrado has ample rainfall, and the climate in much of the cerrado is warm enough to grow two crops per year. Yet, the cerrado remains largely underutilized for agricultural production. One study estimates that 137 million hectares of the cerrado are "well suited to large-scale mechanized farming" (Wallis 1997). As of 1990, only 12 million hectares were being used to grow crops and another 35 million hectares were used as pasture (Schnepf, Dohlman, and Bolling 2001).

Two things have held back development of the cerrado: soil quality and transportation capacity. The soil of the cerrado is deep, but has chemical properties that are not conducive to crop growth: soil acidity is high, aluminum content is high, and soil availability of nitrogen and phosphorus is low. But these shortcomings can be overcome. Spreading lime will reduce the acidity of soil. Applying fertilizer will increase nitrogen and phosphorus. And new plant varieties have been developed that can tolerate soils with high aluminum content. Transportation infrastructure that provides a way to ship output from the cerrado to urban or international markets is limited. There is a "chicken and egg" problem here: farmers will not expand production if there is no way to move the output to market; roads and railroads will not be expanded until the need for commercial transport exists.

effect on agriculture worldwide. Second, as we will discuss in more detail in the next chapter, there is concern that global warming may result in expansion of ocean areas and flooding of coastal areas. Third—and this is the factor of most concern to experts—land currently in production may be "degraded" through soil loss or contamination to such a degree that it can no longer be used to grow crops. This aspect will also be discussed in more detail in the next chapter.

On the other hand, there is undoubtedly some potential for increasing production without increasing yields *or* acres. Most significant here is likely to be expansion of double or triple cropping—where a single plot of land is planted with two or three crops sequentially during a year. Double cropping becomes more feasible if agronomists develop crop varieties that require a shorter growing season. Other new technologies may increase the importance of non-land-based food production—most immediately, fisheries and aquaculture, but potentially including hydroponics, food from the sea, and food from space.

Taking all of these factors into account, some experts are notably more pessimistic than the FAO regarding the future potential for adding or maintaining land devoted to food production. Kendall and Pimentel (1994: 205) cite lack of arable land as "one of the most urgent problems facing humanity . . . [and also] perhaps the most neglected." In another study, Pimentel calculates that nearly one-third of the world's cropland (1.5 billion hectares) has been abandoned during the past forty years because erosion has made it unproductive (Pimentel et al. 1995). Gary Gardner of WorldWatch Institute also concludes that there is little room for large-scale expansion of cropland:

> Replacing lost land is likely to be more difficult than many officials think. . . . Optimistic officials often overestimate the potential for expansion by including marginal land, where cultivation may not be sustainable. Indeed, the world's major grain producers have all overexpanded into marginal land in recent years, damaging large areas of land in the process. Many are now pulling back to the land that can be [sustainably] cultivated, with a resulting loss of grain production. (Worldwatch Institute 1996b)

■ The Importance of Water

Of course, finding new agricultural land is useless unless we also have sufficient water for agricultural production. As Table 12.3 shows, agriculture is a huge user of water, especially in the developing world. Table 12.4 shows that the amount of land that is irrigated has grown steadily over time. Irrigation is especially important in growing rice. This fact is evidenced by the fact that irrigated land produces 80 percent of the food in Bangladesh, 70 percent of the food in China, and over 50 percent in India

Table 12.3　Water Use by Continent, 1995

Continent	Africa	Asia	Former USSR	Europe	North & Central Amer.	Oceania	South America	World
% water used in agriculture	88	86	65	33	49	34	59	69
% water used for domestic	7	6	7	13	9	64	19	8
% water used in industry	5	8	28	54	42	2	23	23
Total use cubic km per year	144	1,531	358	359	697	23	133	3,240
Total runoff cubic km per year	4,570	14,410	348	3,210	8,200	2,040	11,760	44,538

Source: FAO, World Food Summit, Background Paper No. 7, 1997.

Table 12.4　Irrigated Land

Year	Arable & Permanent Cropland (thousands of hectares)	Irrigated Land (thousands of hectares)	% of Cropland That Is Irrigated (%)
1961	1,356,722	139,134	10.3
1966	1,377,127	153,460	11.1
1971	1,405,053	171,807	12.2
1976	1,425,302	192,851	13.5
1981	1,442,386	213,552	14.8
1986	1,490,018	228,202	15.3
1991	1,504,117	248,724	16.5
1996	1,519,853	264,513	17.4
2001	1,532,090	273,052	17.8

Source: FAOSTAT (year?)

and Indonesia (FAO 1996b). Worldwide, irrigated land provides about 40 percent of total food. Yields on irrigated land range from 30 to 200 percent higher than on nonirrigated land. Irrigation raises corn yields from 1.7 to 3.9 metric tons per hectare in Latin America and from 1.2 to 3.1 in Africa, and raises wheat yields from 1.8 to 4.1 in Latin America and from 1.4 to 2.4 in North Africa/Near East; vegetable yields rise from 5.1 to 14.2 in East Asia.

Will it be possible to continue increasing irrigation? The FAO is quite optimistic on this question: "Half or even two-thirds of future gains in crop production are expected to come from irrigated land" (FAO 1996b). A World Bank/UNDP study estimated that an additional 110 million hectares of land could be brought under irrigation, producing enough more grain to feed 1.5 to 2 billion people. Tables 12.3 and 12.4 allow us to calculate that total water use in agriculture was about 2,200 cubic kilometers, amounting to 0.0088 cubic kilometers of water per 1,000 hectares of irrigated land. If 110 million hectares of newly irrigated land was irrigated at this rate, the total additional water requirement would be 968 cubic kilometers, about 30 percent of current water useage.

However, other experts are more pessimistic about future water availability. Alan Wild (2003:217) concludes, "Shortage of water . . . is probably the biggest biological and physical limitation to agricultural development in developing countries." Sandra Postel concludes that agriculture cannot increase water use much beyond current levels without causing substantial environmental problems. She argues that the 44,500 cubic kilometers of water reported in Table 12.3 as total runoff greatly overstates available water. First, she argues, about 20 percent of that is geographically so remote that it is not available for human use. Of the remaining 32,900 cubic kilometers, about 75 percent occurs during floods, and therefore is not available for irrigation during dry periods. The actual quantity of useable water is then around 12,500 cubic kilometers. "The problem is that water use tripled between 1950 and 1990 as world population soared by some 2.7 billion. . . . Worldwide demand for water cannot triple again without causing severe shortages for crop irrigation, industrial use, basic household needs, and critical life-supporting ecosystems" (Postel 1997). She notes that water shortages are already appearing as depletion of groundwater. She cites evidence that water tables are falling 20 centimeters a year in India's Punjab. (See Box 12.2 for a discussion of irrigation in China.)

Others belittle this talk of water shortages as "doomsaying." Julian Simon of the University of Maryland was one of the most outspoken optimists about future resource availability. He based his optimism on a confidence in human ingenuity:

> Usable water is like other resources, however, in being a product of human labor and ingenuity. People "create" usable water, and there are large opportunities to discover and utilize new sources. Some additional sources are well-known and already in partial use: transport by ship from one country to another, deeper wells, cleaning dirty water, towing icebergs to places where water is needed, and desalination. . . .[In addition,] huge new supplies of groundwater have been found in the Red Sea Province of eastern Sudan, Florida, and elsewhere. (Simon 1996: Chapter 6)

The FAO makes some small-scale, practical recommendations of ways that water can be used more efficiently, such as water harvesting (collecting runoff and saving it for periods of need) and drip irrigation (delivering irri-

---

Box 12.2   Irrigation in China

The evidence of the impact of irrigation is striking in China, as described by Brown and Halweil. The Yellow River flows through a dry part of China, and farmers draw water out of the river to irrigate their crops. In the years prior to 1972, the Yellow River always had sufficient water flow to reach the sea. Then in 1972, as more and more water was drawn for irrigation, the river ran dry, failing to reach the ocean for fifteen days. Beginning in 1986, not a year has passed in which the Yellow River has not run dry. In the drought year of 1997, the river failed to reach the sea for 227 days. In places like this, irrigation has grown to its limit; irrigation might continue at current rates, but is unlikely to grow any further. In other parts of China, water is used for irrigation at rates that cannot be sustained indefinitely. A study cited by Brown and Halweil found that in many parts of the North China Plain where irrigation water is pumped from below ground, the water table was dropping by 5 feet per year. However, in February 2003, scientists reported discovering a large new aquifer under the Taklamakan desert in northwest China.

Source: U.S. Water News Online 2003.

---

gation water directly to the roots of plants). In addition, agricultural scientists have developed crop varieties that require less water to thrive and have developed chemicals that promote water retention in soil.

As we will see in the next chapter, water use in agriculture is a major source of environmental concern related to agricultural production. Increased irrigation carries the threat of increased soil erosion, increased chemical runoff and resulting water pollution, and increased threat of global warming from paddy-rice production.

13

Agricultural Production and the Environment

The last chapter discussed the potential for increasing land and water use for future food production. In this chapter, we explore the issue of the degree and significance of environmental damage. The issue has two faces: environmental quality is an important determinant of agricultural output; and agricultural production has a significant impact on the environment. We deal first with the interaction of agricultural production and the local environment (the environment near to the place where the agricultural production takes place). Then we discuss the interaction of agricultural production and the global environment—especially global warming.

■ Agricultural Production and the Local Environment

Agriculture uses natural resources—soil and water—to produce food. This can lead to deterioration in the quality of the natural resources and the ability of the natural resources to support food production.

Land Degradation

The environmental issue with the greatest potential for influencing future food production is land degradation. Land can become unsuitable for agricultural production in the following ways (UN/POPIN 1995):

- Soil can disappear from land through erosion.
- Soil can become chemically unsuitable for agricultural production.
- Land can be come physically unsuitable for agricultural production.

Erosion. Wind or water can pick up soil particles from one area and move them. This can harm agricultural production in four ways. The eroded soil may contain nutrients needed for plant development. The remaining soil may be so dense that it is difficult for plant roots to develop. Erosion may reduce the capacity of the soil to retain water needed for plant growth. Finally, erosion may result in uneven terrain that makes cultivation more difficult.

Soil erosion is to a degree caused by agricultural production. Land used for agricultural production may be bare of vegetation for months at a time. The absense of roots to hold the soil in place makes the soil more easily erodible. Plowing the soil in preparation for seeding exposes it to wind and rain and increases the rate of erosion. Irrigation can contribute directly to water erosion.

Chemical characteristics of the soil.   Land may become chemically unsuitable for agricultural production for several reasons. The nutrients of the soil may be depleted because of past agricultural production, especially if the same crop is grown year after year. "Salinization" of soil occurs when the salt content of the soil increases to levels unsuitable for agricultural production. Salinization can be caused by irrigating land with water that contains low levels of salts, which are left on the soil when the water evaporates. In some areas, this problem occurs because irrigation depletes the naturally occurring fresh groundwater, and causes seawater to intrude into the groundwater system. A third chemical problem with soil is "acidification." This can occur when too much fertilizer of certain types is applied, or when there are drainage problems on certain soils. Finally, other pollutants such as oil or excessive pesticides can reduce the ability of soil to support agricultural production.

Physical characteristics of the land.   Agricultural land can also become unsuitable for production because of changes in the physical characteristics of the land. Soil can become less porous through compaction—when heavy machines or animals pack the soil down—or through the action of raindrops that seal the soil. Nonporous soil makes it difficult for seeds to emerge. Waterlogging occurs when water sits in the root zone of plants, and thus impedes their development. Waterlogging occurs when drainage is poor, or when a field is overirrigated.

The Extent and Impact of Land Degradation Worldwide
The Global Land Assessment of Degradation, or GLASOD, study done by the United Nations (ISRIC/UNEP 1991) estimated that 22 percent of agricultural land worldwide (and 38 percent of cropland) has been subject to one or more of the kinds of degradation described above. Of the 2 billion hectares of degraded land, according to this study, 83 percent was degraded by erosion, 12 percent by chemical degradation, and 5 percent by physical degradation. Seventy million hectares are so badly degraded that the damage cannot be repaired. Other studies report that the amount of degraded land increases each year by an additional 5 to 10 million hectares (Scherr and Yadav 1997). Pimentel et al. (1994) estimate that "each year, more than 10 million hectares (24.7 million acres) of once-productive land are degrad-

ed and abandoned." This bears directly on the question of how much land can be devoted to agricultural production in the future. However, as we saw in the last chapter, agricultural land has increased steadily despite these reports of degradation.

A related possibility is that land degradation will reduce yields per hectare. This can occur for two reasons. First, when land becomes so severely degraded that it is no longer capable of supporting agricultural production, new land may be added to agricultural production to take the place of the degraded land. The new land is likely to be of relatively poor quality—otherwise, it would already have been in use. Second, when the land is degraded, but remains in agricultural use, yields on that land drop.

There is a lack of agreement among agricultural scientists about the severity of the drop in yields attributable to land degradation. Pimentel and Giampietro (1994) point to evidence that corn yields are about 20 percent lower on severely eroded lands in many parts of the United States. Mitchell, Ingco, and Duncan (1997:54) cite other studies that estimate that soil erosion was responsible for yield declines of 3–4 percent over one hundred years. Scherr and Yadav (1997) report yield losses of 5–15 percent attributable to land degradation. See Crosson (1996b) for a review of the debate.

Water Quality

In the last chapter, we discussed the importance of water in agricultural production, and cited one report that expanded irrigation will be a substantial source of increased food production in the future. Expanded irrigation requires a supply of useable water. But agricultural production can lead to degradation of water quality.

Irrigation itself is the main culprit. Irrigation in China and India has caused water tables to drop signficantly. In coastal areas, depletion of groundwater reserves can result in salt-water intrusion into the groundwater system. In some soils, irrigation leeches certain salts from the soil, and carries those salts back into the groundwater, contaminating it and making it unsuitable for future irrigation. Irrigation or rainwater runoff can also carry residues from fertilizers and chemical pesticides. This also creates water quality problems. In addition, as noted, irrigation can contribute to land degradation, contributing to erosion, waterlogging, salinization, and acidification.

Problems Associated with Agricultural Input Use

We have already discussed how agricultural chemical use can lead to land degradation or water pollution. In addition, chemical use can create health problems for farm workers. The manufacture of agricultural chemicals can also create environmental hazards. The 1984 explosion at a chemical plant in Bhopal, India, provided a tragic example of this. The poison gas released by the explosion is used primarily in production of insecticides. Thousands were killed and tens of thousands were seriously injured (Baylor 1996). In laboratory experiments, some pesticides have been shown to affect hormone levels—which could cause cancer, abnormalities in newborns, or reproductive problems. However, evidence is weak that this effect can be found outside the laboratory (Kamrin n.d.).

As there is increasing use of mechanization and petrochemicals in agriculture, there may be concern that energy use in agriculture will become an environmental problem. However, R. S. Chen (1990) reports that agricultural production accounts for only 3.5 percent of commercial energy use in developed countries and 4.5 percent in developing countries. In developed countries, food processing and distribution uses more energy than food production.

Other Environmental Problems

Water quality is not only a concern when it impinges on agricultural production. People drink water, and reduced water quality can directly harm public health. Of special concern here is the possibility that water becomes contaminated with pesticides—chemicals that are deliberately developed to be toxic. Rachel Carson's *Silent Spring* pointed out the impact that agricultural chemicals could have on the environment. This affects not only humans, but also birds, fish, and other wildlife. Water contamination from runoff containing animal wastes has been implicated as a source of problems in commercial fisheries in the United States.

A second environmental concern associated with agricultural production is the issue of maintaining genetic diversity. Especially with the increasingly widespread use of improved varieties of cereals, there is concern that the genetic material contained in traditional varieties will be lost. For example, in 1949 there were 10,000 wheat varieties in use in China; by the 1970s only 1,000 remained in use. The loss of genetic diversity can make the food supply more susceptible to disease, and may foreclose the option of future technological improvements based on genetic characteristics of the "lost" varieties.

Environment and Future Prospects for Agricultural Production

Are these interfaces between the environment and food production likely to create critical constraints on future food production? Some ecologists are very alarmed about this. (See Cohen 1996a,b for a review.) David Pimentel of Cornell University states that the world's resources can support a high standard of living for fewer than 2 billion (compared to today's actual population of over 6 billion). This pessimistic view of the future is based on the belief that the world has already expanded agricultural production into areas that cannot sustain it and has achieved yields per hectare by using production methods that cannot be continued for very long. Pimentel cites studies that show that agricultural methods that do not use chemical fertilizers will result in cereal yields of between 0.5 metric tons per hectare (in semiarid regions with no fertilizer) and 2 metric tons per hectare (in humid regions using animal manure for fertilizer) (Pimentel and Giampietro 1994). Compare these to the average current yield of about 3 metric tons per hectare worldwide and over 5 metric tons per hectare in the United States.

Technology and the Trade-off
Between Production and the Environment

If David Pimentel represents one extreme in the debate about how many people the world can feed, Julian Simon represents the other. He describes a commercial vegetable farm in Illinois, and uses that as a basis for his optimistic calculations:

> In DeKalb, Illinois, Noel Davis's PhytoFarm produces food—mainly lettuce and other garden vegetables—in a factory measuring 200 feet by 250 feet—50,000 square feet, one acre, 0.4 hectares, 1/640 of a square mile—at a rate of a ton of food per day, enough to completely feed 500 or 1000 people. . . . At the current efficiency of PhytoFarm, the entire present population of the world can be supplied from a square area about 140 miles on a side—about the area of Massachusetts and Vermont combined, and less than a tenth of Texas. . . . PhytyoFarm techniques could feed a hundred times the world's present population—say 500 billion people—with factory buildings a hundred stories high, on one percent of present farmland. (Simon 1996: Chapter 6)

Simon's attitude reflects an enormous confidence in the ability of technology to solve problems. Technological progress is all about getting more from less. A good deal of agricultural research in the last decade has been devoted to the problem of maintaining or improving agricultural yields while doing less damage to the environment. For example, new plant varieties are being developed that are naturally resistant to pests and thus require less pesticide use. Tilling and landscaping methods to reduce soil erosion have been widely adopted in parts of the world. "Drip irrigation" that delivers water directly to the plant roots reduces water used in irrigation without causing any reduction in the effectiveness of irrigation. The new technology of aquaculture has made "fish farming" a rapidly growing source of food, as Table 13.1 shows. Nonmarine fish production has increased tenfold over the period shown. The huge increase during the 1980s and 1990s reflects in part the introduction of aquaculture. (Table 13.1 also shows a source of environmental concern: natural ocean—or marine—fisheries have increased production to such a degree that they are

Table 13.1   Fish Production Worldwide, 1950–2000 (in metric tons)

	Freshwater fish	Marine fish	Total fishery production
1950	2,001,583	14,053,370	19,272,820
1955	3,232,501	20,309,790	27,928,800
1960	3,528,471	27,074,260	35,482,890
1965	4,428,228	39,280,980	49,724,460
1970	5,185,769	52,785,080	65,405,130
1975	5,966,062	51,486,110	65,923,600
1980	6,346,598	55,442,810	72,412,450
1985	9,032,671	64,678,350	87,110,550
1990	12,558,730	69,211,340	98,586,180
1995	18,766,880	72,537,990	116,677,400
2000	26,501,480	72,816,750	130,927,000

Source: FAOSTAT Statistical Database 1998.

in danger of being overfished so that the breeding stock is depleted and the total ocean fish population begins to fall.)

Another aspect of agricultural research is to develop technology that relaxes the constraints that environment imposes on agricultural output. For example, scientists are working to develop plants that can survive in brackish water. "Researchers have transferred a gene for salt tolerance from an Old World ice plant into three plants lacking salt tolerance . . . all of which then displayed significantly increased capability to grow with their roots exposed to salt. . . . [This] will contribute to the effort to engineer plants with improved ability to withstand adverse growing conditions such as under seawater irrigation" (National Science and Technology Council n.d.). Other examples of technological ways to relax the environmental constraint to agricultural production are chemicals that increase the ability of soils to retain moisture and seed varieties that are more drought-resistant (so the crops can be grown in more arid regions). Box 13.1 describes an effort to reclaim degraded land in China.

■ Agricultural Production and the Global Environment

Agricultural production also interacts with the environment on a global scale, especially on the issue of global warming. Global warming refers to the phenomenon by which water vapor, carbon dioxide, methane, and other trace gases in the atmosphere trap heat on the earth's surface. As the quantities of these gases (the so-called greenhouse gases) in the atmosphere increase, the amount of heat trapped will increase, and the average temperature of the earth will increase. On these matters there is a high degree of consensus among scientists. There is some disagreement about the extent to which global warming has already occurred, and about the

---

Box 13.1 Reclaiming Degraded Lands in South China

The five southernmost provinces of China have been farmed for over a thousand years, primarily with slash-and-burn techniques that cleared forests, but left the soil exposed to severe erosion. The process of land degradation here is described by Parham (2001):

"When vegetation is removed in these regions, the exposed soil . . . reaches temperatures so high that seeds and sprouts are killed. . . . Since new vegetation cannot be established easily, soil organic matter is reduced, and the soil becomes desiccated. . . . Even small decreases in soil organic matter have a pronounced negative effect on the soil's fertility. . . . When the original topsoil is removed by erosion, the surface becomes a mixture of aluminum-rich clays and quartz sand that contain very few minerals useful to plant life. . . . The loss of vegetative cover and soil organic matter leaves the soil subject to damage from intense tropical rainfall. With little organic matter in the soil, clay particles are moved by raindrops and plug soil pores, thus inhibiting water infiltration and increasing runoff and erosion. . . . The finer-grained eroded sediments damage aquatic productivity and bury what were once freshwater and near-shore marine aquatic breeding grounds. The remaining coarser, sandy material of the weathered granite yields soils of low fertility. Stripped of vegetation that would otherwise have absorbed or slowed the flow of water, the water pours rapidly into streams and rivers, cutting deep ravines in the soft, deeply weathered granite."

By the end of the last century, an estimated 45 million hectares (over 20 percent of the agricultural land of South China) was degraded. Use of commercial fertilizers was unsuccessful in replacing the nutrients lost with eroded soil, because the remaining coarse soil was a poor medium for holding the nutrients provided by the fertilizers.

Recent research suggests that it may be possible to restore most of the degraded lands to agricultural production within two years. One research project planted fast-growing ground cover amidst alternating rows of rubber trees and tea bushes. The ground cover shields the soil from the hot sun and reduces evaporation of soil moisture. The roots of the plants help reduce soil erosion, and the plant residue provides organic material to the soil. The rubber trees provide shade for the tea bushes, and the tea bushes help moderate the temperatures near the roots of the rubber trees. Experimental plots indicate that this type of agriculture is profitable and can restore soil quality while reducing water runoff and flooding.

---

extent to which human activities are responsible for the buildup of greenhouse gases.

The Impact of Agriculture on Global Warming

Agricultural production is a significant source of greenhouse gas emissions worldwide. The three greenhouse gases that are means by which human activity may cause global warming are carbon dioxide, methane, and nitrous oxide. Carbon dioxide comprises nearly 80 percent of greenhouse gases, nitrous oxide 15 percent, and methane 6 percent. Carbon dioxide is created when carbon atoms released from plants (as the plants decompose or burn) join with oxygen atoms. Deforestation in tropical areas is thought to contribute about 25 percent of the human-made carbon dioxide released into the atmosphere (FAO 1997a). Methane is created by cattle as they digest food. In addition, paddy-rice production is believed to be a major source of methane emissions as decomposing fertilizer reacts with crop residues. It is estimated that of methane generated by human activity, 15–25 percent is attributable to animal agriculture and 10–30 percent is attributable to rice production (Neue 1993; Lashof and Tirpak 1990). Release of nitrous oxide into the atmosphere can be promoted by the use of nitrogen fertilizers.

The lesson to be drawn from these data is that agricultural production is a substantial source of greenhouse gases; if agricultural production grows to keep pace with food demand, that will add noticeably to the greenhouse gas problem. Furthermore, any realistic program to reduce greenhouse gas emissions must address the agricultural component; and there is an unavoidable tension between raising agricultural output and reducing greenhouse gases. Perhaps this tension can be reduced by technological innovations, but the tension is there.

The Impact of Global Warming on Agricultural Production
Obviously, when the average temperature in an area changes, the agricultural capacity of the area changes—it may become better for some crops and worse for other crops. Unfortunately, global warming—if it does become a real problem—is not expected to result in a gradual increase in temperature in every area of the globe. Some areas may become much warmer; some only a little warmer; some possibly colder. And the global climate change (if and when it occurs) will not simply mean changes in temperature. It is almost certain to change rainfall patterns, making some areas dryer and some wetter. And it will also change the incidence of severe weather, making some areas more prone to hurricanes, tornadoes, and droughts.

There are huge uncertainties about future climate change. Will the changes be dramatic or nearly imperceptible? Even if the *average* global temperature increases significantly, what will that mean for climates in different geographical areas? Because of these uncertainties, there is a wide variety of opinions among scientists about the possible future impacts of global warming on agricultural production. This debate has centered on two questions: (1) Will global warming cause flooding of coastal areas and loss of agricultural land? and (2) What will the impact of climate change be on average crop yields worldwide? (See Box 13.2 for a related debate—two hundred years old—on the impact of sunspots on wheat prices.)

If the average temperature of the earth increases, the volume of water

---

Box 13.2   Sunspots, Crop Yields, and Wheat Prices

In 1801, British astronomer William Herschel had a theory: sunspots influenced wheat prices. Sunspots are vortices of gas on the surface of the sun. Herschel hypothesized that sunspots would result in "copious emission of heat and therefore mild seasons" on earth. Mild seasons would improve crop yields, which would in turn lead to lower crop prices. Herschel reported that the facts supported his theory: during five prolonged periods of low solar activity (few sunspots), wheat prices were higher. The Royal Society ridiculed Herschel's theory as a "grand absurdity." By the 1840s, astronomers had discovered that sunspots followed a cycle peaking every eight to seventeen years, with an average cycle length of about eleven years. In the late 1800s, economist William Jevons suggested that this might be an explanation of business cycles (alternating periods of economic growth and recession).

A 2003 paper (Pustilnik and Din) examined the link between wheat prices and sunspot activity, and discovered that for all of the ten solar cycles in the 1600s and 1700s, high sunspot activity was associated with low wheat prices. The explanation, say Pustilnik and Din, is somewhat different than the Herschel "mild seasons" theory: in periods of high solar activity, it is more difficult for charged particles from deep space to reach the earth's atmosphere; since these charged particles contribute to cloud formation, skies over England are less cloudy; this reduces threats to wheat production by frost and extended rainfall; better wheat harvests result in lower wheat prices.

See Baliunas (1999) for a report relating this to the current global warming debate.

---

in oceans will increase. This is not primarily (as the popular belief has it) because of melting polar ice caps, but because the volume of water expands as its temperature increases. Rosenzweig and Hillel (1995) report that the sea level is likely to rise from 4 to 20 inches by the middle of this next century. The risk from higher sea levels is not only that land will be flooded, but that drainage problems will increase, and seawater intrusion into freshwater sources will occur. However, Rosensweig et al. (1993) point out that in some areas, global warming may result in new land becoming suitable for agricultural production, because of an extended growing season or changes in rainfall pattern. There is general agreement that rising sea levels would be a huge problem in some geographical areas (see Parry, Magalhaes, and Nih 1992; Ibe and Awosika 1991). But what will be the impact worldwide? Pimentel (1993) reports estimates that global warming will reduce cropland by 10 to 50 percent. On the other hand, Wittwer (1995:165–166) concludes: "Although important for localized regions, [cropland loss from rising sea levels] would be relatively insignificant on a worldwide basis."

Global warming can affect crop yields in a variety of ways (Rosenzweig and Hillel 1995).

Increase in atmospheric CO₂. Atmospheric CO_2 comprises about 80 percent of the greenhouse gases, and increases the efficiency of photosynthesis and thereby boosts plant growth. Wheat, rice, and soybeans are especially responsive to increased atmospheric CO_2. High CO_2 levels also significantly increase water-use efficiency. This fact may actually increase demand for irrigation water, as farmers discover that irrigation has a larger impact on yields. In addition, high CO_2 levels increase plants' resistance to salinity and drought, and increase nutrient uptake. Finally, noxious weeds are (for the most part) less responsive to CO_2 than crops (Wittwer 1995).

Higher temperatures. As higher temperatures will on average increase the length of the growing season, agricultural production may become feasible in areas (closer to the North and South Poles) that are currently too cold. Soils in some of these areas (Canada and Russia) are less fertile than other soils; thus bringing these lands under cultivation could cause a drop in average yield. In addition, some crops (notably rice) show yield declines when the temperature is too high. Finally, increased temperatures make plants mature faster. But plants that mature faster have lower food yields. On the other hand, the faster maturation combined with the longer growing seasons may extend the areas in which double or triple cropping is feasible.

Extreme meteorological events. Hurricanes, tornados, heavy rainstorms, or droughts disrupt crop production and tend to lower yields. (See Box 13.3

Box 13.3   El Niño and Food Production

Every few years, the surface of the Pacific Ocean becomes warmer. Peruvian fisherman named this phenomenon "El Niño" (the boy-child) because it coincided with Christmas (or the coming of the Christ-child). In 1997, the warming was especially large, and this has caused worldwide changes in weather patterns. In Washington, D.C., for example, the winter of 1997/98 was exceptionally mild, with virtually no snowfall. In Los Angeles, rainfall in early 1998 was nearly twice the usual level. The winter also saw March blizzards in the Midwest, and icestorms in New England that left people without electricity for days. The United States was not the only country to feel the effects of El Niño. South America and East Africa experienced heavier rainfall than usual; parts of South Asia were unusually dry.

Because of this "weird" weather, 37 countries were facing food emergencies in early 1998. But the problems are limited to certain areas. Worldwide, cereal production for 1997/98 was slightly above the record levels of 1996/97. FAO scientist Rene Gommes concludes, "It is important not to minimize risks but also to remember that there have been El Niños without any catastrophes and catastrophes without any El Niños."

for a discussion of a meteorological event that is not related to global warming.)

Pests and diseases. Insect pests and crop diseases thrive in higher temperatures. Thus global warming may increase the incidence of pests and disease, and lower yields.

Scientists disagree about the overall impact on yields. An important determinant of this impact is the extent to which farmers adapt their production decisions to the new climatic conditions. For example, suppose we are analyzing production in an area where rice is the predominant crop. Suppose, further, that we conclude that global warming will result in rice yields dropping by 30 percent in this area. A simplistic analysis would conclude that food production would drop by 30 percent in the area. A more sophisticated analysis would recognize the likelihood that many farmers in the area will stop growing rice, and will switch to some alternative crop. The actual drop in production may be much less than 30 percent, depending on the alternative crops available and the extent to which farmers change their cropping decisions.

Rosensweig et al. (1993) estimate that if temperatures increase 2 degrees centigrade, wheat and soybean yields will increase 10–15 percent, and maize and rice yields will increase about 8 percent. However, if temperatures increase 4 degrees centigrade, yields would decline. (According to a UNEP Factsheet [1990], climate models predict an increase of 1.5 to 4.5 degrees centigrade over the next one hundred years.) Wittwer believes that these estimates may underestimate the yield growth from global warming because they ignore some of the possible benefits from increased levels of atmospheric CO_2.

Other prognoses for crop yields are less optimistic. For example, the UNEP (1990) reports: "Mid-latitude yields may be reduced by 10–30 percent due to increased summer dryness," though it admits that "higher yields in some areas may compensate for decreases in others." Pimentel (1993:54–57) reports: "Under the projected warming trend in the United States, farmers can expect a 25 to 100 percent increase in losses due to insects, depending on the crop. . . . U.S. crop losses due to weeds are projected to rise from 5 to 50 percent. . . . In North America, projected changes in temperature, soil moisture, carbon dioxide, and pests associated with global warming are expected to decrease food-crop production by as much as 27 percent." However, Pimentel sees some reasons for hope. He projects that yields in North Africa may improve 10–30 percent as a result of global warming.

Finally, it should be noted that if global warming causes agricultural production to shift from one geographical area (say, North America) to another (say, North Africa), there can be problems establishing the institutions and infrastructure needed to move the food from the production areas to the consuming areas. "While the overall, global impact of climate change on agricultural production may be small, regional vulnerabilities to food deficits may increase, due to problems of distributing and marketing food to specific regions and groups of people" (Rosenzweig and Hillel 1995).

The Ozone Layer

Depletion of the ozone layer permits more ultraviolet radiation to reach the earth. This in turn can affect agricultural production. Pimentel (1993) reports a potential drop in soybean yields of 30 percent due to this. (Soybeans are particularly sensitive to ultraviolet radiation levels.) Wittwer (1995) reports studies that also show substantial yield declines as a response to increased ultraviolet radiation. However, in studies that simultaneously increased both CO_2 levels (the greenhouse gas effect discussed above) and ultraviolet radiation levels, yields were basically unchanged.

14

Increasing Yields

In Chapter 12, we introduced the basic equation of food supply. In Chapters 12 and 13, we discussed one aspect of that equation: the availability of land and water, and the interactions of resource quality and agricultural production. Now we turn to the second part of the equation: yields.

■ Crop Yields Since 1960

It may not be an exaggeration to say that increases in crop yields in the last half of the twentieth century is one of the great accomplishments of human history. To put the yield growth in context, consider the historical record of wheat yields in Britain shown in Table 14.1. It took 350 years for wheat yields to triple from their 1450 levels; it took 300 years to triple from their 1550 levels; it took 250 years to triple from their 1700 levels; then they nearly tripled again in the last 50 years. An acre today produces fifteen times as much wheat as it produced 500 years ago.

Worldwide, cereal yields have more than doubled since the early

Table 14.1   Wheat Yields in Britain, 1600–2000

Year	Approximate Yields (kg/hectare)
c.1450	500
c.1550	600
c.1600	750
c.1650	900
c.1700	1,100
c.1750	1,300
c.1800	1,500
c.1850	1,800
c.1900	2,100
c.1950	3,100
2000	8,000

Sources: Overton 1996:77; Cooke 1967:191 and 463; FAOSTAT.

1960s. As shown in Table 14.2, this growth is seen in all three of the most important cereal crops, and in most geographical areas of the world. (A "percentage change" of more than 100 signals that yields have more than doubled.) Yield growth is lowest in sub-Saharan Africa, and in the transition economies of the former Soviet Union and Eastern-bloc countries. Worldwide cereal yields are illustrated in Figure 14.1, and the consistent growth is demonstrated by the upward trend. Figure 14.2 looks at these data in a little different way; it shows growth rates in yields rather than the yields themselves. To eliminate year-to-year fluctuations caused by weather and other temporary conditions, we show average annual growth rate in yields over a seven-year period, rather than for a single year. The dotted trend line in Figure 14.2 is a logarithmic curve fitted to the data. That trend line suggests that yields are growing (notice that average growth rates are positive at every point), but are growing at a slower rate. The 3-plus percentage point growth rates of the 1960s have been replaced with average growth in the 0.5–2 percent range.

Figure 14.1   Worldwide Cereal Yield, 1961–2002

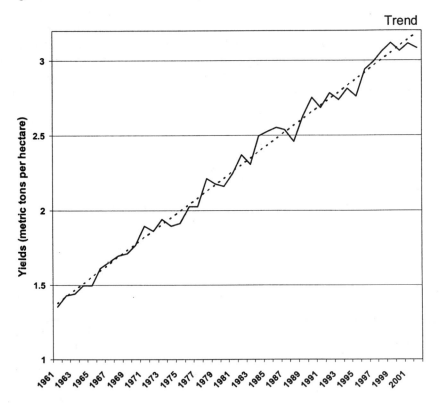

Table 14.2 Yields of Wheat, Rice, and Maize for Various Geographical Areas, 1961 and 2001 (in hectograms per hectare)

	Maize			Rice			Wheat		
	1961	2001	% change	1961	2001	% change	1961	2001	% change
Africa South of Sahara	8,879	12,546	41.3	11,757	16,128	37.2	7,832	16,062	105.1
East & Southeast Asia	10,344	26,457	155.8	17,481	36,638	109.6	6,781	10,563	55.8
Latin America & Caribbean	12,132	31,388	158.7	18,004	38,409	113.3	11,905	23,677	98.9
Near East	17,510	55,871	219.1	29,505	57,624	95.3	9,119	20,739	127.4
Oceania	21,533	55,739	158.9	42,529	89,828	111.2	11,569	21,641	87.1
South Asia	10,437	19,631	88.1	15,802	31,609	100.0	8,447	25,908	206.7
Transition Markets	20,877	38,676	85.3	21,188	27,562	30.1	10,794	23,478	117.5
United States	39,184	86,722	121.3	38,227	72,777	90.4	16,070	27,062	68.4
World	19,435	44,176	127.3	18,671	39,528	111.7	10,889	27,485	152.4

Source: FAOSTAT Statistical Database 2003.

Figure 14.2   Growth Rates of Worldwide Cereal Yields

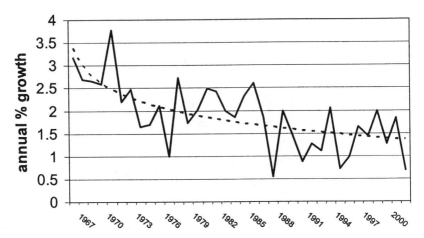

Note: Average annual growth rate in cereal yields for 7-year period ending in the year
shown

■ What Makes Yields Increase?

Yields per acre increase for three principal reasons:

- Productive inputs (labor, fertilizer, machinery, for example) are
  used more intensively on each acre of land.
- New technology increases the output obtainable without increasing
  inputs.
- Farmers increase their efficiency so that less potential output is lost
  to poor farming practices.

These three ways are illustrated in Figure 14.3, which shows a "production function." The production function shows the maximum quantity of
output that is obtainable from any given quantity of input. (To review why
production functions are shaped this way, review Box 7.2.) Here, we will
define output as food production per acre, and we will define input as input
use per acre, and will illustrate with the example of a farmer growing corn
on a plot of land using nothing except his own labor.

An increase in input will move production up along an upward-sloping
production function, such as from point B to point C in Figure 14.3. As the
farmer puts more and more hours into caring for the field, weeding more
frequently, or removing insect pests from the plants, more corn plants will
survive, the ears will be bigger, and the yield of that plot of land will

Figure 14.3   Different Ways of Increasing Output per Acre

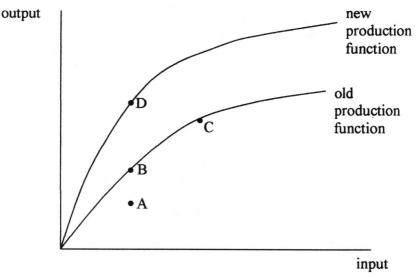

Note: Increase input and move from B to C; advance technology and move from B to D; eliminate inefficiency and move from A to B.

increase. This source of increasing yields will be discussed in the first part of this chapter.

A new technology—broadly defined as new information about how to obtain output from the input—will cause an upward shift in the production function. For any given level of input, a larger output can now be achieved, such as the move from point B to point D in Figure 14.3. Perhaps the farmer is using an improved seed variety that produces bigger ears of corn, or perhaps the farmer has learned that weeding in the first month of growth is especially effective, so that without increasing the number of hours of weeding, he can increase the effectiveness of weeding, and therefore the crop size. This source of increasing yields will be discussed in the second part of this chapter.

An improvement in efficiency is illustrated by the move from point A to point B in Figure 14.3. At point A, the farmer was failing to obtain the maximum possible output using the old technology. Perhaps the farmer was stepping on his corn plants as he worked in the field, or perhaps his hours of work were less effective because he was weakened by hunger or sickness. This source of increasing yields will not be discussed in this chapter; we discussed in Chapter 5 how undernutrition can contribute to reduced economic productivity; in Chapter 15 we will examine the interaction of undernutrition and health in more detail.

Yields and Input Use: Purchased Inputs

In Chapter 12, we saw that yields on irrigated land can be twice as high as yields on similar unirrigated land. This is a dramatic example of how yields can be increased by adding more inputs to the land. The term "inputs" as economists use it refers to factors or goods that contribute to production. Water, labor, chemicals, and machinery are all examples of inputs. As a general rule, when we increase the intensity of input use on plot of land, we increase the output of that plot. In this part of the chapter we look at patterns of use of fertilizer, tractors and animal traction, and agricultural labor.

Fertilizer. Fertilizer use—especially the application of nitrogen fertilizer—has mushroomed around the world over the past forty years, growing to over four times its 1961 level (see Table 14.3). One way to see the impact of fertilizer is to compare countries based on their fertilizer use and their cereal yields. Figure 14.4 shows a scatter plot of 113 countries' fertilizer use and yields for the year 2000. The line fitted to these data points is upward-sloping: especially notable is the large grouping of countries near the origin—countries that have low fertilizer use per hectare and low yields.

Many experiments have verified the effectiveness of fertilizer in increasing crop yields. Two of these are described in Box 14.1. Several general conclusions can be drawn from these experiments.

- Fertilizer use can have quite dramatic impact on yields, ranging from 20 percent improvement to over 1,000 percent improvement.
- For low levels of use, increasing fertilizer application increases yield, but at a decreasing rate, giving a yield response curve that has the same general shape as the production function illustrated in Figure 14.3.

Table 14.3   Worldwide Fertilizer Use, 1961–2001

Year	Fertilizer consumed (metric tons)
1961	31,182,244
1966	52,329,285
1971	73,310,242
1976	95,434,760
1981	115,147,224
1986	133,417,168
1991	134,606,391
1996	134,579,335
2001	137,729,730

Source: FAOSTAT.

Figure 14.4   Fertilizer Use and Yields per Hectare, 2000

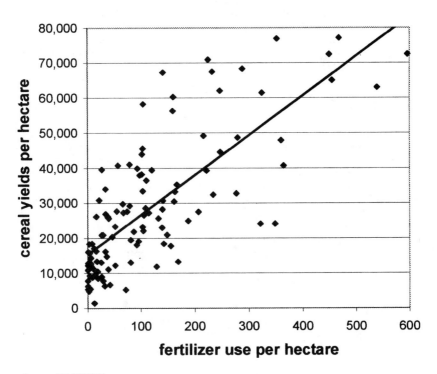

Higher Fertilizer Use increases Crop Yields
113 countries, 2000

Source: FAOSTAT.

- At some point, further increases in fertilizer application actually reduce yields.
- The impact of fertilizer on yields depends on a number of other factors, such as whether the crop is irrigated, the timing of fertilizer applications, and other farming practices used (weeding, types of crop rotation).

Despite the dramatic growth of fertilizer use, there appears to be potential for additional fertilizer use in many parts of the developing world, especially sub-Saharan Africa. This can be seen by comparing fertilizer use (per hectare of permanent crop and arable land) in a developing country to fertilizer use in a more developed country in the same region. For example, average fertilizer application rates in the Democratic Republic of Congo

Box 14.1   Fertilizer Increases Crop Yields: Experimental Evidence

The best evidence about the impact of fertilizer on crop yields is not comparisons between different countries' fertilizer rates and yields, or analyses of changing use and yield patterns over time within a country or region. The best evidence is gathered from individual plots on which carefully controlled experiments are carried out holding all variables constant except the uses of fertilizers.

In the mid-1800s, the British Experimental Station in Rothamsted carried out experiments that first demonstrated that applying nitrogen, potassium, and phosphate to crops could increase crop production. In a series of experiments there between 1848 and 1919, average barley yields were 1,210 pounds per acre when grown without fertilizer, and 2,061 pounds per acre when grown with fertilizer; average wheat yields increased from 1,434 pounds per acre to 1,994 pounds per acre when fertilizer was applied (Cooke 1967:191). The Rothamsted experiments "have often been interpreted as demonstrating that high levels of inputs of inorganic fertilizers . . . can maintain and increase yields for more than a century and a half. While this is true of wheat grown on the soil of the Broadbalk field, it is not always true" (Greenland, Gregory, and Nye 1998:45).

Alan Wild (2003) reports on two fertilizer experiments in Africa. In one experiment in Tanzania, cotton yields were 1,000 kg per hectare when grown with compost and phosphate, but no nitrogen. When nitrogen was applied at a rate of 37 kg per hectare, yields increased to 1,500; when nitrogen application was increased to 112 kg per hectare, yields increased further to 2,000 kg per hectare. (Notice how this path of increased input use traces out a curve of the same general shape as that in Figure 14.3.) In a second experiment in Nigeria, fertilized fields had maize yields of 4,369 kg per hectare compared to yields of 56 kg per hectare in unfertilized fields.

are less than 1 percent of application rates in South Africa; in Nigeria application rates are 6–7 percent of application rates in South Africa. The experience in Asia is instructive. In 1961, application rates in China, India, and Indonesia were 1–3 percent of application rates in Japan. Today, application rates in China are nearly as high as those in Japan and those in Indonesia and India have risen to 25–30 percent of the Japanese level. If sub-Saharan Africa can follow in the next thirty to forty years the path taken by Asian countries during the last thirty to forty years, fertilizer use in sub-Saharan Africa will grow substantially.

Table 14.4 shows two different projections about future fertilizer use, one from a paper for the FAO by Daberkow et al. (1999), and the other from a paper for the International Food Policy Research Institute (IFPRI) by Bumb and Baanante (1996). Both papers estimate that fertilizer use will continue to increase, but the rates of increase will slow substantially. The highest growth rate is expected in sub-Saharan Africa.

Table 14.4 Two Estimates of Projected Fertilizer Use in the Future

	Actual use 2000 (millions of metric tons)	Annual growth 1961–2000 %	Projected use 2015 (millions of metric tons)	Annual growth 2000–2015 %	Projected use 2020 (millions of metric tons)	Annual growth 2000–2020 %
East Asia	43.7	8.7	49.2	0.7	55.7	1.2
South Asia	21.3	9.9	22.2	0.3	33.8	2.2
Latin America	12.3	6.5	12.3	0.0	16.2	1.3
Near East and North Africa	6.1	7.0	6	-0.1	11.7	3.1
Sub-Saharan Africa	1.2	5.2	1.7	2.0	4.2	6.0
Developing countries	85.2	8.2	91.4	0.4	121.6	1.7
Developed countries	50.0	1.5	60.8	1.2	86.4	2.6
World total	135.2	3.7	152.2	0.7	208	2.1

Sources: Actual use: FAOSTAT. Projections in 2015: Daberkow et al. 1999. Projections in 2020: Bumb and Baanante 1996.

Fertilizer use may be less than the economic optimal rate in the poorest countries because farmers are unable to borrow money and are unable to save enough money to buy as much fertilizer as they would like. In addition, states the FAO, "In sub-Saharan Africa, where fertilizer use is still very low, consumption is hampered by high distribution costs, the lack of markets for output, lack of a domestic fertilizer industry and poor yield response, and the high risk of using fertilizer in traditional agricultural settings" (FAO WFS Background Paper No. 10, 1996a).

Animal traction.   Another important input in agricultural production worldwide is "animal traction"—the use of draft animals to pull equipment or transport goods. There are an estimated 400 million draft animals worldwide. About half of the land in agricultural production in the world is farmed with draft animals; another quarter is farmed with hand tools only; and the remaining quarter is farmed with mechanized equipment (Gifford 1992).

A draft animal can do the work of three or four adult humans (Stout 1998:76). By using animal traction rather than hand tools, a farmer is able to farm a greater area of land. This increases the self-produced food supply for the farmer's family and increases the likelihood that the farmer will produce a marketable surplus. In addition, use of animal traction may increase crop yields for two reasons: (1) plowing with animals breaks up the soil more deeply and more completely, and thereby aids in plant growth; and (2) animal manure is a source of fertilizer for the soil. In addition, animals provide other benefits to subsistence farmers: milk from cows, goats, and sheep are an additional food source; animal hides are used for clothing and shelter; animal manure is used as fuel for cooking and heating. (See Box 14.2.)

Pingali (1987) conducted a review of twenty-two published studies about the impact of animal traction on agriculture in various parts of the developing world. He found:

• Seventeen of the twenty-two studies examined the effect of animal traction on the area farmed. All seventeen found that farmers who used animals had larger farms than nearby farmers who farmed with hand tools.
• Nineteen of the studies examined the effect of animal traction on the use of land to produce crops that could be sold, rather than crops to be consumed by the farm household. Twelve of the nineteen studies found that farmers who used animals devoted more land to market crops.
• Fourteen of the twenty-two studies examined the effect of animal traction on yields. Four of these studies found a positive effect on yields; two found a negative effect; eight found no statistically significant effect.
• Sixteen of the studies found that farmers who used animal traction

> **Box 14.2   Sacred Cows**
>
> Why is the cow venerated in India? Wouldn't it be better nutritionally to devote scarce agricultural resources to feeding humans rather than to feeding cows—and, at that, cows that will not even be slaughtered for human food? The anthropologist Marvin Harris has an intriguing answer to this. Cattle contribute in three important ways to improved life in rural India. First, they are a source of power for crop cultivation. "The shortage of draft animals is a terrible threat that hangs over most of India's peasant families. . . . The main economic function of the zebu cow is to breed male traction animals" (Harris 1974:10–11). Second, cows provide milk. "Even small amounts of milk products can improve the health of people who are forced to subsist on the edge of starvation." Third, cattle produce manure. "India's cattle annually excrete about 700 million tons of recoverable manure. Approximately half of this is used as fertilizer, while most of the remainder is burned to provide heat for cooking. The annual quantity of heat liberated by this dung . . . is the equivalent of . . . 35 million tons of coal. . . . Cow dung has . . . one other major function. Mixed with water and made into a paste, it is used as a household flooring material" (p. 13).

had higher farm incomes than nearby farmers who farmed with hand tools.

Pingali also identifies impediments to the more widespread use of animal traction in the developing world.

- Cattle in sub-Saharan Africa succumb to a disease—trypanosomiasis—spread by the tsetse fly. Trypanosomiasis occurs in thirty-seven sub-Saharan African countries and threatens 50 million head of cattle. About 3 million cattle die from the disease each year, and another 35 million are treated for the disease. (For more information, see FAO's Programme Against African Trypanosomiasis, n.d.)
- Many famers in developing countries lack necessary experience and training in care of animals and equipment.
- The initial cost of animals and equipment is high, making animal traction impossible for farmers with limited access to credit.
- Using draft animals only makes sense when the farmer can expand the land under production. In some situations, all available land is being farmed by individuals who cannot or will not transfer the land to another farmer. In other situations, the land is too steep or rocky to be suitable for animal traction.
- Increasing production beyond what is needed for the farmer's family only makes sense if the farmer can sell surplus production. This requires

adequate transportation and access to reliable markets for agricultural goods.

Tractors and machinery. For the poorest farmers of the world, a major turning point may be the move from hand cultivation to animal traction. For a smaller group of slightly less-poor farmers, the replacement of animal traction with mechanized farming equipment represents a major change. Worldwide data on use of tractors and agricultural machinery are shown in Table 14.5.

The arguments presented above in the context of fertilizer may also apply to machinery—poor farmers with limited access to credit may not be able to buy as much machinery as they would like. But we should be cautious in assuming that machinery can be as efficiently used in the developing world as it is in the United States and other "rich" countries. Agricultural production in the United States tends to be done on large-scale farms using a lot of machinery and relatively little labor. Because the United States is a rich country and a large agricultural exporter, there is a tendency to regard this kind of capital-intensive farming as the "modern" and "efficient" method to which all farmers in all countries should aspire. This type of farming *is* efficient in the United States because of the relative prices of inputs that prevail there. Labor is relatively scarce in the United States, so labor wages are high. Capital markets are well developed, so farm credit is widely available at relatively low interest rates. Gasoline and equipment prices are also relatively low.

Consider the fact that farm laborers in the United States earn over $6 per hour, while gasoline costs $1.20 per gallon. Thirty days of labor costs the same as 1,200 gallons of gas. In some developing countries, thirty days of rural labor costs the same as 30 gallons of gas. Now consider a simple example in which a farmer trying to decide whether to adopt a method of

Table 14.5   Worldwide Use of Tractors and Machinery, 1961–2001

Year	Agricultural Tractors	Harvesters and Threshers
1961	11,318,243	2,230,968
1966	14,528,021	2,333,362
1971	16,524,147	2,648,527
1976	19,282,814	3,136,580
1981	22,311,077	3,655,983
1986	25,200,682	4,089,294
1991	26,248,089	4,049,710
1996	26,475,962	4,243,987
2001	26,854,002	4,121,569

Source: FAOSTAT.

production that uses machinery more intensively—weeding between crop rows with a tractor rather than by hiring people with hoes. The method will allow the farmer to use less hired labor (suppose it would save thirty days of hired labor per year), but will require the farmer to use more gasoline (suppose it would require 500 more gallons of gasoline each year). For a farmer in the United States, adopting the new method is sensible and efficient. The farmer saves enough money (in reduced labor costs) to buy 1,200 gallons of gas, but he only needs to buy 500 gallons. For a farmer in a developing country such as that described above, adopting the new method is not sensible and is inefficient. That farmer only saves enough money (in reduced labor costs) to buy 30 gallons of gas, but he needs to buy 500 gallons.

Of course, "machinery" does not *have* to be the giant large-scale tractors and equipment we find in the United States. In developing countries, farmers are more likely to use smaller-scale farm machinery, or machinery that relies more on human or animal power.

■ Population, Labor, and Agricultural Productivity

In Chapter 9, we saw that under any reasonable assumptions population will grow substantially over the next fifty years. As population grows, there are more people available to work in agricultural production. Of course, it is possible that the future population growth will occur only in the cities. In fact, Mundlak, Larson, and Crego (1996) found that agricultural labor dropped in 40 percent of countries worldwide over the period 1967–1992. However, it appears likely that population growth will lead to increases in average labor per hectare in many parts of the developing world. Table 14.6 shows trends in agricultural labor force. In Africa, Asia, the developing world, and the world as a whole, the number of agricultural workers per unit of agricultural land has increased steadily. (Not shown in the table, workers per hectare are decreasing in the developed world and in Latin America. In the United States there are about .007 workers per hectare— the average farm worker tends over 340 acres. Compare that to Asia at 4 acres per worker, or Africa with 13.5 acres per worker.)

Adding labor to each hectare of land will increase yield as long as there is productive work for the additional workers to do. Economists describe this situation as one where there is a "positive marginal productivity." One can imagine a situation where existing workers are already doing all that is possible and adding another worker to a plot of land causes a decline in production as workers begin to get in each other's way ("negative marginal productivity of labor").

In those areas that are already under cultivation, what is the marginal productivity of labor in agriculture? That is, by how much would the addi-

Table 14.6 Agricultural Work Force and Workers per Hectare of Agricultural Land, Selected Regions, 1961–2001

	Africa		Asia		Developing Countries		World	
	Economically Active Agricultural Population (in thousands)	Workers per hectare of Agricultural Land	Economically Active Agricultural Population (in thousands)	Workers per hectare of Agricultural Land	Economically Active Agricultural Population (in thousands)	Workers per hectare of Agricultural Land	Economically Active Agricultural Population (in thousands)	Workers per hectare of Agricultural Land
1961	101,697	0.096195	612,500	0.579808	735,238	0.280146	849,711	0.188633
1966	110,172	0.104074	653,484	0.604339	788,840	0.293539	890,157	0.195037
1971	119,642	0.112178	707,840	0.640968	856,948	0.311594	944,308	0.203838
1976	128,911	0.120415	773,487	0.68708	936,619	0.334422	1,017,307	0.217072
1981	140,040	0.130657	829,588	0.714074	1,008,039	0.353157	1,081,481	0.228163
1986	153,978	0.142284	896,068	0.716603	1,089,755	0.366824	1,157,293	0.238655
1991	168,818	0.153741	963,465	0.737378	1,172,453	0.383463	1,233,252	0.250795
1996	184,303	0.167509	1,013,676	0.613821	1,230,956	0.393386	1,284,339	0.257156
2001	200,439	0.180847	1,045,945	0.622618	1,280,042	0.402712	1,326,642	0.264184

Source: FAOSTAT.

tion or subtraction of one worker change farm production? In the years before World War II, a considerable literature developed that assumed such a large pool of unemployed and underemployed labor languished in third world agriculture that substantial amounts could be withdrawn for the industrial labor force with no diminution in agricultural production—in other words, that the marginal product of labor in agriculture was zero (Lewis 1954; Fei and Ranis 1964).

Gary Becker (1975) called that thesis into question with a powerful argument that people attach at least some value to their leisure time. If this is the case, then they will not work their fields up to the point that another minute spent farming yields no product at all. They would rather spend those few minutes at leisure.

Still, we see considerable evidence that the marginal product of labor in agriculture is below the wage rate. A number of studies have shown that yields on small holdings in India, so small that all labor is supplied by the farm family, are significantly higher than yields on large farms where a substantial proportion of the labor force is hired (Berry and Cline 1979). Studies in other locations have arrived at similar results (see Figure 14.5).

Farmers who hire labor are unwilling to hire so much that the product for the last hour worked by the laborer is less than the cost of hiring him for that hour. But when labor is all from the family, for those last few hours worked family members may be willing to work for something less than the going wage, because the family will benefit from those last few hours and because they may have no higher-valued use for their time (Mazumdar 1965, 1975; Sen 1964, 1966). (Enslaving agricultural workers is not unknown. See Box 14.3.)

All this argues that the marginal productivity of labor in agriculture is low, and comparisons of wages in agriculture versus nonagricultural activities in the third world support this thesis. The International Labour Organization (ILO 1987) lists the daily wage rate for agricultural activities in the Philippines in 1985 as P 23.74 per day (just over one U.S. dollar), but the daily rate for nonagricultural activities is P 56.48 per day, or 2.4 times the agricultural rate. The ILO lists the daily rate for farm labor in India at about half a dollar and shows the manufacturing wage to be over five times that amount.

Given the low wage rates in third world agriculture relative to work outside of agriculture, it is difficult to make a case for enough of a labor shortage in agriculture to make the typical farm family better off with many, rather than few, children. If farm productivity is the main consideration, it appears that the typical developing-country farm family would be better off spending more on fertilizer for high-yielding seeds and less on raising extra children.

Figure 14.5   Farm Size and Production per Unit of Land in Less Developed Nations

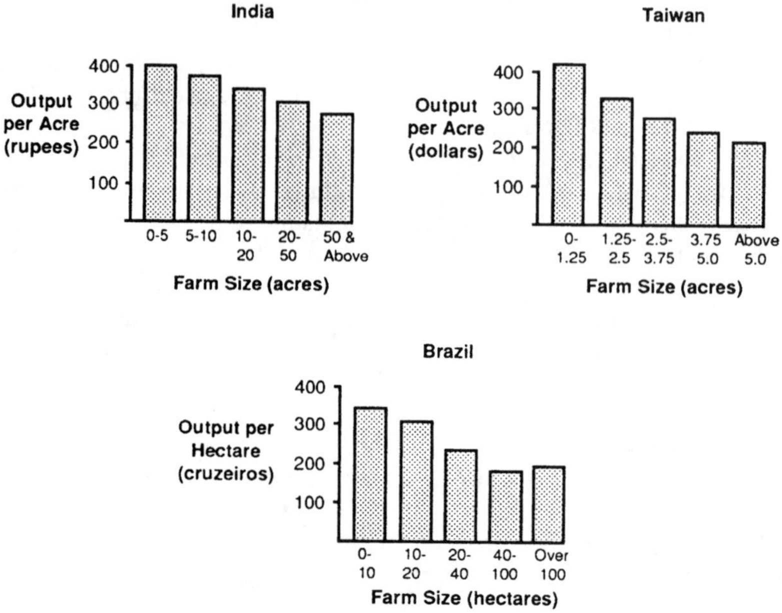

India

Taiwan

Brazil

Source: Adapted from Stevens and Jabara 1988:68.

AIDS and Agricultural Productivity

Chapter 9 discussed the problem of AIDS and the high incidence of HIV infection in some sub-Saharan countries. HIV infection and AIDS will reduce labor productivity in the following ways:

- As people fall ill to AIDS, their capacity for work is reduced.
- The labor of healthy family members is diverted from agricultural production to caretaking.
- Premature deaths of AIDS victims removes a source of expertise and experience from the household.
- Fear of AIDS and its spread may make HIV-infected people unemployable even when they are capable of working.
- Orphaned children receive less education and care than children with living parents; thus these orphans grow up to be less productive as adults.

Several reports verify the effects of AIDS on agricultural production. In Thailand, one-third of rural families affected by AIDS saw their agricul-

---

Box 14.3   Slavery in Modern Agriculture

When we say, "slavery in agriculture," students in the United States are likely to think of antebellum cotton plantations. But the practice of slavery in agricultural production worldwide is still alive.

In Côte d'Ivoire, cocoa farmers lured workers—many from neighboring countries—with promises of high wages. Once the workers arrived at the cocoa plantation, the farmers "refused to pay their laborers, and instead kept them working without pay through beatings, intimidation, and threats of magical spells," according to ABC News (see Chang 2001).

In India, an estimated 15 million children work as "bonded laborers." Destitute parents in need of cash borrow money—usually small sums of between $20 and $200—from unscrupulous lenders. The parents pledge their children to work for the lenders until the debt is paid off; but high interest rates and low wages keep the children in servitude for years. In some cases, the labor burden is passed from older siblings to younger siblings, as the family debt remains unpaid. The great majority of bonded child laborers work in agriculture—tending cattle, picking tea, and working in the sugarcane fields. (See Human Rights Watch 1996.)

In Florida in 2002, two men were convicted of holding seven hundred men as slaves. These were undocumented workers from Central America, smuggled into Florida by the two men, and put to work in the orange groves of Florida until they had earned enough money to buy their freedom. (See Maxwell 2002.)

---

tural output drop to less than one-half of earlier levels. A study of Tanzanian households found that a woman married to an AIDS patient spent 60 percent less time on agricultural activities. A study in Uganda found that two-thirds of households who had lost a family member to AIDS produced less food than before.

Population Growth as a Stimulant to Productivity

A number of thinkers have argued that population growth in and of itself is a stimulant to productivity. One of the writers in this school (Clark 1973) capsulized one of its chief arguments in the title of his article: "More People, More Dynamism." That is, society is better off with a large population than with a small one "as a result of there being more knowledge creators" in a large population (Simon 1986:169).

Critics of this argument note that in today's high-tech world large numbers of people create little assurance of a high level of knowlege creation. If they did, then India and China, with over a third of the world's population between them, should account for a greater share of the world's technological development than do Germany, France, Great Britain, the United States, and Japan, which collectively account for only 10 percent of the world's population. In the third world, many Einsteins may be undiscovered for want of a proper education.

Ester Boserup, in her book *Population and Technological Change* (1981:5), argues that population growth creates a kind of crisis situation that stimulates the invention of new technology: "Shrinking supplies of land and other natural resources would provide motivation to invent better means of utilizing scarce resources or to discover substitutes for them." Note that in this "necessity is the mother of invention" argument, it is population growth that drives the creation of technology, and not the creation of technology that expands the capacity of the economy to support more people.

Boserup argues that farming is most intense in the densely settled regions of the world (not that people have tended to gather in those regions of the world where soils are most productive). She argues that, because periods of technological innovation and expanding productivity have usually been accompanied by increases in population, growth of population must have caused the increase in technology and production. Critics of this thesis argue that it is just the other way around, i.e., that it is the technological innovation and expanding productivity that have, in fact, made possible the associated increase in population.

Because productivity is related to income, and income is so closely related to food consumption, those who argue that population growth of itself is a stimulant to productivity imply that population growth would help alleviate the world hunger problem, or at the least impose no threat to a solution. This school of thought has to contend with a series of arguments that claim population growth has a detrimental impact on the nutrition of the poor.

Kahkonen and Leathers (1997) suggest an additional reason why increasing population density may be beneficial to agricultural development. If transactions costs—the costs associated with setting up an exchange of goods—decline with the number of transactions, then areas with high population density are more likely to have established markets (or other means of exchange); this in turn gives farmers incentives to produce marketable surplus.

Partial Productivity Measures

Yield per unit of land is a "partial productivity measure"—it measures output per unit of input for a single input. Work by economists Craig, Pardey, and Roseboom (1994 and 1997) analyzes differences in partial productivity measures across different countries. Some of their data are shown in Tables 14.7 and 14.8.

Table 14.7 shows two partial productivity measures: the value of agricultural output per hectare and the value of agricultural output per worker.

Table 14.7   Value of Agricultural Output per Agricultural Worker and per Hectare of Agricultural Land, 1986–1990

Region or Country	Average value of output per worker (in US$)	Average value of output per hectare (in US$)
Sub-Saharan Africa	412	123
China	324	300
Asia and Pacific	817	955
Latin America and Caribbean	3,260	239
West Asia and North Africa	2,608	534
Australasia	38,580	216
Western Europe	18,088	1,231
Southern Europe	6,662	652
Eastern Europe	5,324	703
Former USSR	4,432	150
North America	32,948	224
Japan	3,103	2,589
South Africa	3,812	72

Source: Craig, Pardey, and Roseboom 1994.

Notice how the numbers here reinforce a concept presented above in the section on machinery use: efficient agricultural practices conserve on use of the scarcest resource. In densely populated parts of the world (Japan and Asia) returns per hectare are approximately equal to returns to worker; agricultural practices in these parts of the world use relatively high amounts of labor on each plot of land in order to extract the most from the scarce resource—land. In parts of the world where population density is low (Australasia and North America), returns per worker are 150 times that of returns per hectare; agricultural practices in these parts of the world use relatively low amounts of labor on each plot of land in order to extract the most from the scarce resource—labor.

Table 14.8 illustrates how increased output per unit of land is associated with more intensive use of other inputs. In this table, the countries and areas have been sorted according to value of output per hectare. The other tables show per hectare use of labor, fertilizer, and horsepower (both mechanized and animal traction). The countries at the top of the list attain high outputs per acre by using a lot of inputs per acre. The countries at the bottom of the list have low output per acre, but also low inputs per acre. (The data shown are input and output per unit of agricultural land. The fertilizer application rates discussed above for countries such as China and Japan were fertilizer use per hectare of arable and permanent crop land. This accounts for the difference in numbers presented earlier in the text and the numbers in Table 14.8.)

Table 14.8   Output and Input Use per Hectare, 1986–1990, Selected Countries and Regions, Sorted by Output per Hectare

Country	Output	Labor	Fertilizer	Tractors	Animal Traction
	$/ha	Workers/ 1,000 ha	Kg/ha	HP[a]/ha	HP[a]/ha
Japan	2589	834	373	13095	4
Western Europe	1231	70	186	4222	17
Asia & Pacific	955	1289	80	173	230
Eastern Europe	703	147	171	1632	32
Southern Europe	652	118	82	1955	23
West Asia and North Africa	534	292	63	519	116
China	300	925	48	177	70
Latin America& Caribbean	239	179	21	121	71
North America	224	7	35	629	9
Australasia	216	5	13	188	4
USSR (former)	150	34	43	274	11
Sub-Saharan Africa	123	354	2	14	18
South Africa	72	19	8	107	3

Source: Craig, Pardey, and Roseboom 1994.
Note: a. HP = horsepower.

■ Yields And Technology

The previous three sections show that yields per hectare can be increased by using productive inputs more intensively on each hectare of land. Next, we turn to an alternative way of producing higher yields—improved technology. As described at the beginning of this chapter, technological improvement allows us to gain more output from the same quantity of inputs (or the same output using fewer of the inputs).

The Green Revolution

There can be no doubt that the centuries-long climb in yields reported in Table 14.1 is the result of better agricultural techniques: improved knowledge about crop rotations, timing and levels of fertilizer applications, and selective animal breeding. Much of the new knowledge came from trial and error by farmers themselves, but the scientific experiments (such as those reported in Box 14.1) also played a role. Since the 1960s, the most highly publicized new technology has been the new seed varieties developed in the so-called green revolution (described in Box 14.4).

The green revolution began with the work of crop scientist Norman Borlaug in Mexico in the 1940s. (For his efforts, Borlaug was awarded the 1970 Nobel Peace Prize.) At that time, wheat yields in Mexico were severely depressed by a fungus disease ("wheat rust") that shrivels the wheat

Box 14.4 What Is the Green Revolution?

Dana Dalrymple

In October 1944, about a year before the close of World War II, the Rockefeller Foundation brought to Mexico a young plant scientist to join a team of agriculturalists that had recently started work to assist in the agricultural development of that country. In a few months, the new man, Norman Borlaug (who was later to be awarded a Nobel Prize for his work in Mexico), was put in charge of the wheat program. He and his team set out to develop new varieties of wheat that would do better than the local varieties. Disease resistance (e.g., resistance to the fungus causing the disease rust) was particularly important at first. In the mid-1950s increased emphasis was given to increasing yields and within a few years varieties had been developed which could produce much more than the traditional ones.

Encouraged by this success, in the 1960s the Rockefeller Foundation joined with the Ford Foundation to establish two permanent research stations for the development of high-yielding cereals, the International Rice Research Institute (IRRI) in the Philippines and the International Maize and Wheat Improvement Center (CIMMYT) in Mexico. The success of these centers in developing high-yielding varieties led to such enthusiasm for the idea of international agricultural research centers that by the late 1980s thirteen centers, treating various aspects of improving third world agriculture, had been set up worldwide, and sponsorship had spread to a consortium of donors worldwide including both foundations and government agencies.

The high-yielding varieties of wheat and rice have spread more widely, more quickly, than any other technological innovation in the history of agriculture in the developing countries. First introduced in the mid-1960s, they occupied about half of these countries' total wheat and rice area by 1982–1983 (Dalrymple 1985). Figure A shows the remarkable growth in adoption of high-yielding varieties in South and Southeast Asia.

Figure A

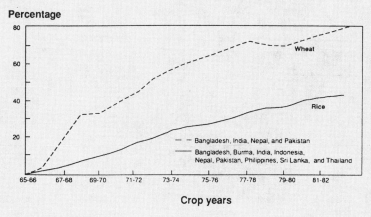

(*continues*)

Continued

Struck by the remarkable speed with which high-yielding varieties of wheat and rice were being developed for the third world and by their potential to alleviate world hunger, William S. Gaud, who was then administrator of the U.S. Agency for International Development, referred, in a 1968 speech, to the phenomenon of their development and spread as "the green revolution" (Dalrymple 1979:724).

Actually, the green revolution's wheat and rice varieties, also known as high-yielding varieties (HYVs) or modern varieties (MVs), do not do much better than the traditional varieties (they can even do worse) unless they have appropriate amounts of water and fertilizer. In fact, it is largely tolerance of and response to substantial amounts of fertilizer that makes them so successful.

The traditional varieties of wheat and rice were not tolerant of significant amounts of fertilizer. When third world farmers attempted to increase rice or wheat yields by adding fertilizer—especially nitrogen fertilizer—to their fields, their plants would grow so tall that they would fall over. The technical term for this is lodging. What the plant scientists at the international institutes did was to locate plant varieties with genes for shortness and breed these genes into plants that had other characteristics desirable for the third world. The new plants, called semidwarfs, borrowed dwarfism genes from Japan (for wheat) and China (for rice). When used with fertilizer, they grew taller than without the fertilizer, but not excessively so. Thus they were much more resistant to lodging (Figure B).

Figure B

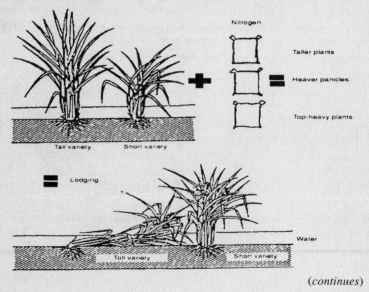

(continues)

Continued

Plant scientists did not stop merely with the development of nonlodging plants. They bred into their new varieties a host of other characteristics such as disease resistance.

One of the more intriguing changes in plant design that they accomplished involved rearranging the location of the seed cluster on the plant. Traditional rice plants sent their cluster of seeds (the panicle) high into the air. The seeds themselves store energy, but they do not make it. Photosynthesis is concentrated in the leaves. It did not make sense for the seed cluster to shade the highest leaves on the plant, so the scientists bred rice plants whose topmost leaf, the flag leaf, extended well above the panicle, thus taking maximum advantage of the available sunshine (Figure C).

Figure C

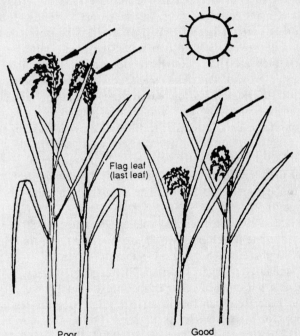

Flag leaf (last leaf)

Poor   Good

The green revolution, then, is a whole complex of innovations, such as those described above, that combine to make up new plant varieties. The modern plant varieties, when used with a package of appropriate inputs such as fertilizer and water and good management, are dramatically raising crop yields in the third world.

(For more about the green revolution, see Brown 1970; U.S. Department of State 1986a, b; Stackman, Bradfield & Mangelsdorf 1967.)

grain. In his search for a rust-resistant variety of wheat, Borlaug collected 8,500 varieties of wheat being grown in different parts of Mexico; two of these 8,500 varieties proved to be rust-resistant. Borlaug and his associates, using tweezers and a magnifying glass, bred these rust-resistant varieties to other high-yielding varieties using the technique of crossing. Year after year, Borlaug experimented with new crosses, searching for varieties that gave higher yields. By 1957, the wheat rust problem in Mexico was solved, and average wheat yield had nearly doubled from 11 to 20 bushels per acre. In the meantime, Borlaug was working to solve another problem: as yields increased, the heavier grain caused plants to tip over ("lodge," as illustrated in Fig. B in Box 14.4). Crossing with "dwarf" varieties of wheat—wheat with shorter and stronger stems—solved this problem. By 1963, Mexican wheat yields had grown to 30 bushels per acre, and experimental plots showed yields of 105 bushels per acre (Paarlberg 1988:102–105).

The shorter and stronger stems of the dwarf varieties meant that the plants could support a heavier crop of grain. The new seed varieties achieved this improved yield in two ways: they were more responsive to fertilizer and they used the photosynthetic energy of the plant more efficiently for grain growth. The traditional seed varieties responded to fertilizer at a rate of 10 kilograms of increased grain output for each kilogram of increased fertilizer use. The new varieties responsed at a rate of 25 kilograms of grain for each kilogram of fertilizer. This made use of commercial fertilizers much more attractive for farmers who used the new seed varieties. The old seed varieties allocated about 20 percent of the photosynthetic energy of the plant to grain production and the remaining 80 percent to growth of roots, stems, and leaves. The new seed varieties improved this ratio to about 50:50.

By the late 1990s dwarf wheat varieties accounted for 80 percent of the wheat planted in the developing world. In Asia and Latin America, the figure is over 90 percent, while in sub-Saharan Africa about 65 percent of wheat land is planted in dwarf varieties. Borlaug's methods were adapted to developing new varieties of other crops; most notably rice for Asia. The International Rice Research Institute (IRRI) has been the leading institutional support for this research. In the early 1960s, average rice yields in Asia were 1–2 metric tons per hectare. By 2002, IRRI could claim in their project report: "The adoption of improved varieties that have a yield potential of 10 tons per hectare is almost complete."

Criticisms of the Green Revolution

The green revolution is not without its critics. As already described, the new seed varieties encourage farmers to use more fertilizer; the green revolution also brought increased use of irrigation and pesticides. For these reasons, the green revolution has been criticized as potentially damaging to the environment. A second criticism centers on whether the green revolution varieties have crowded out traditional varieties and led to a loss of species diversity. But perhaps the most widespread criticism of the green revolution is the fear that it might increase inequality of income; indeed, it might make the poor absolutely worse-off in regions where it was adopted. After all, it has been common for new agricultural technologies to be adopted earlier by the leading farmers in a region, who are often those with the biggest or best farms, the best education, and the greatest willingness to take a risk by trying something new. Furthermore, a tendency exists for public services to be more available to the big farmers than to the small, for technology to carry with it a labor-saving bias that reduces labor's share of the product, and for technological innovations to be more appropriate to some geographical areas than to others. Would not wealthy landlords use the benefits from green revolution technology as a stepping-stone to increasing the size of their holdings at the expense of small farmers, thus increasing income inequality?

Some of the above fears turn out to have been justified, but most have not. Early adopters did tend to be the bigger, better farmers, but this has not prevented smaller farmers, who are often slower to change, from adopting green revolution technology.

Still, the benefits of the green revolution have accrued more to farmers in regions where water, especially irrigation water, is plentiful. Growers of lowland rice (rice that spends much of its early growing days with its stalks standing in a few inches of water) benefit more than growers of upland rice. Wheat and rice farmers, who predominate in tropical regions with 40 inches or more of annual rainfall, benefit more than sorghum and millet farmers, who farm the semiarid tropics where rainfall is usually less than 40 inches per year.

The high-yielding fine grains (wheat and rice) grown with adequate water are far more responsive to fertilizer than are even the best varieties of the coarse grains (sorghum and millet) grown in the dry regions where irrigation water is scarce to nonexistent. The fertilizer subsidies that third world governments frequently provide to their farmers therefore benefit the fine-grain producers more than the coarse-grain farmers. Thus, the benefits of the green revolution have concentrated mainly in the wetter tropics and especially on the flatter lands where irrigation and water management are easier. This phenomenon may well have increased income inequality between regions.

Nevertheless, within regions "the benefits from adopting modern varieties have been remarkably evenly distributed among farmers differing in size of holding and tenure status." This is the conclusion of a major study commissioned to examine the impact of the international agricultural research centers (Anderson et al. 1985:4).

In a detailed study of the economy of a northern Indian village where modern varieties had been widely adopted, Bliss and Stern (1982:291) found no strong association between size of holding and the intensity of use of inputs associated with the adoption of green revolution technology. In fact, "the adoption of various newer varieties and intensive practices seemed to be particularly associated with the younger educated farmers."

How is it that the benefits could be so evenly distributed among farms of different sizes and farmers of different tenure status? For one thing, the capital requirements of the green revolution are minimal. Unlike hybrid corn, which has done so much to increase corn yields in the United States and Europe, the green revolution fine-grain seeds breed true (i.e., produce offspring almost identical to the parent plant). Hybrid seed corn must be produced annually under technically demanding conditions on specialized farms and sold to farmers each year. A farmer who planted the grain from his hybrid corn crop as seed would be most disappointed in the yield results. Green revolution rice and wheat, although the result of complicated crosses, are not true hybrids. You can plant a little one year, take the resulting grain as seed for next year's crop, and rapidly and cheaply multiply your seed stock. Thus, a handful of green revolution seed is all you need to begin farming—and it usually does not cost any more than traditional seed.

On the one hand, green revolution varieties do require capital in the form of commercial fertilizer. On the other hand, fertilizer, like seed, is almost infinitely divisible, and a farmer need purchase only as much as he needs for his particular plot. Unlike capital investment in a tractor, the capital investment in the green revolution is not "lumpy"—that is, it does not come only in large, indivisible clumps.

A second reason for the evenly distributed benefits is that the green revolution technology is not labor-saving. To the contrary, it turns out to be labor-using (Hossain 1988b:12; Ranade and Herdt 1978:103; Pinstrup-Andersen and Hazell 1985:11). Much of the third world grain crop is harvested and threshed by hand, and the increased crop yield requires more labor for harvest. More important, though, the fertilizer applied to the crop turns out to stimulate the growth of weeds as well as grain. Farmers are finding it profitable to remove these weeds and, in the third world, weeding a field is labor-intensive (weeds are pulled by hand or chopped with a blade, for example).

Because the poor spend a greater proportion of their income on food than do the rich, the benefits from price drops associated with increased production following the adoption of green revolution technology favor the poor over the rich. Because of the very low overall elasticity of demand for cereals, consumers benefit substantially from the price drop caused by increased production, but farmers as a whole experience a decline in total revenue (see the last part of Chapter 7 for a review of why this happens).

In a study of the social returns to rice research, Evenson and Flores

(1978:255) found that in the Philippines, during the period from 1972 to 1975, the annual loss to producers from the adoption of the high-yielding rice varieties was $61 million, while the annual gain to consumers was $142 million, yielding a net annual gain to society of $81 million. Similarly, working with Colombian data, Scobie and Posada (1984) concluded that, during 1970–1974, Colombian rice producers lost $796 million, while consumers benefited by over $1.349 billion, for a net gain to society of $553 million. Furthermore, they concluded that "while the lower 50 percent of Colombian households received about 15 percent of household income, they captured nearly 70 percent of the net benefits of the [rice] research program" (p. 383).

The cereal production increases that, because of demand elasticities of well below one, result in the loss of revenue for commercial rice growers may, at the same time, result in an increase in total revenue to the semi-subsistence farmer. A semisubsistence farmer is defined as one who purchases less than 50 percent of his food supply in the marketplace. (Almost no one is a subsistence farmer, purchasing no food supplies, not even spices, in the marketplace.)

Consider a semisubsistence farmer who consumes, say, 90 percent of his rice crop. He has a small amount left over for sale in the market. He sees his neighbors on larger farms, who sell most of what they grow, practicing green revolution technology, and copies them, purchasing some seed and fertilizer and irrigating his crop as usual. His yield increases by the same percentage as that of the larger farmers, but, if he consumes the same amount of rice as he used to, the size of the surplus that he has left to sell grows by a much greater percentage than the percentage growth in his total production. Thus, even in the face of sharply declining rice prices, he may experience a gain in total revenue whereas his more commercially oriented neighbors are experiencing losses.

Impact of the Green Revolution on Yields

Whatever one makes of the criticisms of the green revolution, there can be no doubt that it has led to increased yields. How much of the yield increases are attributable to increases in inputs described in the previous section, and how much to new technology? This question is hard to answer because of the nature of the new seed varieties. As we have seen, the new varieties achieved their higher yields in part by being more responsive to fertilizer; in addition, the new varieties were often more sensitive to drought, and thus have been frequently grown on irrigated land. Therefore, the higher observed yields are the result of a complex interaction between technological improvement and additional levels of inputs.

Several researchers have attempted to unravel this complexity. The Consultative Group on International Agricultural Research (CGIAR 1997) reports that "22 percent of the developing world's [wheat] production increase resulting from higher yields is attributed to the gradual spreading of modern or high yielding varieties." A study of Syrian wheat found the increase in wheat yields (which more than quadrupled from the 1950s to the early 1990s) was due to several factors: new varieties accounted for about 35 percent of the increase; better management and increased fertilizer use accounted for 23 percent each; and irrigation accounted for 19 percent of the increase (CGIAR 1995). Peter Oram (1995), in an IFPRI paper, writes: "It is estimated that about 50 percent of the gains in farm yields have resulted from plant breeding and the balance from the application of other improved practices." These suggest that of the average yield growth of 2 percent per year from 1968 to 1997, new technology accounts for between 0.5 and 1 percent per year, and input growth accounts for the remaining 1 to 1.5 percent per year.

The technological improvements shift out the aggregate supply curve for food and cause food prices to be lower than they would otherwise have been. CGIAR reports that in developing countries, prices for crops targeted by CGIAR have dropped more than the prices for non-CGIAR crops. The U. S. Department of Agriculture (USDA 1991) estimates that research into improvements in agricultural production methods has reduced the average yearly food bill in the United States by $400 per person.

Total Factor Productivity

One systematic way to quantify the impact of all different kinds of technical change is to calculate *total factor productivity* (TFP). Recall the discussion above of partial factor productivity, such as growth in output per unit of land or per unit of labor. When looking at growth in partial factor productivity, it was not readily apparent what part of that growth was attributable to technical change and what part was attributable to growth in use of other inputs. Total factor productivity is calculated by first constructing two indexes: an index of output that is a single number that reflects changes in levels of all outputs, and an index of input use that reflects changes in levels of all inputs (or at least all inputs on which data are available). Total factor productivity is the ratio of these two indexes: outputs divided by inputs. (See Box 14.5 for an example of how index numbers can be constructed.) Therefore (referring again to Figure 14.3), an increase in TFP means that output can be increased without increasing input, either because inefficiency has been eliminated (moving from A to B) or because a technological improvement has caused an upward shift in the production function (moving from point B to point C).

Pingali and Heisey (1999) review TFP estimates from fifteen separate studies, covering thirty-two different countries, for a variety of time periods. They report seventy-two total measurements of annual percentage

Box 14.5   Index Numbers

An index number is essentially a weighted average of quantities, scaled to reflect the level of that average compared to some base period. Suppose a farm produces wheat and corn. In 2002 the farm produces y^1_{corn} units of corn and y^1_{wheat} units of wheat. In 2003 the farm produces produces y^2_{corn} units of corn and y^2_{wheat} units of wheat. Let p_{corn} be the price of corn and p_{wheat} be the price of wheat. To construct an index of output, first choose a "base year." This is arbitrary, so we could choose either 2002 or 2003; for this example we will choose 2002. The index number for each year is:

$$\text{Output index year t} = 100 \times \frac{p_{corn} \, y^t_{corn} + p_{wheat} \, y^t_{wheat}}{p_{corn} \, y^{2002}_{corn} + p_{wheat} \, y^{2002}_{wheat}}$$

where t can be 2002 or 2003.

The sample outputs and prices in the following table show how the index is constructed:

Year (t)	Corn output (y^t_{corn})	Wheat output (y^t_{wheat})	Corn price (p_{corn})	Wheat price (p_{wheat})
2002	125	50	3	5
2003	150	45	3	5

For 2002, the sum of price x quantity is 125 x 3 + 50 x 5 = 375 + 250 = 625. For 2003 the sum is 150 x 3 + 45 x 5 = 450 + 225 = 675. The index numbers are therefore

$$2002: 100 \times \frac{625}{625} = 100$$

$$2003: 100 \times \frac{675}{625} = 108$$

A number of points should be obvious:

- For the base year, the value of the index is 100 by definition.
- If all outputs increased by exactly 10 percent from 2002 to 2003, the index number for 2003 would be 110. If all outputs decrease by exactly 10 percent, the index number would be 90.
- In the example, the increase from 100 to 108 reflects an average of the 20 percent increase in corn production and the 10 percent decrease in wheat production. The weight assigned to the different commodities depends on the price of those commodities.
- This concept is easy to extend to more than two outputs, or more than two years. It can be applied to output of a single farm, or a state, or a nation, or a combination of nations.

(*continues*)

Continued

If the farm used three inputs—land, seed, and labor—we could construct an index of input use in a similar fashion.

Year (t)	Land input (x^t_{land})	Seed input (x^t_{seed})	Labor input (x^t_{labor})	Land price (r_{land})	Seed price (r_{seed})	Labor price (r_{labor})
2002	2	50	10	30	2	40
2003	2	55	12	30	2	40

For 2002, price times quantity is 2 x 30 + 50 x 2 + 10 x 40 = 560.
For 2003, price times quantity is 2 x 30 + 55 x 2 + 12 x 40 = 650.
The input index numbers are therefore

$$2002: 100 \times \frac{560}{560} = 100$$

$$2003: 100 \times \frac{650}{560} = 116$$

Total factor productivity is the ratio of the output index to the input index. The total factor productivity measures are therefore:

$$2002: 100 \times \frac{100}{100} = 100$$

$$2003: 100 \times \frac{108}{116} = 93$$

In this example, even though output increased (as indicated by the increase in the output index from 100 to 108), input use increased faster (as indicated by the increase in the input index from 100 to 116); so total factor productivity declined by 7 percent.

growth in TFP; sixty-six are positive and six negative; seventeen of the estimates are greater than 2 percent per year. To put this in perspective, worldwide production of all cereal crops has growth at an annual rate of 2.16 percent from 1961 to 2001; total calories worldwide have increased by 2.24 percent per year over the same period.

In a 2003 article, Nin et al. used FAO data on 115 countries and country-groups for the period 1965–1994 to estimate TFP separately for crops and animal products. The results of that study are summarized in Table 14.9. TFP for all countries is estimated at 0.51 percent per year for livestock and 0.63 percent per year for crops. This is one-quarter to one-third of growth

Table 14.9   Annual Percentage Growth in Total Factor Productivity

	Livestock	Crops
Middle East–North Africa	0.01	0.2
Sub-Saharan Africa	–0.01	–0.32
South America	0.52	0.98
Central America	0.83	0.03
Eastern Europe	0.63	1.55
China	1.8	0.69
India	0.83	–1.74
Western Europe	1.19	2.5
All	0.51	0.63

Source: Nin et al. 2003.

rates in worldwide output reported in the last paragraph. This is consistent, at the low end, of the discussion in the last section about the extent to which yield growth is attributable to new technology and the extent to which it is attributable to increased input use.

Prospects for Future Yield Growth
Can crop yields continue to grow? And if so, at what rate? The answers to these questions go a long way to determining whether the future food supply will keep pace with demand. Above, we reviewed the different opinions about the prospects for adding irrigation, fertilizer, and labor to agricultural production. Even the most optimistic projections see input usage growing more slowly than in the past. But what about technology? Can technological advances pick up the slack caused by slower growth in input use? We find optimists and pessimists on this question.

Reasons for concern.   The pessimists point out that growth in yields has been slowing (see Figures 14.1 and 14.2). Imagine (say the pessimists) that crop yields are growing according to an S-shaped curve; we have gone through a period of rapidly rising yields, but we are now reaching the top, where yields become flat: "Countries that have doubled or tripled the productivity of their cropland since mid-century are the rule, not the exception. But with many of the world's farmers already using advanced yield-raising technologies, further gains in land productivity will not come easily" (Brown and Kane 1994:132). An IRRI 2002 project report warns: "Yield at the farm level is approaching a plateau."

Some pessimism about yields is based on a belief that scientists cannot discover new ways to increase yields. "Rising grain yield per hectare . . . must eventually give way to physical constraints. . . . Yields may now be pushing against various physiological limits such as nutrient absorption capacity or photosynthetic efficiency" (Brown and Kane 1994:138). Thomas Sinclair, a horticulturist at the University of Florida, Gainesville, explained to *Science* magazine: "To grow corn, . . . you have to have leaves, stalks, and roots, so there's got to be mass committed to what you don't harvest. . . . At the beginning of this century, . . . many crops had harvest indexes on the order of 0.25 of their weight in grain, and now many crops are approaching 0.5. . . . Maybe you could go up to 0.6 or 0.65, but beyond that you can't have a viable plant" (quoted in Mann 1997:1042). (For alternative views, and discussions of other factors affecting yield growth, see Box 14.7 on p. 241.)

Another source of pessimism about yields is concern about whether they are "environmentally sustainable." According to this school of thought the current high yields have been obtained by putting extreme pressure on the natural environment. As discussed in Chapter 13, the environment can stand this pressure for only a short time; yields then naturally begin to decline.

A second green revolution: research efforts to reduce environmental degradation. Perhaps in response to these legitimate concerns about the environmental impact of agricultural production, the emphasis of international agricultural research shifted during the 1990s from increasing yields to reducing environmental impact. Some of the new production techniques developed include low-till and no-till cultivation methods that reduce soil erosion, and drip irrigation techniques that improve the efficiency of delivery of irrigation water to the plants.

Not all of the innovations rely on high-tech solutions. One example comes from China, where a fungus was destroying rice fields. Wherever the fungus emerged, windblown spores would spread the fungus from row to row until the entire field was affected. Scientists discovered a low-yielding wild variety of rice that was resistant to the fungus. By alternating rows of the high yielding but fungus susceptible rice with rows of the lower yielding but fungus resistant rice, scientists were able to halt the spread of the fungus. Spores would be blown from the infected rows to the neighboring resistant rows, which stopped the spread of the fungus. This research simultaneously pursued the objectives of improved yields and reduced stress on the environment, since it found an alternative to chemical fungicide.

Some research into indigenous farming practices also has found ways to increase agricultural production in an environmentally friendly way. For example, some indigenous populations use fish or anthill waste as a source of fertilizer. In the Sudan, planting millet under the acacia albida tree improved millet yield. The tree roots drew nutrients from deep in the soil and the dropping tree leaves transferred those nutrients to the top of the soil. Furthermore, the timing of the leaf growth and decay allowed the millet plants to receive sun and shade at crucial times in the life cycle of the millet plants.

A possible application of biotechnology to sustainable aquaculture is described in Box 14.6.

Reasons for hope. The change in focus of agricultural research from increasing yields to reducing environmental impact may help explain why yields in experiment stations (the laboratories of crop production) have leveled. A related explanation is that international crop research has been underfunded (Pardey and Alston 1995). Alexandratos (1995) argues that the slowdown in yield growth is less a result of technological feasibility and more a result of low farm-level prices. Finally, worldwide average crop yields have been brought down during the 1990s by a large drop in yields

---

Box 14.6   Genetic Engineering to Save Fish Species

The original problem was overfishing the ocean's supply of salmon. For economists this is a textbook example of the "tragedy of the commons." Because the fish population does not belong to any individual or group of individuals (property rights are not defined), and because anyone is free to catch fish (there is no way to exclude users), no one has the appropriate incentive to watch out for the long-run health of the fish population, and to ensure that enough fish are left this year to replenish the fish stocks for next year. (The same argument explains why wild species may be hunted to extinction, and why communally owned pastures may be overgrazed.)

The introduction of aquaculture, or fish farming, provided a way to grow salmon in cages or in ponds. Under these conditions, the fish population was no longer a common resource: the fish in the cages or ponds are owned and no one can remove them without permission of the owner. The owner's future profitability depends on maintaining a healthy fish population.

But a new problem emerged. Fish farms feed their salmon a diet of fish meal made of ground up herring and anchovies. This fish meal is high in omega-3 fatty acids, which is an important nutrient in the diets of salmon. As fish farming grew, it put more and more pressure on wild populations of herring and anchovies, which were being overfished to provide the fish meal.

Scientists at Montana State University discovered that a plant called carpetweed produces omega-3 fatty acids. Unfortunately, the salmon had trouble digesting carpetweed meal; fish require low-fiber diets, such as a meal made of hulled sunflower seeds. Scientists are now attempting to modify sunflower genes to incorporate the omega-3 gene from carpetweed. If they are successful, the new feed will reduce the pressure on wild fishing populations.

Source: John Baden 2003.

in the former Soviet Union, probably a temporary phenomenon. If you accept any of these explanations about the slowdown in yield growth, you may be more optimistic about future growth in yields.

Many analysts are more optimistic about future yields. The FAO projects cereal yields will grow at 1.4 percent per year between 1990 and 2010, compared with a 2.2 percent growth rate between 1970 and 1990. A World Bank study estimates that grain yields will continue to grow at a 1.5–1.7 percent annual rate. An IFPRI report on food supply and demand in the year 2020 presents a base scenario in which yields continue to grow at the rate observed in the late 1980s and early 1990s. Rejesus, Heisey, and Smale (1999) review a number of studies that project annual growth rates for wheat yields of between 1.4 percent and 1.9 percent for developing countries during the first decades of the new millenium, and slightly lower growth rates for developed countries. For a criticism of these projections, see WorldWatch Institute (1996). For an FAO defense, see FAO *Food Watch* (1996d). For an analysis of the debate about future yields, especially focusing on China, see Crosson (1996a). To put the debate in perspective consider this: In 1989, CIMMYT projected that wheat yields between 1987 and 2000 would grow at a rate of between 1.5 percent per year (the "realistic" estimate) and 2.3 percent per year (the "optimistic" estimate); the actual growth rate was 1.85 percent. (CIMMYT, Centro Internacional de Mejoramiento de Maize y Trigo, is the division of the Consultative Group on International Agricultural Research that focuses on wheat and maize research.) Box 14.7 presents some optimistic evaluations by crop scientists.

The optimistic beliefs cited above are based on several observations. A European study (see Penning de Vries et al. 1995 for a description) concludes that potential yields of cereal crops are close to 10 metric tons per hectare, compared to current yields of about 3 metric tons per hectare. Some dramatic reports about new technological breakthroughs have been published. A "super rice" developed in 1994 by the IRRI has potential yields of 15 tons per hectare, compared with current yields of about 5 tons per hectare. A new cassava strain promises yields that are ten times higher than current yields.

Biotechnology and genetically modified food. One source of optimism about future yield growth are the scientific advances in the field of genetic engineering and biotechnology. In the past few years, the issue of genetically modified food has become a subject of public debate and discussion. Genetic engineering creates new seed varieties that contain specific genetic characteristics. Genes from one organism can be inserted into the DNA another organism to create certain characteristics. To date, the most common types of genetic changes are the following:

- Plants are modified so that they contain a bacterium (Bacillus therogensis, or Bt) that is a natural pesticide. Thus these plants are protected from pest damage without being sprayed with a commercial chemical pesticide.
- Plants are modified so that they are particularly resistant to certain

---

Box 14.7   Agronomists' Perspective on Potential for Future Yield Growth

A 1998 symposium (Waterlow et al. 1977) heard a number of papers reviewing the scientific literature on specific ways that crop yields could be increased. The tone of the papers was optimistic.

"The rapid rise in yield potential and response to inputs . . . seems unlikely to be maintained beyond the next two decades . . . unless crop growth rates can be enhanced. Although these may . . . be limited by the photosynthetic rate, other process . . . may also have a significant effect. . . . Even in the absence of any further rise in genetic yield potential, crop yields could continue to rise with improvements in climatic adaptation, pest and disease resistance, and agronomic support." (Evans)

"I have no hesitation in stating that . . . plant biotechnology can bring major progress to tropical agriculture." (Van Montagu)

"Before writing this article I approached 10 or more leading exports on photosynthesis research throughout the world. . . . All agreed that the efficiency of photosynthesis in the field is far from the theoretical maximum and is restricted by environmental factors. . . . [Research into ways of] enhancing . . . protective and repair mechanisms [of plants] will help us to approach levels of photosynthetic efficiency observed under optimal/nonstressed conditions." (Barber)

"The possible prize for successful engineering of Rubisco [an enzyme that reduces photorespiration in plants] in the world's major . . . crops—an increase of 20% in the potential yield in temperate regions and of 50% in the tropics—must surely justify increased effort toward this single charge." (Long)

"Metabolic engineering of source-sink relationships is a promising approach to increase . . . genetic yield potential of cereal crops. . . . By combining the expression of several different transgenes . . . a significant increase in . . . crop yields may be achieved." (Choi et al.)

"With the availability of biotechnological tools . . . procedures for breeding genetically diverse parental lines and hybrids can be made more efficient." (Khush, Peng, and Virmani)

Other papers at the symposium discuss research efforts to promote tolerance to salinity and drought (Verma) and resistance to disease (Lamb).

weed killers. Therefore, the weed killers can be applied more heavily to kill weeds without killing the crop.

- Plants are modified to thrive in adverse conditions: for example, to be more resistant to disease or pests, or to be more tolerant of frost, drought, or saline soil.
- Plants are modified so that the crop has certain nutritional characteristics: for example, a potato that is rich in protein.
- Salmon grown in fish farms have been genetically modified to change their inbred eating habits and increase weight gain.
- Genetically modified microbes can be applied to soil to assist in nitrogen fixation.
- Genetically modified animals may produce more milk, less manure, and use feed more efficiently (CAST 2003).
- Pharmaceutical drugs can be produced in genetically modified plants and animals.

Genetically modified (GM) crops have been adopted by farmers in growing numbers since they were commercially introduced in the mid-1990s. Figure 14.6 shows the growth in worldwide acreage planted to GM crops. In 2002, 58.7 million hectares of land were planted in GM crops. Seventy-three percent of this land is in developed countries (almost all of it in the United States and Canada), and 27 percent is in developing countries (led by Argentina with 23 percent of the total GM land). Soybeans, corn, and cotton account for most of the GM land. Table 14.10 shows that more than half of the land planted to soybeans worldwide is planted with GM varieties. It is estimated that 60 percent of the food supply in the United States contains GM products either directly or indirectly, as when GM crops are fed to animals (James 2000).

Adoption of genetically modified varieties is growing faster in developing countries than in developed countries. One explanation for this is found in a 2003 paper by Qaim and Zilberman. They showed that some genetically modified crops that reduce pest damage may be especially effective in boosting yields in developing countries, where farmers are unable to afford commercial pesticides. The study examined cotton yields in India and found that Bt cotton had yields 80 percent higher than non–genetically modified varieties. However, the advantages of Bt to the farmer evaporate if the price of the genetically modified seed is too high. In a study of Bt cotton adoption in Argentina, Qaim and de Janvry (2003) found that the cost of the seed was twice as high as the average expenditures on chemical pesticides by farmers who adopted non-GM cotton.

Concerns about GM crops, especially food crops, have been so strong that many countries, notably those of the European Union, have banned their use. The EU ban on GM imports has been challenged in the World

Figure 14.6   Land Planted to Genetically Modified Crops, 1996–2002

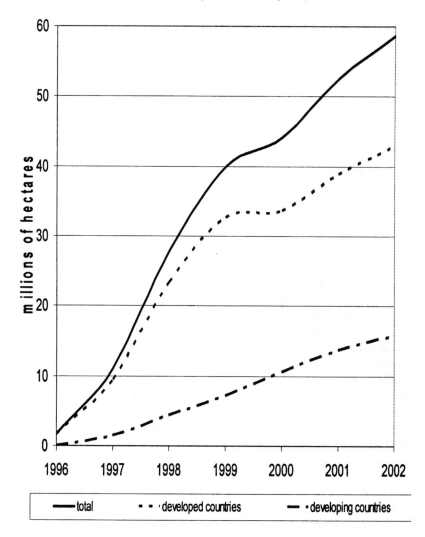

Source: James 2002.

Trade Organization as a violation of the EU's commitments to free trade. During the 2002 famine in southern Africa, some countries felt pressure to refuse food aid from countries that permitted GM crops, or refused to distribute GM food to their starving citizens. What are the concerns that drive opposition to GM crops?

Human health concerns about GM foods focus especially on allergies.

Table 14.10   Area Planted to Genetically Modified Crops, by Crop, 2002

Crop	Million hectares planted in GM crops	GM area as percent of total area in that crop
Soybeans	36.5	51
Maize	12.4	9
Cotton	6.8	20
Canola	3	12

Source: James 2002

For example, one kind of GM soybean includes a genetic sequence derived from the Brazil nut. Will a person who is allergic to Brazil nuts have an allergic reaction if exposed to the GM soybeans? How can a person who is assiduously avoiding foods with Brazil nuts know that he must also avoid this other food containing soybeans? To date no verified cases of allergic reaction to GM food have been found, but scientists do not fully understand the mechanisms of allergy, so the possibility of hidden allerginicity cannot be eliminated (see Haslberger [2003] for a recent discussion). The concern about allergies erupted into front-page headlines when the StarLink brand of GM maize, which had been FDA approved for animal feed but not for human food, was mistakenly used to make tortilla chips for a fast-food chain. In response to the publicity and a multimillion-dollar recall effort, twenty-eight people reported that they had possible allergic reactions to the products containing StarLink corn. However, further lab tests found that none of the twenty-eight were allergic to StarLink (Centers for Disease Control 2002).

A second human health concern arose out of experiments with rats in the United Kingdom. Researchers found that, when fed a diet of GM pota- toes the rats developed weakened immune systems (Ewen and Pusztai 1999). The research was criticized by the Royal Society for poor experi- mental design. The Royal Society review of the research found "no con- vincing evidence of adverse effects from GM potatoes" (Royal Society 1999:1). A further Japanese study on the effect of GM soybeans found no effect on the immune system (Teshima et al. 2000).

A third human health concern about GM foods is that they may pro- mote the evolution of diseases that are immune to antibiotics. One common method of genetic engineering is to introduce a virus containing the foreign gene into the host organism. The virus is constructed to contain an antibiotic- resistant marker gene to allow scientists to select the transformed cells. Thus, according to some scientists, "The urgent question which needs to be addressed is the extent to which genetic engineering biotechnology, by facilitating horizontal gene transfer and recombination, is contributing to the resurgence of infectious, drug-resistant diseases" (Ho et al. 1998:36). Other research (Jackson et al. 2001) shows that it may be possible to genetically engineer viruses to overcome the natural immune responses. The concern here is that the introduction of human and animal genes into field crops may lead to production of insect viruses bearing these human genes; in turn, these new viruses could be able to overcome natural immune responses in humans.

Other human health effects continue to be studied. The website *Biotech Info* (http://www.biotech-info.net/health_risks.html) carries up-to-date news on recent research.

Several environmental concerns about GM crops have been raised. The inclusion of the natural insectide (Bt) gene raises the possibility that non-target insects could be harmed by the GM crops. One of the earliest studies to raise this possibility suggested that monarch butterflies could be exposed to the Bt because they eat milkweed plants that grow near cornfields. However, a review of the findings by USDA's Agricultural Research Service (2003) found that "there is no significant risk to monarch butterflies from environmental exposure to Bt corn." However, other studies have shown possible impact of Bt crops on nontarget insect populations (see Wolfenbarger and Phifer [2000], table 2, for a review).

A second environmental concern is the possible development of a "superweed" that is resistant to insects and to commercial herbicides. If the genetic material that makes crops resistant to insects or to herbicides "escapes" into the genetic material of weeds, it may make the weeds difficult or impossible to get rid of (Snow 2002).

A third environmental concern is that GM organisms will upset the current ecological balance. For example, herbicide-tolerant crops lead to heavier application of herbicides and more complete elimination of weeds; but animals that feed on those weeds may be adversely affected. Also, genetic modifications can enhance an organism's ability to become an invasive species. GM crops may interbreed with wild relatives, ultimately leading to the extinction of the wild varieties (Wolfenbarger and Phifer 2000). More broadly, the concern that GM organisms may lead to an erosion in species diversity has been discussed, for example in Schaal (2003).

The above discussions suggest that there is a degree of uncertainty in the scientific community about the effects of biotechnology. The "precautionary principle" has been proposed to urge policymakers to oppose use of GM organisms until the scientific uncertainty is resolved and the organisms have been proven to be safe. Of course this raises the possibility that unscrupulous or ideological scientists could deliberately create or perpetuate uncertainty in order to achieve their own policy goals.

Not all environmental impacts of GM organisms are negative. Bt crops allow farmers to use less insecticide. Herbicide-resistant crops allow application rates and chemicals that may in the aggregate be less stressful on the environment. GM fish may reduce pressure to overfish wild stocks. The Council on Agricultural Science and Technology (CAST) convened a colloquium of agricultural scientists to discuss the overall environmental impact of GM organisms. They concluded that "biotechnology-derived [crops] . . . are consistent with improved environmental stewardship . . . [and] can provide solutions to environmental . . . problems" (CAST 2002:2).

Some opposition to GM organisms is based on political or ethical arguments rather than on scientific evaluations. Some doubt whether any social benefit can be derived from multinational corporations whose primary motivation is to increase their own profits. "The vast majority of scientific research being undertaken today is driven more by the goal of being first in line at the patent office than that of meeting profound social needs" (Dawkins 2003:39). A related argument is that GM crops put small subsistence farmers at a disadvantage and force farmers to deal with giant corporations on terms of unequal power. Other critics question whether our laws should permit a genetic sequence to be "owned," patented, and sold. Finally, some are uneasy about biotechnology for religious reasons, questioning whether the scientists are "playing God" with their experiments.

Balanced against the health, environmental, and other concerns about biotechnology are the benefits of increased yields. A panel of experts reporting to the World Bank and the Consultative Group for International Agricultural Research in 1997 concluded that GM crops could boost world crop yields by 25 percent. Nigeria's minister of agriculture, writing on the op-ed page of the *Washington Post*, states: "We do not want to be denied this [GM] technology because of a misguided notion that we don't understand the dangers or the future consequences. . . . The harsh reality is that, without the help of agricultural biotechnology, many will not live" (Adamu 2000).

■ Postproduction Food Losses

Before leaving the subject of food production, we should recognize that food consumption theoretically can be increased *without* increasing food production—if we can reduce losses between the field and the consumer (FAO, WFS Background Papers Nos. 4 and 8, 1996a). These losses are estimated as high as 30 percent (Erlich and Erlich 1991). In developing countries, postharvest food losses have been attributed to pests (Angé 1993), poor facilities for storage and transportation (James and Schofield 1990), and on-farm handling (FAO, WFS Background Paper No. 8, 1996a). One might think that postharvest food losses would decline as countries develop economically, because of improvements in roads, credit, and information. However, a study in the United States estimates that over 25 percent of food is lost in retailing, restaurants, and at-home consumption. So in rich countries there may be less food lost to pests and poor storage facilities, but more food is wasted by consumers or thrown away by restaurants.

15

Health-Related Causes of Undernutrition

All infectious diseases have direct adverse metabolic effects.
—Scrimshaw, Taylor, and Gordon 1968:12

Complex interactions among diet, disease, and physical characteristics determine the health and nutritional status of people, which in turn affects their enjoyment of life and ability to work.
—Bouis 1991:1

■ The Synergisms Between Nutrition and Health

A healthy person has a good appetite, likely has a good diet, digests his food well, and makes efficient use of it in his body. A well-nourished person can keep his immune system functioning at a high level and is likely to be healthy.

A sick person is likely to lose her appetite, have a poor diet, digest her food poorly, and use some of her nutrients to fight infection. A poorly nourished person suffers a weakened immune system and is susceptible to infections.

We see a positive feedback loop: Good health promotes good nutrition; good nutrition promotes good health. But when you look at it the other way around—poor health leads to poor nutrition and poor nutrition leads to poor health—you are more likely to call it a vicious circle.

Just as there are strong synergistic relationships between health and nutrition, infection exacerbates malnutrition and malnutrition exacerbates infection. This interrelationship is so important that the definitive review of the literature (Scrimshaw, Taylor, and Gordon 1968:267) concludes: "Where both malnutrition and exposure to infection are serious, as they are in most tropical and developing countries, successful control of these conditions depends upon efforts directed equally against both."

■ Infection Exacerbates Malnutrition

Infection increases the potential for and severity of malnutrition. Most common infections have a heavy impact on nutritional status in three important ways: (1) through loss of appetite or intolerance for food (e.g., vomiting); (2) through cultural factors (e.g., relatives of the sick individual substitute less-nutritious diets for the regular diet and administer purgatives, antibiotics, or other medicines that reduce absorption of specific nutrients); and (3) through loss of body nitrogen (protein).

This last pathway to malnutrition through infection (loss of nitrogen) is complex enough that it deserves separate discussion. What happens is that protein tissue in the body is used up to fight the infection. To manufacture such disease-fighting materials as interferon, white blood corpuscles, and mucus, the body needs amino acids, which it acquires in part by breaking down previously existing protein—chiefly from the muscles. This borrowing of muscle tissue for fighting infection is one of the reasons you feel so weak following a serious illness. It might seem reasonable to try to keep up the body's supply of protein during an illness through pushing food, but this is usually impracticable. Sick people often have little appetite. During convalescence, with an appropriate diet, the lost body protein is usually replaced.

Infection Promotes Dietary Deficiency
A reasonably healthy person who is presently on the borderline of nutritional deficiency may not show clinical signs of nutritional difficulties. But, owing to the above problems associated with infection, an illness can increase his nutritional deficiency, and he can then develop any one or more of a number of conditions caused by dietary deficiency (Scrimshaw, Taylor, and Gordon 1968:265):

- Keratomalacia (a softening and ulceration of the eye's cornea) caused by a shortage of vitamin A; if the shortage continues long enough and is severe enough, xerophthalmia (a dry, thickened, lusterless condition of the eyeball resulting in blindness) may ensue
- Scurvy (spongy gums, loosening of the teeth, and a bleeding into the skin and mucous membranes) caused by lack of ascorbic acid (vitamin C)
- Beri-beri (inflammatory or degenerative changes of the nerves, digestive system, and heart) caused by lack of thiamine (vitamin B_1)
- Pellagra (a condition marked by dermatitis, gastrointestinal disorders, and disorders of the central nervous system) resulting from insufficient niacin (one of the B-vitamins)
- Macrocytic anemia (anemia associated with exceptionally large red blood cells) caused by a deficiency of vitamin B_{12} or folic acid (one of the B-vitamins)

- Microcytic anemia (anemia associated with exceptionally small red blood cells) caused by a shortage of iron

In addition to the above, a number of studies show that low-birth-weight babies suffer more health problems as adults than do normal-birth-weight babies. These problems include high blood pressure, too much cholesterol and sugar in the blood, cardiovascular disease, and diabetes. Also, cataracts were significantly less likely to develop in elderly people who took vitamin supplements (or beta-carotene, or riboflavin and niacin). There is also evidence that undernutrition can increase the possibility that a person who is HIV-positive will graduate to full-blown AIDS. A study that followed HIV-positive men for seven years found those who consumed three to four times the RDA of niacin and vitamin A had a 40–50 percent lower chance of developing AIDS (Tang et al. 1993).

Diarrhea and Nutrition

The serious conditions noted above result from a specific dietary deficiency exacerbated by infection. But the most common instance of an illness seriously affecting nutritional status is that of undernutrition induced or exacerbated by a gastrointestinal infection (gastroenteritis) that causes diarrhea or, in its more extreme form, dysentery. An outstanding feature of kwashiorkor, for instance, is the frequency with which it is precipitated by an attack of acute diarrheal disease (Scrimshaw, Taylor, and Gordon 1968:27).

For the world as a whole, diarrhea is not as ubiquitous as the common cold, but in many third world localities it comes in a close second in frequency of occurrence. Diarrhea particularly affects children under five years old, and childhood fecal matter is a main source of the infective material. Food and water are key transmission routes. Children often make their first contact with diarrheal disease organisms through weaning foods (Martorell, personal comm.). In fact, an outstanding feature of diarrheal disease in the third world is the concentration of cases among children during and immediately after weaning (Durand and Pigney 1963), illustrated in Figure 15.1.

In poor countries, the onset of diarrhea at weaning time (so common that it has sometimes been called by the special name of *weanling diarrhea*) is typically acute and rapidly progressive, with liquid or semi-liquid stools, varying from three to as many as twenty a day. About one-fourth of patients have blood or mucus in the stools and, frequently, pus. Fever may be absent, but low-grade fever is usual, along with malaise, toxemia (buildup of toxic substances in the blood), intestinal cramps, and tenesmus (a distressing but ineffectual urge to evacuate the rectum or bladder). The usual clinical course runs four to five days. Repeated episodes can result in

Figure 15.1   Third World, Age-Specific Diarrheal Morbidity Rates

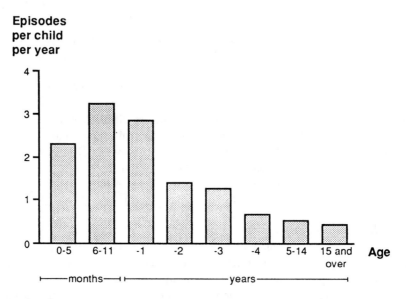

Source: Adapted from de Zoysa et al. 1985:8 using data from Snyder & Merson 1982.

a month or more total time spent fighting diarrhea during a year's time (Figure 15.2). In malnourished children a low-grade indisposition often continues for a month or more, sometimes as long as three months, with irregularly recurring loose stools, a progressively depleted nutritional state, and occasional recurrent acute episodes (Scrimshaw, Taylor, and Gordon 1968:220).

Although there are some twenty-five different organisms (bacteria, viruses, and parasites) that can cause diarrhea, all cases result in a shortage of water and salts (electrolytes) in the body. This dehydration of the body can be the most serious consequence of diarrhea. By the time a weanling child is seriously dehydrated from diarrhea, it is lethargic; its eyes are dulled and when it cries there are no tears; its skin is wrinkled like an old man's; it stops urinating; the fontanel (soft spot at the top of an infant's skull) is sunken. If you pinch the child's skin, it only slowly returns to the normal conformation (Goodall 1984). At best, this dehydration stands in the way of a quick recovery from the diarrhea. At worst (if the child loses more than 15 percent of his body fluids) it is fatal. A baby may well die within twenty-four hours of the arrival of these signs of serious dehydration. Some 60 to 70 percent of the 5 million annual diarrheal deaths are caused by this associated dehydration (WHO 1985c:6).

For generations, it was thought that the only way to replace these elec-

Figure 15.2   Diarrheal Illness, Developing Regions and Selected U.S. Sample

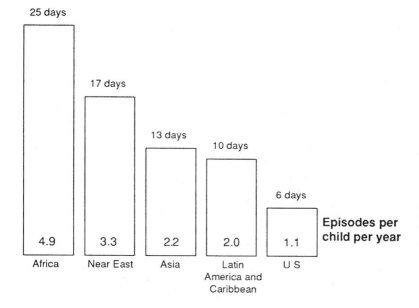

Average number of days per year with diarrhea

Source: Adapted from de Zoysa et al. 1985:11.
Note: An average episode of diarrhea is expected to last five days.

trolytes was through intravenous injection. Oral replacement using the salts alone simply did not work. In the late 1960s researchers in India and what is now Bangladesh found that merely adding common cane sugar to the missing salts produced a formula that worked by mouth. Called *oral rehydration therapy* (ORT), this simple technology was first used to fight cholera (the most virulent form of dysentery) in an epidemic in India in 1971. Since then it has become a third world public health mainstay and is being vigorously promoted by both the United Nations International Children's Fund (UNICEF) and the WHO. UNICEF (1987:8) has called ORT the cheapest and most effective health intervention that can be implemented in the home to decrease childhood mortality. UNICEF estimates that 1 million deaths per year are prevented by ORT. A brief explanation of how it works is provided in Box 15.1.

■ **Malnutrition Exacerbates Infection**

Malnutrition often amplifies the impact of infection. An example from the Philippines is illustrative. Severely undernourished children admitted to a

Box 15.1   Oral Rehydration Therapy (ORT)

Roger M. Goodall

The discovery that sodium transport and glucose transport are coupled in the small intestine so that glucose accelerates absorption of solute and water was potentially the most important medical advance this century.
—*Lancet* 1978, no. 2:300

In the normal healthy intestine, there is a continuous exchange of water through the intestinal wall. Every twenty-four hours, up to 20 liters of water is secreted and very nearly as much is reabsorbed. This mechanism allows the absorption into the bloodstream of the soluble breakdown products of digestion.

In a state of diarrheal disease, this balance is upset and much more water is secreted than is reabsorbed, causing a net loss to the body that can be as high as several liters in a day. If more than 15 percent of the body's fluid is lost, death occurs.

In addition to water, sodium is lost. The body's store of sodium is almost entirely in solution in body fluids and plasma. By contrast, 98 percent of the body's total potassium is held within cells.

For the proper functioning of the body, the concentration of sodium in the blood has to be held to within close limits (which perhaps correspond with the salinity of the archaic seas from which our evolutionary ancestors emerged eons ago). This sodium concentration is normally precisely controlled by the kidneys. However, in a state of dehydration water is conserved by the reduction or even complete absence of urination, and the kidneys cannot do their normal job of regulating sodium concentration. Continued diarrhea causes rapid depletion of water and sodium.

Simply giving a saltwater solution by mouth has no beneficial effect because, in the diarrheal state, the normal mechanism by which sodium ions are absorbed by the healthy intestinal wall is impaired, and if the sodium is not absorbed, the water cannot be absorbed either. In fact, excess salt in the intestinal cavity causes increased secretion of water into the intestine (through osmotic pressure), and the diarrhea worsens!

If glucose (also called dextrose) is added to a saline solution, a new mechanism comes into play. The glucose molecules are absorbed through the intestinal wall—unaffected by the diarrheal disease state—and in a process called cotransport coupling, carries sodium through the wall at the same time. This occurs in a one-to-one ratio: one molecule of glucose cotransporting one sodium ion. Glucose does not cotransport water. Rather it is the now increased relative concentration of sodium across the intestinal wall that pulls water through.

It was the discovery of the mechanism of cotransport of sodium and glucose that Dr. Kathleen Elliott, in an editorial in the prestigious British medical journal *Lancet,* described as potentially the most important medical advance of this century. *ORT is, in fact, the practical realization of this potential.*

While common table salt and ordinary white sugar are the dominant constituents of the recipe for oral rehydration salts (ORS) recommended jointly

(continues)

Continued

by the WHO and UNICEF, two other constituents are included: potassium chloride and sodium citrate.

Although 98 percent of the body's potassium is held within the cells, prolonged diarrhea will result in a loss of potassium. The loss of potassium from repeated diarrheal attacks over a period of time causes muscular weakness, lethargy, and anorexia. The typical distended abdomen of a chronically undernourished child is caused by loss of muscle tone in the abdominal wall largely attributable to chronic depletion of potassium.

Potassium is not involved in any way in the sodium-glucose cotransport mechanism. But restoring a potassium deficit promotes a feeling of well-being and stimulates the appetite. Although potassium is not absorbed as dramatically as is sodium during ORT, the effectiveness of the recipe is enhanced by its inclusion, especially for a child who has suffered repeated diarrheal attacks.

The loss of body salts and fluid leads to an inappropriate pH level in the blood, called acidosis, that is corrected by the addition of a base such as sodium citrate to the recipe. When account is taken of the different molecular weights of glucose and sodium and the needs of the body for the depleted salts, the completed recipe typically comes out as:

Sodium chloride, 3.5 grams
Sodium citrate, 2.5 grams
Potassium chloride, 1.5 grams
Glucose, 20.0 grams

The above to be dissolved in 1 liter of clean drinking water.

Research is going on at many centers around the world to develop new and improved versions of ORS. Other effective recipes are now in use. Some, for instance, substitute starch for sugar. In the intestine, starch is metabolized to glucose and therefore has the same properties of enhancing sodium absorption. However it has the added advantage that it has less osmotic effect (through this process sugar has some limited tendency to pull water back into the cavity of the intestine).

Although diarrhea always produces at least some dehydration, some of the more than twenty-five pathogens that cause it may strip the tips of the villi from large patches of the intestinal wall, leaving the inside of the intestine looking rather like a piece of velvet that has lost its nap. This decreases the surface area and can lower by more than 50 percent the specific absorptive capacities of the intestine. The result is malabsorption, which can cause or exacerbate undernutrition, most especially in a child already nutritionally compromised by repeated previous attacks of diarrhea.

Withholding food, even for one or two days, greatly exacerbates the undernutrition. This, coupled with anorexia, caused partly by chronic potassium depletion, results in a vicious circle: diarrhea causing undernutrition and undernutrition causing ever more frequent and severe diarrhea.

Source: More detail on this subject is available in the UNICEF information papers of Roger Goodall (1984). Goodall was formerly senior advisor on oral rehydration therapy and essential drugs to UNICEF. He is currently an independent consultant.

hospital for acute respiratory infection are found to be thirteen times as likely to die from the disease as children whose nutrition is normal (see Figure 15.3).

Malnutrition is almost always synergistic with intestinal diseases caused by worms or protozoa and with any disease caused by bacteria (Scrimshaw, Taylor, and Gordon 1968:263–264). That is, malnutrition aggravates the course of the disease, and the disease, in turn, intensifies the malnutrition.

A wide variety of nutrients have been demonstrated to have an impact on the competency of the body's immune system (Gershwin et al. 1985: 2; Phillips and Baetz 1980). The impact of nutrition on infection begins at birth and lasts throughout life. Not only is breast milk loaded with the appropriate nutrients for an infant's diet, but it carries with it a load of substances that help protect the infant against disease: immunoglobulins, macrophages, lymphocytes, neutrophils, components of the complement system, and so on (Rivera and Martorell 1988). (The complement system

Figure 15.3   Acute Respiratory Infection Mortality by Nutritional Status, Philippine Hospital Cases

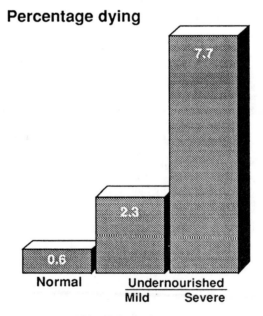

Percentage dying

7.7

2.3

0.6

Normal   Undernourished
                Mild   Severe

Nutritional status

Source: Adapted from Galway et al. 1987:23 using data from Tupasi 1985..

involves a set of more than eleven proteins normally found in the blood-stream. These proteins act in conjunction with the blood's antibody system in fighting infection, complementing the work of the antibodies.) Under-nutrition increases the duration of infections, especially diarrhea. Unequivocal evidence shows that the immune response is reduced in severe undernutrition, and some evidence suggests a diminished immune response in moderate undernutrition, particularly in wasted children (Rivera and Martorell 1988).

Worldwide, malnutrition is the most common cause of deficiencies in the immune system, even among adults. Two examples will help to illustrate this point: (1) Nutritional supplements given to the elderly have been found to improve their response to the influenza virus vaccine; and (2) among individuals given a vaccine to protect them from tuberculosis, a positive correlation between better nutrition and resistance to the disease was observed (Chandra 1988). Malnutrition interferes with various bodily mechanisms that attempt to block the multiplication or progress of infectious agents (Figure 15.4). The list of ways it can do this is long, but significant among them are a decrease in the response and activity of white blood

Figure 15.4   Protective Factors Instrumental in Health Maintenance

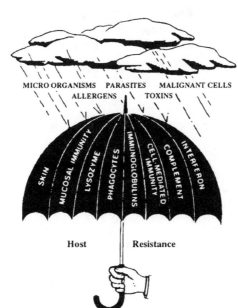

Source: Adapted from Chandra 1980.

corpuscles; a reduction in the production of interferon; a decrease in the integrity of the skin, the mucous membrane, and other tissues that serve to bar the entrance of infection; and interference with normal tissue replacement and repair (Scrimshaw, Taylor, and Gordon 1968:263–264).

The exploration of the mechanisms by which undernutrition affects the immune system has only just begun, but already we have enough information to provide interesting clues as to what is happening. For instance, the mucous membrane not only provides a physical barrier against the entrance of foreign particles that might cause infection (bacteria, viruses), but provides a chemical barrier as well. Mucus contains a variety of biochemical and immunological disease fighters, one of which is an enzyme called *lysozyme,* which has the capacity to attack the cell walls of invading bacteria. Colombian children suffering from protein-energy malnutrition were found to be producing reduced levels of lysozyme. In a process called cell-mediated immunity, T-lymphocytes play a key role attacking disease-causing microbes. Children with protein-energy malnutrition (PEM) are also likely to suffer an atrophied thymus, the organ primarily responsible for the "education" and proliferation of T-lymphocytes, and at the same time to produce fewer of these lymphocytes than expected when their bodies are challenged with invading disease organisms (Sherman 1986).

A final point we must remember: not only does malnutrition reduce resistance to infection, but it decreases stamina, which in turn decreases the capacity to cope with life and to perform on the job, making it more difficult to earn money to pay for transportation to healthcare centers, to pay for the services themselves, and to pay for appropriate drugs for combating infection.

PART 3

Policy Approaches to Undernutrition

In Part 2, we looked at the causes of undernutrition—vehicles by which undernutrition is delivered to families—and identified economic, demographic, agricultural, environmental, and health factors. The central focus of Part 3 is to explore public policy alternatives of interest to nutrition planners.

16

Philosophical Approaches to Undernutrition

In this section of the book, we consider policies that can be adopted to reduce the degree of worldwide hunger. Before proceeding, we spend a few pages exploring philosophical approaches to the issue. What motivates governments, societies, individuals, or groups of individuals to concern themselves with the issue of undernutrition? How does the motivation influence the policy decisions?

■ From the Standpoint of a Moral Philosopher

Charity or Concern for the Poor and Hungry
Our first chapter opened with a reference to starving Ethiopian babies— babies with bloated bellies, spindly arms and legs, and bodies too weak to sit up. The device is a standard technique for grabbing the attention of people attuned to Western culture and making them stop to think about the world food problem.

Those who live in the Western world are exposed to repeated appeals to conscience, asking them to join the battle to end hunger. In 1980, the Presidential Commission on World Hunger urged that the United States "make the elimination of hunger the primary focus of its relations with the developing world." Commenting on this in a paper written for a religious audience, McLaughlin (1984) said that "the moral and humanitarian reasons for such a policy seem self-evident."

A common argument in favor of studying and solving the world hunger problem is the moral dictate that each of us should help individuals who are less fortunate than ourselves. The pope's statement to the World Food Summit, for example, contains the following:

> In the analyses which have accompanied the preparatory work for your meeting, it is recalled that more than 800 million people still suffer from malnutrition and that it is often difficult to find immediate solutions for improving these tragic situations. Nevertheless, we must seek them together so that we will no longer have, side by side, the starving and the

261

wealthy, the very poor and the very rich, those who lack the necessary means and others who lavishly waste them. Such contrasts between poverty and wealth are intolerable for humanity.

It is the task of nations, their leaders, their economic powers and all people of goodwill to seek every opportunity for a more equitable sharing of resources, which are not lacking, and of consumer goods; by this sharing, all will express their sense of brotherhood. It requires "firm and persevering determination to commit oneself to the common good; that is to say, to the good of all and of each individual, because we are all really responsible for all" (Sollicitudo rei socialis, no. 38). This spirit calls for a change of attitude and habits with regard to life-styles and the relationship between resources and goods, as well as for an increased awareness of one's neighbour and his legitimate needs (Pope John Paul II 1996).

This is a matter of religious conviction or personal ethics. The motivation comes from within the individual. I may believe that I "owe" compassion to the hungry, but that debt is a product of my beliefs, something generated from within myself. In that regard, it is quite different from the debt I owe to the government as taxes.

Food as a Right

This distinction (between being motivated by personal ethics and being motivated by an obligation to society) is important as we consider a second type of moral argument about why we should be interested in the problem of world hunger. That is the issue of "food as a right." Some eighty-five countries have endorsed the International Covenant on Economic, Social and Cultural Rights (adopted by the United Nations General Assembly in 1966), which defined and formalized the right to food as a basic human right. The right to food was widely discussed in preparation for and during the World Food Summit of 1996 (Pinstrup-Andersen, Nygaard, and Ratta 1995; Alston 1997).

If food is a right, then hunger is a violation of that right, and we have a second ethical motivation to be concerned about hunger—the moral requirement that we seek justice and oppose violations of rights. There is a difference between the "charity" motivation (we have an ethical obligation to help the hungry) and the "justice" motivation (food is a right). That difference is illustrated by the following:

• If you accept the view that there is a fundamental right to food, then you are motivated to address the hunger problem even if you do not believe that you have a moral duty to help the poor and hungry. Your motivation here is simply to ensure the protection of that fundamental right.

• If you believe that you have a moral duty to help the poor, then you are motivated to address the hunger problem even if you do not believe that there is a fundamental right to food. Your motivation here is your duty to be charitable.

To illustrate this difference, consider the right to religious freedom. A Christian who embraces the concept of this right could simultaneously believe (1) that people have a right to worship as a Jew or Muslim, and (2) that nobody ought to exercise that right, because those religions deny the divinity of Christ. Or consider the right to "free speech." A person might simultaneously believe (1) that people have the right to read pornographic books, and (2) that nobody ought to exercise that right.

The assertion that people have a right to food is in this sense stronger than the assertion that people have a moral responsibility to help the poor and hungry. The latter is an assertion of a principle that will guide the speaker's behavior, and a plea to others to adopt the same principle. The former is an assertion that other people have a responsibility to help the poor and hungry even if those people do not choose to adopt the moral principle that would motivate that behavior. In other words, a coercive element is embedded in the "rights" assertion that is absent from the "moral principle" assertion.

The assertion that food is a right (or that people have a fundamental right to food and other necessities or "basic needs") is highly controversial. Let us consider some of the sources of controversy by means of analogies.

Consider a right that we accept as fundamental in the United States: the "right to remain silent" or the right not to incriminate oneself. We accept the existence of that right even when we disapprove of its exercise. For example, if a kidnapper refuses to tell where he has hidden his victim, we may doubly abhor the kidnapper for his silence as well as his violence. Furthermore, we do not seriously argue about whether we should adopt rules permitting police to torture suspects. The widespread acceptance of the right to remain silent sets this issue beyond the reach of political debate. It simplifies decisionmaking; we don't need to consider the pros and cons of any action, we need only to answer the question, "Does the action violate the right?"

This may explain why activists have pushed to have the right to food accepted as a fundamental right. They may hope to eliminate debate over the costs and benefits of various programs; the existence of the right trumps all other arguments. The FoodFirst Information and Action Network (FIAN 1997) fact sheet on "Twelve Misconceptions About the Right to Food" states that "governance is negotiable; rights are not." A panel of constitutional experts supporting the concept of economic rights stated: "Fundamental needs such as social welfare rights should not be at the mercy of changing governmental policies and programmes, but must be defined as entitlements." The intention of advancing the "right to food" concept is to force acceptance of more active government programs to combat world hunger without having to justify those programs economically.

The strongest objection to the concept of food as a right is that unlike traditional civil rights, which require government *not to act* in certain ways, economic rights appear to require the state *to act* in certain ways. Traditional civil or political rights do not require government to act. Consider the right to religious freedom, or the right to worship as one chooses. This right imposes on the state the restriction that it cannot pass laws or take actions that interfere with an individual's right to worship. Suppose you want to attend a Zoroastrian temple for weekly worship; but suppose the nearest such temple is in Chicago, and suppose further that you cannot afford to travel to and from Chicago each week. Does the government have any obligation to buy a weekly plane ticket for you? No, at least not as the right to religious freedom is interpreted in the United States.

Economic rights do not only require the government to avoid actions that would interfere with any individual's ability to obtain food; they additionally require the government to take actions to increase the ability of hungry people to obtain food.

The most extreme objections to the concept of economic rights assert that these rights are immoral themselves because they require government to limit the freedom of some members of the society. It is hard to conceive of any effective assertion of economic rights that does not require extensive redistribution of income from rich to poor. If we accept the argument that government limits on freedom are immoral, then any taxation is immoral, since the taxation itself is coercive, restricting individual liberties. But isn't taxation required to guarantee other civil rights? To ensure the right to be free of "cruel and unusual punishment," the government must use tax revenue to build new prisons. As long as it is costly to guarantee individuals their civil rights, some element of government coercion through the taxation system is necessary.

The word *rights* in the traditional sense refers to entitlements that are in most applications absolute. The U.S. government cannot censor a newspaper, or ban a religion, because those rights are absolute. Of course, it is easy to find examples of ways in which "absolute rights" are not absolute. The right of free speech does not extend to cover the right to yell "FIRE" in a crowded theater. The right of freedom of association (the right to choose your own friends) does not mean that an employer has the right to hire individuals of only one race. Absolute rights become limited only when the exercise of the right interferes with another person's exercise of his or her rights. The false yell of "FIRE" interferes with other people's right to congregate safely in a theater. Racial discrimination interferes with employees' rights to be free of discrimination. When one right conflicts with another, as in these cases, it is impossible to guarantee both rights absolutely.

On the one hand, what makes the concept of economic rights so controversial is that economic rights inevitably conflict with other rights because economic rights require government expenditures. On the other hand, the assertion that food is a right gives those who favor government intervention an important argument to use against libertarians. The civil libertarian argues: "The government cannot take my money (through taxes) to buy food for a poor person because I have a right to control my own property." (Notice how the assertion of a right is used to trump other arguments about whether a policy is a good or bad idea.) The hunger activist can respond: "You have a right to property; but the poor person has a right to food. This is a conflict of rights and the government has an appropriate role in settling that conflict."

Further, because economic rights are in inevitable conflict with rights to property, economic rights can never be absolute. So a right to food does not mean that as long as a single hungry person exists in the world, the United States cannot devote any government expenditures to defense, or student loans, or drug interdiction, or civil rights enforcement. We have competing social goals that must be pursued with limited resources.

Who decides the priorities for these competing social goals? In the United States, conflicts between rights are typically resolved in the court system, not by democratically elected representatives. This raises the additional question of whether we have a fundamental right to control the level of taxation through a political process. If we have no such right, then courts could require higher and higher taxes to ensure economic rights. If there *is* such a right (to a social contract on taxes), then this right must be balanced against economic and other civil rights.

If we maintain the current system of establishing priorities through a political process, we impose a severe limit on economic rights. The process of simultaneously "guaranteeing" economic rights and property rights is really no different that the process of setting policy goals and balancing competing interests.

■ From the Standpoint of an Economist

The last section started as a discussion of moral imperatives, moved on to the notion that the assertion of a right makes economic policy analysis unnecessary, and ended by raising the question: How should we allocate scarce resources to accomplish competing objectives? This question covers familiar ground for economists. Whether the trade-offs are made by courts, legislatures, or administrators, the economic rule for policymaking is *maximize total benefits minus total costs* (see Posner 1986). Much of the remainder of the book will look at policy from the standpoint of an economist; before proceeding, we lay out some of the basic doctrines of economic policy analysis, and critiques of those doctrines.

Perhaps the questions they ask say more about economists than the way they answer those questions. The two questions that identify the asker as an economist are: (1) What is the right, or appropriate, policy for the society as a whole? (2) How can government best manipulate human greed to achieve its policy objectives?

What Is the Best Policy?

A political scientist wants to know: What do different people or different groups care about? Then: How will those differences in those objectives be resolved? What political processes will be involved in resolving those conflicts? What are the levers of power and who controls those levers?

Economists start at the same place: What do different people want? And in one sense economics is inherently about resolving conflict; after all, the buyer wants to pay a low price and the seller wants to receive a high price. But from the economists' perspective, there is some ideal way of balancing the conflicts. Any decision or choice imposes costs on some people and provides benefits to some people. The economists ideal (at least in its simplest and purest form) says that the best choice is the one that maximizes the extent to which benefits exceed costs.

Policymaking as a rational process.   Economists implicitly view policymaking as a rational orderly process managed by benevolent, well-informed, rational, analytical policymakers. This view tends to be so ingrained in the economics literature that many professional economists may not have even considered that they have adopted this view. If pushed on the subject, few even among economists would say that this is a realistic view—that policies are actually made according to this idealized process. Nor do economists really propound this as the way policy should be made; certainly it would be nice (in the minds of economists) if policy were made like this, and the policy outcomes are likely to be improved if made this way, but no one can conceive of a practical way of implementing such a process, except perhaps through the dictatorship of an enlighted well-trained economist, and no one is striving to have such a process implemented.

Economists do their analytical work in the hopes of tweaking the consciences of the actual policymakers, saying in effect, "Of course you can do whatever you want, but a benevolent, well-informed, rational, analytical policymaker would do the following . . ." The hope here is that actual policymakers who like to think of themselves as benevolent, well informed, etc., will adopt the recommended policy to avoid the shame of doing otherwise.

This idealized view of the policymaking process is that policy debates are more like scientific inquiries than like forensic debates. The scientific method presumes that truth is discovered through a series of interchanges among scientists who share the same objective—uncovering the truth. In jurisprudence, the truth is presumed to be arrived at through an adversarial contest of advocates. The prosecutor presents the very best case as to why the defendant should be found guilty, and the defense presents the very best case as to why the defendant should be found not guilty; the judge or jury, balancing those two cases, comes to a decision (in most cases) in which one side wins and the other side loses; the defendant is found guilty of the charge or not guilty.

An example of a real-world policy decision. Let us consider a concrete policy example. (This is a fictitious example, but closely resembles a policy decision that might be made in the real world.) The government has built a dam and reservoir and every year must decide how much water to release from the reservoir to provide irrigation water for farmers. If the water is left in the reservoir, it will provide a healthy habitat for fish and birds, and be a place where people can enjoy outdoor recreation (hiking, canoeing, sport fishing, and birdwatching). Of course, the policymakers can release none, some, or all of the water from the reservoir.

How does an economist look at the issue? We use this example to illustrate a number of important points.

• *Point 1: Every action has costs and benefits.* There are benefits (to farmers) from releasing the water—the farmers will use the water for irrigation that will increase crop yields and therefore increase the farmers' profits. But there are costs (to fish and wildlife and people who value these) associated with releasing the water.

• *Point 2: "Declining marginal benefits" and "Increasing marginal costs."* As described in Chapter 7, economists make frequent use of the concepts of "marginal costs" and "marginal benefits." Benefits to farmers increase as the quantity of water released increases—but the benefits increase at a decreasing rate. The costs to habitat increase as the quantity of water increases—and increases at an increasing rate.

• *Point 3: The economist's ideal decision: where marginal costs equal marginal benefits.* Just as the boy with the berries in Chapter 7 based his decision on marginal cost and marginal benefit, so too, say economists, should policymakers. To apply this rule to the hypothetical water allocation example above, the ideal water allocation would be to continue to release water until the point is reached where the marginal benefits (the increased value of crops attributable to the last 1,000 gallons released) just equals the marginal costs (the additional value of environmental amenities lost by the last 1,000-gallon release).

• *Point 4: Under certain circumstances, an unfettered free market allocates resources in the optimal way.* One way to reach the optimum is to sell each increment of the water to the highest bidder. If a coalition of hikers, canoeists, conservationists, and environmentalists submits the winning bid, that increment of water stays in the reservoir; if a coalition of farmers submits the winning bid, the water gets released for irrigation. This will result in the optimal allocation of water. If you are unconvinced by our claim, consider the following action during the auction. The auction of the first unit of water is won by the environmentalists; they are willing to pay (in our imaginary example) a lot more than the $23,000 farmers are willing to pay for their first increment. At some point, perhaps after nearly all of the water has already been bought by the environmentalists, they are not willing to pay more than $23,000 for an increment, and the farmers win that. The farmer's win a second increment because they are willing to pay $20,000 and environmentalists are willing to pay only $9,000. A third increment will end in a tie, with both groups bidding $15,000.

This means that if the water were owned by a private owner whose selfish objective was to make as much money as possible, the water would be allocated in a way that is socially optimal. This is an expression of Adam Smith's "invisible hand," and explains why economists do not think of free competitive markets and private enterprise as inherently bad.

But economists recognize that there can be a number of problems with markets that cause the "market solution" to be different from the social optimum. Some of those problems are discussed in the next section.

■ Criticisms and Extensions of the Simple Policymaking Rule

Having laid out the general tenets of how economists define an "optimal policy," we now explore some finer points, including criticisms of the simple rule as laid out above.

Objectivity and Prejudices and the Role of Economics in Policymaking

In the simple example, there is a clear, apparently objective, answer to the question "What is the best policy?" If we provided the above example of marginal costs and benefits and asked twenty randomly chosen economists to identify the optimal policy, most likely all twenty would come to the same conclusion.

But does this mean that economists never disagree with each other about policy? Clearly, the answer to this question is a vehement "NO." Economists have prejudices or opinions about policy that influence their evaluations. An economist knows how to undertake an objective analysis, but if that analysis arrives at a conclusion that contradicts her prejudice, she may decide that her prejudice needs to be reexamined, or she may decide that there was some mistake in the analysis.

Of course, an easy way to cleave to the economist's dictum ("the optimal choice is where marginal cost equals marginal benefit") and come to a different conclusion about the optimal policy is to dispute the empirical basis of the decision. An economist with an environmentalist prejudice may say, "Release 2,000 gallons?!?!?! That can't be right; it's much too high. How did my analysis lead me to this conclusion? Oh, I see. The numbers are clearly skewed in a pro-farmer way." We will examine some of the ways that numbers can be wrong in their basic development below. For now, suffice it to say that if we raise our estimate of the value of environmental amenities, then the "optimal" water release drops. In exactly the same way, an economist with a pro-farmer prejudice may be shocked that the analysis leads to a recommendation of such a small amount (in his opinion) of water being released, and may find "mistakes" in the underlying data—"Farmer benefits from water are grossly understated," might be this economist's claim.

On the one hand, this recognition of how economists actually analyze and debate policy undercuts their claim to scientific objectivity. However, this also illustrates a major strength of the economics approach: people on different sides of an issue (people with different prejudices) are forced to think in a careful and orderly way about what their opinions are based on; they are forced to define terms clearly; they are forced to produce and to defend empirical data supporting their position. In a policy debate among economists, sincere conviction and clever phrasing count for little.

Comparability of Costs and Benefits
and the Dollar Valuation of Intangibles

You have read the above description of how economists think about policy. If you read it uncritically, you may not have noticed that we slipped something by you—we put the costs and benefits in dollar terms so that they could be compared to each other. This is the aspect of economic analysis that is most nettlesome to many thoughtful noneconomists. Suppose, at some level of water release from the reservoir in our example, a species of fish that lives only in that reservoir dies off and becomes extinct; how do you put a dollar value on that species? Or suppose that the food produced with the water used for irrigation saves ten people who otherwise would die of undernutrition; how do you put a dollar value on those lives?

For many items, economists measure costs and benefits by prices determined in a competitive market. So, in our example, the value of increased production from irrigation can be measured using the market price of the crops grown. Even this has a controversial side, as we will discuss in more detail below. But for other goods that are not traded in markets, the problem of valuation is trickier. What, for example, is the value of a species of fish that might become extinct under certain policy choices? Economists have developed ways to assign dollar values to these nontraded commodities by conducting surveys that ask, for example, "How much would you be willing to pay to protect this fish from extinction?" or "How much would we have to pay you to compensate you for the loss of this species of fish?"

The underlying assumption that everything can be valued in dollar terms is troubling to many people. For example, there are those who would say to the fish extinction survey question: "It is wrong to take an action that would deliberately lead to the extinction of a species. In one sense, the value of protecting the species is very high to me; to compensate for the loss of the species you would have to pay me an infinite amount (or some arbitrarily high number). But I am opposed to the idea that I should be required to pay money to preserve the species; therefore I am not willing to pay anything to preserve the species."

The issue of putting a dollar value on things is especially troubling when it comes to human life. What is a human life worth? That may seem at first a horribly crass question to ask. But government policy has to deal with that question in many different contexts (the numbers in the examples below are entirely made up for the purposes of illustration).

- Requiring every car to have a seatbelt and an air bag will increase car prices by $800 (or $800 million over the 1 million cars sold each year), but will save twenty thousand lives in auto accidents; do the benefits from the law exceed the costs?
- Requiring all cars to drive no faster than 10 miles per hour will reduce national output by $1 trillion, but will save five thousand lives in auto accidents; do the benefits from the law exceed the costs?
- Requiring all vegetables sold to be tested for pesticide residues will cost $50 billion per year, but will save fifteen lives; do the benefits exceed the costs?

Even more difficult are cases where lives are saved by restricting people's liberty, or by forcing them to take actions they believe are wrong—for example, forcing parents to immunize their children when the parents have religious beliefs that prohibit immunization.

Market Prices, Market Allocations of Resources, and the Distribution of Income

The market works, as described above, in allocating resources among their various alternative uses. Over the past hundred years, a lot of the labor force in the United States shifted from farm work in the early 1900s to factory work in the mid-1900s, to producing services and entertainment by the end of the century. This shift in resource allocation was driven largely by market forces. As profitable opportunities developed in manufacturing, the market directed more resources into factories. As profitable opportunities developed in the health services sector, the market directed more resources into hospitals.

If we take a step back, a troubling question arises: Why did the market direct resources toward the production of a television show or a sporting event, rather than toward the production of more food in a world where millions of people are undernourished? If you think of the market as a election in which goods are produced in levels that depend on how many votes they get, the people with more dollars to spend get more votes than the people with fewer dollars to spend. Theoretical economists recognize that the "social optimum" achieved by perfectly competitive markets is an optimum that can be defined for a given distribution of income and that draws no conclusions about what distribution of income is appropriate.

Externalities and the Optimum

There is one set of circumstances that economists recognize as a common reason why competitive markets may not lead to a social optimum: when a decision made in the market by a buyer and a seller have benefits that accrue to or costs that are borne by others. Because these costs and benefits go to people outside the market transaction, they are referred to as "externalities" or "external costs" and "external benefits."

To return to our reservoir-water example, suppose that farmers bought a certain amount of water and it was released out of the reservoir; homeowners along the river between the reservoir and the farmers would get an external benefit from the release: they would be able to swim or boat or fish, and they would get these benefits without paying for them, but the benefits only exist because someone else (the farmers) *did* pay for the water release. In measuring the costs and benefits of water release, the market has taken into account only the private benefits of the farmer (who participates in the market), and not the full social benefits (that would include the benefits to the river users). In a case where there are external benefits, the amount that is bid for the good is lower than its true social value and the market price is "too low" and quantity provided is "too low" compared to what would be a social optimum.

An external cost might occur if someone who never visited the reservoir enjoyed watching birds who summered in the reservoir and then migrated many miles away to where the bird watcher lived. Releasing water imposes a cost on this distant bird watcher that would not be reflected in the bids for water by the reservoir users. In this case the social costs would exceed the private costs.

■ Economic Incentives and Human Behavior

A second insight of economics is that personal materialistic satisfaction is a strong motivation of human behavior.

Of course, if you think about your own behavior, you will be able to identify a lot of other motivations: a sense of honor or a sense of duty, a desire to be liked, or to be admired, etc. Some of these motivations are appealed to by advertisers: to get people to buy more of our product, we will run ads to convince people that if they buy our product others will think that they are "cool." But even marketing experts recognize that people respond to materialistic motivations: to get people to buy more of our product, we will lower the price.

In our study of the problem of world hunger and policies to deal with that problem, this insight will enter in at least three ways:

• We will see how economic incentives can be and have been used to achieve policy objectives. For example, policies that make it more expensive to have children have been successful in reducing population growth, and policies that make it more expensive to degrade the environment have been successful in reducing environmental degradation. In this context, we will see that assigning and enforcing property rights are often an integral part of creating economic incentives.

• The production of goods also responds to economic incentives; the more you materially reward people for producing a certain good, the more that good will be produced. The implication of this is that the distribution of goods influences the quantity of goods available for distribution.

• The third aspect of incentives and human behavior that will be important in our study of the world food problem has to do with the dynamic nature of production. As a commodity or resource becomes more scarce, or as increased demand for the commodity or resource bids its price up, people respond by finding ways to use the resource more efficiently, by finding ways to produce the commodity or make the resource available more cheaply, and by finding alternatives to the commodity or resource.

On the second point, a mistake that noneconomists frequently make in discussing policy options is to conceive of the policy problem as one of how to distribute a fixed stock of goods. For example, we noted that there is sufficient food available for human consumption in the world so that every person could consume his/her caloric requirements. Many people when they hear this think, "So the problem is just one of distribution. If people in developed countries just consumed less, the extra food could be used in the developing world, and the undernutrition problem would be solved." The first sentence is true: the problem can be thought of as a distribution problem. But the second sentence is false, or at least grossly misleading.

The amount of food that is available for human consumption depends on the amount of food that farmers worldwide produce. And the amount that farmers produce depends on the economic incentive—the price farmers receive for their output. If people in rich countries made a concerted effort to consume less food—if they spent less money on food and more on items other than food—then the price farmers receive would drop and farmers would produce less food; in the world economy as a whole, resources would move from production of food into production of nonfood items. There would be a positive effect on the undernutrition problem in poor countries, but the effect would be much smaller than imagined by those who think, "If I consume 1,500 fewer calories each day, then that food can be given to people in poor countries, and three people there can each have an extra 500 calories per day."

In order to get this kind of a redistribution to work, the rich person would have to continue to buy the food (or at least to pay for its production in some way) and then donate the 1,500 calories per day to the poor people.

The energy crisis of the 1970s provides excellent examples of the human responses to economic incentives. During the 1970s oil prices shot up dramatically. Many people perceived this as an inevitable result of growing demand for a fixed resource, and therefore predicted that prices would continue to rise. But the high prices for petroleum products caused a number of reactions over time. People began to use the resource more efficiently: auto gas mileage increased, and people began to insulate their homes more effectively. Oil exploration companies discovered new sources of oil and developed ways to pump more of the oil out of the ground. Alternative energy sources—nuclear, solar, and wind power— grew. As a result of these reactions, prices of oil and gas did not continue to rise.

■ Economics and the World Food Problem

How do these economic insights apply to the problem of worldwide undernutrition? What is the "optimal" nutrition policy? What kinds of government programs can be used to achieve the objective of reducing undernutrition?

Optimal Policy to Reduce Undernutrition

The benefits of reducing undernutrition are obvious: lives saved, health improved, productivity increased. For an individual case, the costs of achieving adequate nutrition are remarkably low. In countries with an average calorie deficit (see Table 6.5 for a partial list), 250 calories per person per day would erase the deficit. (Though derived in a different way, this is consistent with the FAO estimates of average calorie deficits among people who are undernourished, ranging from about 100 to 500 calories per person per day [see FAO, SOFI 2001].) Two hundred and fifty calories is about the equivalent of a peanut butter sandwich (two slices of bread and 2 tablespoons of peanut butter is 370 calories). The cost of a peanut butter sandwich is 35 cents. $6,400 invested at 2 percent interest would pay interest of 35 cents a day. Thus, we can conclude that there are a substantial number of people whose lives could be saved at a cost of $6,400. Compare this to an estimated "value of human life" of $150,000 to $360,000 found in a study of Indian manufacturing workers (Simon et al. 1999).

Or, compare this $6,400 figure to the estimated costs of saving a life implicit in policy choices made in the United States, shown in Table 16.1. Saving lives by means of improved nutrition is an incredible bargain. Economic analysis here serves only to raise the question: If the benefit-cost ratio is so favorable, why haven't policymakers leapt to make the investments necessary to substantially eliminate undernutrition?

There are a couple of possible answers. The first has to do with targeting. The calculation above assumes that the peanut butter sandwich actually gets eaten by a person who is undernourished. But in reality food donations are sometimes diverted to people who are not undernourished. A January 2004 report (Strategy Page 2004) on the situation in North Korea states:

> The current food crisis is a result of foreign donors refusing to contribute food for North Korea because the government has not allowed foreigners to observe where the donated food goes. Other witnesses have consistent-

Table 16.1 Dollar Costs per Life Saved of Various Regulations in the United States

Government Action	Cost per Life Saved
Requiring seat belts and air bags in cars	$100,000
Banning flammable sleepwear for children	$1,200,000
Requiring seat belts in rear seats of cars	$3,800,000
Restricting arsenic emissions from glass-manufacturing plants	$40,200,000
Banning asbestos	$329,000,000

Sources: Viscusi and Gayer 2002; Viscusi 1993:1912–1946.

ly reported that the donated food goes to the armed forces and is not sent to areas where there has been unrest, or where the government suspects there might be unrest (because a number of locals have fled to China or Russia). . . . New supplies will not arrive for several months. But after that, the food aid could dry up again if the North Korean government does not become more cooperative.

From a human standpoint, it is natural to want to avoid being "conned"—tricked into making charitable donations to people who do not deserve our charity. From an economic standpoint, however, even if only one in ten of the donations hits its mark, the program would still be more cost effective than any of the policy steps listed in Table 16.1. A more cynical answer is that the people dying from lack of seatbelts or from asbestos are "like us" and therefore it is worth the high cost to save those lives. We can empathize with the people who would die in the absence of the government policy, but we imagine the people dying from undernutrition are "not like us"—we cannot imagine being that poor, therefore our empathy is low. Subramanian and Cropper (1995) cite other unfunded programs that would save lives at a low cost.

Finally, the $6,400 figure above is the cost of saving a single life, without taking into account any impacts on market prices that would occur if the policy were aimed at reducing undernutrition among many of the 800 million suffering from it. As subsequent chapters will explain, a large-scale program would increase food prices and environmental costs associated with increased food production.

Policy Instruments to Reduce Undernutrition

Economic analysis has a lot more to contribute to the question: What kinds of policy actions can contribute to reduced undernutrition? Most of the rest of the book is devoted to some answers to this question. The supply-demand framework helps organize the discussion.

Chapter 8 emphasized the two elements of the food security equation—income and price. For the most part, our policy discussion can be broken down into policies that influence income and policies that influence price.

Policies to raise incomes of the poor. Chapter 18 will discuss policies that raise the incomes of the poor. There are two possibilities: redistributing income from rich to poor, or improving the rate of economic growth.

The main economic rationale for redistributing income from the rich to the poor is the belief in declining marginal utility of income. Above, we discussed the principle that as food consumption increases, unit by unit, declining marginal benefits (or "decreasing marginal utility") accrue from adding an additional unit. Many economists accept the hypothesis that this principle can be extended to cover the consumption of all goods taken together: thus, a decreasing marginal utility of income.

A direct implication of this is that a dollar is worth more to a poor person than to a rich person. On the one hand, the idea is that a couple of more dollars to a poor person will be spent on "necessities"—items that are fundamental to life. On the other hand, taking a couple of dollars away from a rich person will cause that person to consume fewer frivolous things. Therefore, this transfer from rich to poor increases the "common good." This may explain why governments are motivated to adopt programs that have the effect of redistributing wealth from the rich to the poor.

The practical problem is that the "declining marginal utility of income" hypothesis implies that appropriate policy is a total and complete equality of income distribution. If one person in the country (or the world) earns slightly more than another, then dollars should be taken from the former and given to the latter. Most people reject this policy prescription. That rejection raises questions about whether this is the true explanation for policy concern about the poor and hungry.

There is much literature on the subject of what kinds of policies may promote general economic growth. Our discussion in Chapter 18 will give a general overview. In it we will address the issue of "globalization" and whether integration into the global economy can be beneficial to growth rates in developing countries.

Policies to reduce the price of food.   Chapters 19 through 23 will consider a variety of policies that may cause of price of food to be lower than it otherwise would be. Chapter 19 discusses population control policies. If population growth can be reduced, the demand curve for food will not shift out as fast, food supplies per capita will be higher, and food price will be lower than they otherwise would have been.

Chapters 20 through 23 consider policies that target food prices more directly. These policies can be thought of in one of two ways. They can distort the social equilibrium and cause a reduction in economic efficiency, or they can correct a distortion and increase economic efficiency.

If the aggregate supply-and-demand curves represent the true social costs and benefits, then policies that alter the equilibrium price are "distortionary"—they reduce economic efficiency. This is illustrated in Figure 16.1, wherein a government policy creates a wedge between the price that consumers pay and the price that farmers receive. Perhaps the program is one that sells food to consumers at below cost, or perhaps the program pays subsidies to farmers, or perhaps the subsidy is paid to firms in the processing or marketing sector. In any case, the price received by farmers is higher than the price paid by consumers (the difference between the price at point A and the price at point D in the figure).

Figure 16.1   Impact of a Policy that Subsidies Production or Consumption

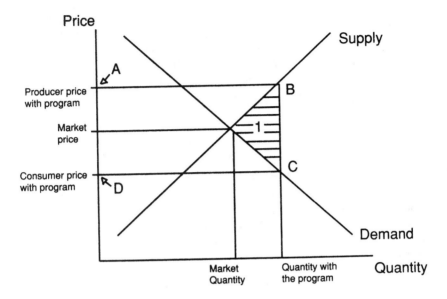

This type of policy achieves the direct objective we are looking for here: quantity increases (from the "market quantity" to the "quantity with the program" in the figure). But the policy reduces economic efficiency. As the quantity produced increases above the market quantity, the cost of producing an additional unit exceeds the value that consumers get from consuming the additional unit. The quantity of this efficiency cost is shown as the shaded triangle in Figure 16.1. Subsidies also have a direct cost paid by the government. This is the amount paid per unit (producer price minus consumer price) times the number of units. This cost is shown as rectangle ABCD in the figure.

But policies that change prices can sometimes be seen as "corrective." For example, we discussed above the possibility that production or consumption of a good might create external benefits that are not reflected in the market supply-and-demand curves. In this case, the market equilibrium quantity will be lower than the optimum, and a government policy to subsidize consumption or production may correct the situation.

Economist Arnold Harberger (1983) suggested that we all (or at least many of us) suffer when any person in the world (or country or ethnic group or family) suffers from undernutrition or failure to meet "basic needs." When a hungry person is fed, a direct benefit goes to that person (which benefit is reflected in the market transaction), but also an indirect benefit goes to us, because we care about human suffering. This indirect benefit is external to the market. Because such a reduction affects our happiness, we would be willing to pay to see the incidence of hunger reduced or eliminated. The reduction of hunger is a good: the more it happens, the better we feel. But there is no market on which we can purchase this good. This is a case of missing markets, or *externalities*. Private action is unlikely to solve this problem. Because we know others also care, we may wait for *them* to take actions to reduce hunger, in which case *we* get the good (reduced world hunger) free of charge. Government action may be justified in creating an artificial market by collecting money from each of us who derives satisfaction from reductions in hunger, and using that money to reduce hunger.

Chapter 22 will examine another kind of corrective action: removing distortive policies that actually *reduce* food output and consumption. Chapter 23 will discuss policies that cause the aggregate supply curve to shift out, increasing output and reducing price. These policies include investments in research and development, where private markets may underinvest. They also include government interventions to correct market failures in the provision of loans to farmers.

17

Policies Aimed at Health-Related Causes of Undernutrition

If we could increase the health spending in the developing countries by only $2 per head, we could immunize all their children, eradicate polio, and provide the drugs to cure all their cases of diarrheal disease, acute respiratory infection, tuberculosis, malaria, schistosomiasis and sexually transmitted diseases.
—Hiroshi Nakajima, director general of the WHO, in WHO 1989:1

This chapter is a companion to Chapter 15. The remaining chapters on policy deal with policies to reduce undernutrition by making food more affordable. But Chapter 15 reminded us that the morbidity and mortality associated with undernutrition are in fact a combination of undernourishment and health problems. Therefore, before proceeding to a discussion of policies designed to improve nutrition, we discuss policies that may improve public health.

■ The Economic Efficiency of Public Health Programs
In Chapter 15 we noted the positive feedback loop between good health and good nutrition: good health promotes good nutrition, and good nutrition promotes good health. In recent years experts have said that, by and large, it is cheaper to maintain good health than it is to make people well after they get sick. This idea is coloring many of the current healthcare developments in the third world, which are emphasizing low-cost delivery of health services to the poor. We see "barefoot doctors" in China, "nutrition huts" in the Philippines, and "health huts" in Haiti.

Actually, we have known of the economic efficiency of public health programs for a long time, and, despite the emphasis in many Western countries on private healthcare, governments have been sponsoring public health services in the West for many years. Modern engineering principles were applied to water-borne sewage disposal systems in the West during the 1840s. By the early 1900s it was common for local governments in the Western world to consider the supply of drinking water properly within their purview. In the twentieth century, public programs promoting the iodization of salt and the fortification of flour with vitamins became routine in the West. (The history of such programs in the United States is outlined in Box 17.1.) Third world countries now sponsor parallel public programs for drinking water, sewage, food fortification, and salt iodization (see Box 17.2).

The present emphasis on publicly sponsored, low-cost primary health-care for the poor is relatively recent. Most common third world illnesses

---

Box 17.1 A Brief History of Food Fortification in the United States

Richard Ahrens

The leading cause of draft deferment in the United States during World War I was the swelling of the thyroid gland called goiter. One problem associated with goiter was that boys who had the condition could not fit into the tight collars of the military uniforms. In 1923 the Harding Commission, appointed by President Warren Harding, recommended a voluntary program for the iodization of salt to combat goiter. A gentlemen's agreement was worked out between the salt companies and the executive branch of the government that there would be no price difference charged between the iodized and uniodized product.

During Word War II a bill was introduced into Congress that would have made it mandatory that all table salt be iodized, but the bill was defeated in committee when a number of medical doctors testified that there were probably some people in the United States who were sensitive to iodine and who would have skin problems as a result of being unable to obtain iodine-free salt.

Fortification of flour arose at the start of World War II, after President Franklin Roosevelt asked the National Academy of Sciences (NAS) to evaluate the nation's readiness for war. As one of their recommendations, the NAS came up with a proposal to ask flour millers to fortify wheat flour with iron, thiamin, riboflavin, and niacin. The flour fortification program became policy in 1940 and was looked after by the U.S. War Department. Later it became the province of the U.S. Department of Health, Education and Welfare, and now it is the province of the U.S. Food and Drug Administration.

A recommendation to increase substantially the iron fortification of enriched flour and bread came out of the 1969 White House Conference on Food, Nutrition, and Health, and in 1973 the Food and Drug Administration proposed to triple the iron-enrichment level in flour. Several experts recommended against this proposal because doing so would exacerbate a problem of iron toxicity (hemochromatosis) among some hundred thousand people, and by 1977 the idea of upping the iron level in flour was dropped.

Source: Richard Ahrens is professor emeritus, of nutrition at the University of Maryland.

Box 17.2 Food Fortification in the Third World

Eileen T. Kennedy et al.

Countries in which a single grain product supplies a disproportionate share of the total dietary intake consistently show a higher prevalence of micronutrient deficiencies. Fortification intervention schemes have been put into effect in order to alleviate this problem.

Fortification is a process whereby nutrients are added to a food to maintain or improve its quality; protein, amino acids, vitamins, minerals, and fat are all fortifications that can be added to a food. In order for fortification to be feasible and effective, a carrier for a particular fortificant must be consumed regularly and in sufficient quantity. As such, staples such as grains, sugar, salt, monosodium glutamate (MSG), and other condiments have been used as carriers in fortification interventions.

To serve as carriers, however, these staples must pass through the market. Thus, fortification of staples produced for consumption on the farm is not usually feasible, and malnourished members of semisubsistence farm households cannot usually be reached by this approach.

Micro-level fortification interventions have been regarded as a relatively easy method of alleviating some forms of malnutrition among food-purchasing households, since micronutrients can be added to food with a minimum of change in the diet and at a relatively low cost.

Vitamin A, iodine, and iron-folate are the three most common micronutrient deficiencies in developing countries. As a result, fortification programs have been focused on these three nutrients.

The most dramatic results have been obtained by the addition of iodine to salt. Iodization of salt has almost completely eliminated goiter and cretinism in the United States and some parts of Latin America and Asia.

The results of vitamin A and iron-folate fortification programs are less clear-cut. Results from a sugar fortification project in Guatemala and an MSG fortification program in the Philippines indicated that serum vitamin A levels were increased as a result of these interventions. The MSG fortification also showed a reduction in the clinical signs of vitamin A deficiency.

A limited number of iron-folate supplementation programs have been successful in improving hematological status in pregnant women. Results of iron-folate supplementation for preschoolers, however, have been less successful. In Tanzania, iron supplementation of the diets of children five to fourteen years old failed to improve hematological status; the prevalence of malaria was then diagnosed as the primary cause of the anemia rather than simply dietary iron deficiency.

Source: Extracted from Kennedy and Pinstrup-Andersen et al. 1983:42–46.

can be successfully treated in the field by paramedical workers using simple equipment and a limited range of medicines. Thus a strong argument develops for placing increased emphasis on preventive medicine carried out by lower-level technicians in clinics close to people's homes, contrasted with curative medicine carried out by highly trained physicians surrounded by a hierarchy of staff in expensive urban hospitals.

Development programs that lean toward emphasizing human capital development (which would include primary healthcare and public health programs) not only serve to improve people's productivity, especially at the bottom end of the income distribution, but may also raise per capita income faster than programs that emphasize physical capital investment (industrialization). So although we are now discussing policies aimed at health-related causes of undernutrition, keep in mind that these policies not only serve to improve simultaneously health and nutritional status, but they also serve to accelerate income growth among the poor and help to reduce income inequality, both of which, in turn, help to reduce third world undernutrition.

One highly effective means of delivering primary health services where costs are very low relative to the benefits is through maternal and child healthcare centers.

■ Subsidizing Maternal and Child Health Services

Providing public subsidies for expanding and improving maternal and child health services is entirely consistent with promoting better nutrition in the third world and can be done within the framework of modestly trained field health technicians working outside the hospital. The success of programs to immunize children against common diseases demonstrates this point.

In 1974, less than 5 percent of children in the developing world were immunized against six common vaccine-preventable childhood killers—measles, tetanus, diptheria, pertussis, tuberculosis, and polio. Today, that number is 80 percent. This enormous increase is due in large part to government policies—in particular the World Health Organization's Expanded Program on Immunization. UNICEF estimates that over 9 million lives per year are saved by immunization. However, the work is not finished. About 36 million infants worldwide are not immunized each year (WHO 2003a).

The World Bank (1993 *World Development Report*) urges public health officials to promote immunization with a new vaccine—for hepatitis B and yellow fever and recommends that this be combined with supplements of vitamin A and iodine, saying such a combination "would have the highest cost-effectiveness of any health measure available today."

In areas where the childhood diet is short on vitamin A, a program for its distribution would be an appropriate activity for maternal and child health centers. This idea is supported by an interesting controlled experiment that was conducted in Ache province in northern Sumatra, where vitamin A deficiency may well be the most severe in the world. During a one-year period, some preschoolers in Ache were given one capsule containing

200,000 international units of vitamin A every six months. Others were given no vitamin A supplement. The vitamin A supplement was shown to reduce dramatically both the risk of xerophthalmia and the death rate (Sommer et al. 1986; Gopalan 1986). Vitamin A pills such as those used in this experiment can be manufactured for less than 5 cents each. The cost of distribution far exceeds the cost of the pills. The presence of an ongoing maternal and child healthcare center permits the cost of a vitamin A supplementation program to be shared among the costs of other health delivery programs.

Such other health delivery programs appropriate to maternal and child healthcare centers include promoting growth monitoring of preschoolers, providing family-planning services, and promoting the use of oral rehydration salts (ORT) for the control of diarrhea.

And, of course, maternal and child healthcare centers are logical vehicles for gaining health and nutrition benefits through promoting breast-feeding. The sanitary and educational conditions prevalent in low-income third world homes can easily lead to a diarrhea disaster for a bottle-fed infant (see Box 17.3). But there are other problems when low-income third world mothers substitute the bottle for the breast. To such mothers, commercial infant bottle-feeding formula can seem exorbitantly expensive. So mothers tend to overdilute the mixture with water or even to mix it with white flour or sugar (after all, it looks very much the same). These practices can lead to marasmus (emaciation). Even in relatively well-off third world households, the knowledge regarding nutrition can be such that substituting the bottle for the breast can lead to marasmus (see Box 17.4). Breast milk also contains anti-infective properties not present in infant formula. Furthermore, lactation prolongs postpartum amenorrhea (the lack of menstruation that reduces fertility following birth). The contraceptive protection from lactation declines with each month of breast-feeding following birth, and about 7 percent of women conceive during this period without having resumed menstruation (World Bank, *World Development Report, 1984*:116). Nevertheless, lower fertility during lactation does reduce the chance that another pregnancy will follow too closely upon the recent birth, and increases the physical, emotional, and economic resources the mother has available for care of her infant.

■ **Public Health Measures to
Interrupt the Transmission of Diarrhea**

Programs to interrupt the transmission of diarrhea are among the important activities that public health services can undertake to promote better nutrition among the world's poor. Leading measures to take here include better handling of fecal wastes, especially those of children; programs to teach cleanliness, especially washing of hands before cooking or eating; improv-

---

Box 17.3   The Difficulties of Preparing Baby Formula in a Third World Low-Income Household

Michael Latham

The reasons for the contamination of baby formula, or milk, in a baby bottle are numerous. Milk is a good vehicle and culture medium for pathogenic organisms. It is incredibly difficult to provide a clean formula, let alone a sterile one when:

1. The family water supply is a ditch or a well, contaminated with human excrement (and few households in developing countries have their own safe supply of running water).
2. Household hygiene is poor and the home environment is characterized by flies and feces.
3. There is no refrigerator or other safe storage place for a mixed formula.
4. There is no turn-on stove and in order to sterilize the bottle or boil some water, someone has to gather fuel and light a fire on each occasion.
5. There is no suitable equipment for cleaning the bottle between feeds or when the bottle used may be a cracked and almost uncleanable soda bottle.
6. The mother, with little access to education, lives in the pre-Pasteur era, having little knowledge of hygiene and no knowledge of the germ concept of disease.

Source: Extracted from Latham 1984:60.

---

ing case management, especially through promoting ORT; promoting breast-feeding; increasing the rate of measles immunization; and improving the local water supply.

Not only do breast-fed infants have a lower morbidity rate from diarrhea, but breast-feeding protects against death from diarrhea. Infants who receive no breast milk are about twenty-five times more likely to die of diarrhea than those who are exclusively breast-fed (Feacham and Koblinsky 1984).

Measles associated diarrhea is more severe and is more likely to lead to death than other diarrheas. One estimate suggests that up to a quarter of diarrheal deaths among preschoolers could be prevented by an effective measles immunization program (Feacham and Koblinsky 1983).

The WHO (2003b) estimates that 1.1 billion people do not have access to improved water supplies. Improving the local water supply in rural areas can involve something as simple and effective as technical assistance and encouragement for the construction and use of rainwater-gathering vats. Use of such vats provides not only a clean but a convenient source of

Box 17.4   Marasmus in a Newly Rich Urbanized Society

Peter Pellett

I was long of the opinion that infantile marasmus would be essentially eliminated when social and political change were accomplished such that abject poverty no longer existed. However, recent experience in Libya, a rich but still developing nation, has caused me to reconsider somewhat this view.

The Libyan Arab Republic was formed in 1969 by a coup d'état led by Colonel Muamar al-Qaddafi against the king. During the eight years between then and 1977, real incomes for ordinary workers in Libya increased fourfold. In 1977 the major food items (flour, rice, tomato paste, meat, olive oil, coffee, tea, and sugar) were subsidized by the government, and baby foods were tax-free. Both gross poverty and inadequate housing were largely eliminated and phenomenal social progress was accomplished.

Despite this, in 1977 infantile marasmus in Libya remained a widespread problem. As elsewhere in the developing world, breast-feeding had declined.

In a study in Tripoli, the capital city of Libya, we compared the family backgrounds of 50 marasmic infants with the backgrounds of 50 essentially healthy infants of similar age. Total income was similar in both sets of families, and major consumer items such as TV sets, cars, and refrigerators were widely present in both groups. However, families with marasmic infants had less-literate mothers who tended to breast-feed for shorter periods and to feed purchased pureed baby foods more frequently. We concluded that the causal factor for marasmus in most of these instances was probably unhygienic infant feeding, despite the availability of clean water and modern kitchen facilities.

Although there were no statistical studies to back them up, some local hospital staff members were of the opinion that the rapid decline in breast-feeding and the accompanying rapid increase in bottle-feeding and in the use of purchased pureed baby foods had combined to increase mortality rates for children during the early period of the very rapid rise in per capita income!

Source: Extracted from Pellett 1977:53–56; for more information on the topic see Mamarbachi et al. 1980.

household water. When a mother does not have to walk so far to get her household supply of water, she has more time available for other activities, including child care.

Providing an ample supply of clean water to the poor in a third world city can be a political as well as an engineering problem. Port-au-Prince, Haiti, provides an extreme example. During 1976, a shortage of water outlets promoted a substantial and profitable private market for what was, ostensibly, a publicly provided city service (see Box 17.5). The issue of whether water should be provided by public utilities or by private companies continues to be a subject of heated debate (World Bank 2001).

Box 17.5   The Political Economy of Drinking Water

Simon M. Fass

An in-depth examination of one small segment of the public service sector in Haiti, specifically water distribution management in Port-au-Prince, highlights the severe consequences which deficient administration can bring to bear upon a relatively large number of people.

In Port-au-Prince, in 1976, about 50 percent of the water input leaked out of the municipal water system. For the most part the loss was due to breaks and leaks in pipes, but much of it occurred because connections to reservoirs in homes and establishments were not equipped with automatic shut-off valves, or sometimes any valves at all. When such reservoirs, including swimming pools, were full, the overflow spilled into the streets. Since there were no metering devices or enforced penalties for not having valves, and the water tariff was on a flat-rate basis, subscribers had little incentive to invest in appropriate valves. The United Nations estimated that control mechanisms at private connections could have reduced losses to a more reasonable rate of 30 to 35 percent.

Individuals installed reservoirs because of irregular distribution and pressure of water flows. Heavy demand fluctuations, variations in rainfall, limited public storage capacity, and high distribution losses caused the irregularities. Subscribers had to be prepared for periods of several days, sometimes weeks, between deliveries through the pipes.

The 30,000 legal and clandestine private connections in 1976 provided direct service to only about 150,000 residents. The remaining 490,000 residents were in theory serviced by the 36 officially designated standpipes [public water outlets employing multiple spigots] that were supposed to exist at the time. In reality only 27 standpipes functioned. The others had long since been destroyed. The total outflow from the operating standpipes on any given day did not exceed 1.4 million liters. Thus under the best of circumstances their total supply could not provide more than 2.8 liters per person each day for the 490,000 residents presumably dependent on them. To put this in perspective, a single flush of a modern toilet facility requires 19 liters.

The extreme scarcity caused by the municipal distribution system led the city's population to adapt in a number of ways. There were a number, something on the order of 40,000, who relied on leaks and breaks in the pipes. It was common to knock a hole in a pipe, if necessary digging into the street to find one, plugging it with a wooden spike when not in use, and attaching a short rubber hose from the hole to a bucket when drawing water from it. Since penalties for this practice could be quite severe, this method of obtaining water was not widespread.

A more common practice, providing water to some 95,000 residents, was sharing among neighbors. In a number of areas, high, middle, and low-income homes are located side by side. In such neighborhoods, the proportion of families with connections tend to be relatively high, and so the number of individuals requesting water from a particular subscriber on any given day, usually in the form of a request to a household servant, is low, typically less than 10 or 12.

(continues)

Continued

The majority of nonsubscribers, however, some 300,000 low income residents who lived in downtown areas with relatively few private connections, were obliged to buy water from fixed and mobile vendors. The shortage of water outlets had in effect given rise to a rather substantial private market for a publicly provided service.

The Private Water Market, 1976.   The private water market in 1976 contained three principal sets of vendors. The first set were tanker truck operators who drew water from the fire hydrants and transported it to industrial and commercial establishments and to about 1,200 higher income homes located in areas without piped service or with very irregular service. Charges for truck supply varied between U.S.\$3.00 and U.S.\$6.00 per m^3. The gross revenues of truckers, who paid nothing for water, whether in the form of user charges or in the form of license fees, amounted from these consumers alone to an average of \$2,700 per day, \$980,000 per year, and an annual return of \$39,000 per truck.

There were substantial profits to be made, and often truckers were known to break pipes in order to create demand for transported water over the extended periods required to locate the breaks and repair them.

The second set of vendors consisted of some 2,000 households which had connections to the system and sold water in lower-income areas to neighboring consumers and/or to mobile sellers who would transport it further afield. The common method was to sell water by the bucketful (about 18 liters per bucket).

The minimum price, in effect during the rainy season if water was flowing in the pipes, was two cents a bucket, or about \$1.10 per m^3. In the dry season the typical price would be ten cents, equivalent to \$5.60 per m^3. During drought periods, as happened in 1975 and 1977, unit prices could reach anywhere from \$10.00 to \$20.00 per m^3 for several months at a stretch.

The third set of vendors were mobile vendors who bought water from connected households and transported it to consumers. They numbered 14,000 or about 4.5 percent of the urban labor force.

The margin charged by the vendors in ordinary circumstances was one cent per bucket, or two if the transport distance was long. These were margins on top of whatever the vendors themselves paid to connected families. For 1976, the aggregate net earnings of mobile vendors came to \$930,000, or approximately \$5.50 a month for each vendor.

Total expenditures by consumers in the private water market thus amounted to about \$3.8 million a year, a quarter being paid largely by a very small group of high-income residents and the balance by some 300,000 low-income families. By contrast, [the municipal water authority's] total annual revenue from the sale of water was \$650,000 during the same period.

Impacts on Low-Income Families.   At a price of \$2.30/m^3 a typical family of five would have to spend about \$4.00 a month in order to consume 11 liters

(*continues*)

Continued

of water per day. In 1976 about 40 percent of urban families had incomes of $20 per month or less.

Given all the various daily demands placed on the use of money, many of these families found it impossible to spend a fifth of their income on water. They responded in a number of ways.

The poorest of them, with incomes of less than $10 per month, used purchased water only for cooking and drinking. They used surface runoff for cleaning themselves. They might also launder and wash less often. A major hazard was that of illness caused by contaminated water or by residence in areas with disastrous sanitary conditions, susceptibility to which was aggravated by the extra energy expended by already malnourished bodies to trudge 20-kilogram buckets of water several kilometers each day. With the risk of illness came the possibility of seriously compromising the capacity to generate income streams. Curative medical services would require such families to curtail other expenditures further, to dig into savings, or to incur heavy debts.

Source: Extracted from Fass 1982.

18

Policies Aimed at Raising the Income of the Poor

The world's hungry are hungry because they are poor. They cannot afford enough food to provide their basic needs. Policies to alleviate their poverty fall into two categories: policies that redistribute income or wealth from rich to poor, and policies that promote general economic growth.

■ Programs that Redistribute Wealth or Income

Progressive Taxation

Taxes that take a greater percentage of income or wealth from the rich than they do from the poor are called *progressive*. Progressive taxation is one way of transferring income or wealth from the rich to the poor. In developed countries the income tax is usually designed to be progressive, and the same features can be incorporated into the tax structure of the third world, as they often are.

Taxes that take a greater percentage of income or wealth from the poor than they do from the rich are called *regressive*. Sales taxes have a reputation for being regressive. In the developed world the poor spend a greater proportion of their income compared to the rich, who save a greater proportion of theirs. However, in the third world the poor are not generally as well integrated into the market economy as are the rich. The poor are much more likely to barter and exchange goods and services and to raise some of their own food. All these activities escape the sales tax. So in the third world a sales tax is generally progressive and can therefore be recommended as another method of reducing income disparity.

Income and sales taxes are attractive alternatives to land reform because they transfer income from the rich to the poor across all sectors of society. We must bear in mind, however, that the method of spending the money in the government tax till can have distributive effects just as surely as does the method of collecting it. A government that taxes some rich people only to provide services to other rich people will do little to reduce undernutrition. Spending public money on programs to increase agricultur-

al production (Chapters 22 and 23) or on programs that subsidize food consumption (Chapters 20 and 21) is what we think of as the expenditure side
of redistribution through progressive taxation. A mere transfer of purchasing power from the rich to the poor may prove less effective as a way of
improving the nutrition of the poor. For example:

> Take a simple case within a developing country, say India. If one rupee of
> purchasing power is taken away from a person in the top 5 percent of the
> income distribution, that will cause a reduction, in constant prices, of 0.03
> rupee in food-grain consumption. That same rupee provided to a person in
> the bottom 20 percent of the income distribution will provide increased
> demand for 0.58 rupee of food grains. The one-to-one equality of finan-
> cial transfers is matched by a nineteen-to-one inequality in the material
> transfers. Thus, a marginal redistribution of income is profoundly infla-
> tionary in driving up food prices. In this case, what the left hand of socie-
> ty gives to the poor, the right hand of the market takes away. (Mellor
> 1988:1003)

This is illustrated in Figure 18.1. Taking income from the rich shifts
their demand for food back, but by a relatively small amount, since income
elasticity of demand for food is low for rich people. Giving income to the
poor shifts their demand for food out, by a relatively large amount, since
their income elasticity of demand for food is large. Therefore, the shift in
aggregate demand (combining the demands of rich and poor) shifts out,
driving up the equilibrium price. This partially offsets the impact of the
income on food consumption of the poor, though the new quantity is still
above the old quantity.

Taxing land according to use-value is another way to implement a
progressive tax. Through a properly executed land-use survey, farmland

**Figure 18.1   The Effect of an Income Transfer from the Rich to the Poor Is
Partially Offset by an Increase in Aggregate Demand and a
Resulting Increase in Food Price**

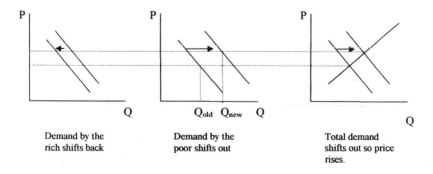

can be classified according to its value associated with its use potential. Often third world taxes on good farming land are so low that large land-holders can afford to keep their holdings while farming them inefficient-ly. By raising taxes and keeping them proportionate to land use–value, farmers who are making poor or inefficient use of their land will be forced to sell out to those who would farm the land better. The beauty of this system is that it readjusts resource use by weeding out the bad farm-ers without uprooting the good farmers, who may be doing a fine job for society.

Minimum-Wage Laws

It is frequently, and often emotionally, argued that minimum-wage laws are an effective way to improve the income of the poor. There is no question that, for those workers covered by minimum-wage legislation and whose wages are higher than they would otherwise be, minimum-wage laws yield a higher level of living. However, effective minimum-wage legislation, as it raises wages at the bottom end of the scale, motivates entrepreneurs to sub-stitute capital for labor. This drives labor out of the economy covered by minimum wage and increases unemployment in the economy generally (Mincer 1976). If credit subsidies are available, the motivation to substitute capital for labor is even greater.

Minimum-wage laws are more easily enforced in urban than in rural areas. So one result of effective minimum-wage laws is an increase in the wage differential between the country and the city. In the third world, the difference in wage rates between farm and city has resulted in mass migra-tions of rural population to the city in search of jobs. Although the proba-bility of an unskilled rural migrant's obtaining an urban job may be small, the decision to migrate may be rational because some, in fact, do get good urban jobs (Todaro 1980). The waiting may take months, years, or even a lifetime; but if enough get jobs, then by and large for most people the wait seems worth it.

Effective minimum-wage legislation increases the ultimate reward from waiting for an urban job. It simultaneously increases the number of people in the queue, increases urban unemployment, wastes labor resources, and increases the number of family members accompanying unemployed migrants who may be subjected to undernutrition.

Land Reform

Historically, in developing countries the most extreme form of redistribu-tion is redistribution of land, or land reform. Since 1960 virtually every country in the world has passed land reform laws (De Janvry 1981:385). Land reform can mean many things, but typically it means at least one of the following:

1. *Redistributing the ownership of private or public land in order to change the pattern of land distribution and size of holding.* At one extreme this might mean creating small plots from large blocks of land and allocating these small plots to the poor. At the other extreme it might mean nationalizing all agricultural land and assigning it to large, state-owned farms.
2. *Changing the rights associated with land.* For instance, tenant farmers or sharecroppers can be made owners of the land they work. Lenders, too, can be prohibited from taking land from smallholders for lack of payment of debt.

Land reform can mean other things, such as consolidation of individual holdings, that is, regrouping fragmented holdings into contiguous blocks of land (World Bank 1975:2–21). In this case there is no objective for wealth redistribution, but only productivity considerations. In most cases of land reform the hope is that the twin objectives of accelerated growth and increased equity can be accomplished.

The hope for land reform.   The land reform program carried out by the U.S. military government in Japan following World War II is widely credited with helping significantly with the reconstruction of Japanese agriculture at the time. Similarly, a land reform program in Taiwan at about the same time is credited with stimulating greater productivity in Taiwanese agriculture.

Given the tendency for land distribution to be skewed in such a manner that relatively few owners control very large shares of this valuable productive resource, land reform presents an attractive tool for redistributing wealth.

In Figure 10.4 we saw the Lorenz curve for the skewed land distribution in 1968 and 1981 for the Indian village we have looked at from time to time in this book. In Table 18.1 the same data are presented in a different form. In 1981, 20 percent of the households owned 76 percent of the land. This, by the way, was after a land reform program that limited farm size to a maximum of 50 acres in India (De Janvry 1981:386). The situation in this village is representative of much of the agriculture of the third world, where landownership typically is concentrated and where a third of the families, more or less, typically own no land. But in some places, concentration of ownership is more intense.

Before Algerian independence from the French in 1962, the good farmland in that country had become concentrated into large estates. In 1960, six thousand French colonists owned one-third of all the agricultural land (the best land) while 2 million Algerian peasants owned the other two-thirds (the marginal land) (Aron et al. 1962). In other words, 0.3 percent of

Table 18.1   Acres of Land Owned, by Ownership Group, Bagbana Village Households, 1968 and 1981

	Land Owned			
	1968		1981	
Quintile	Land Owned	Percentage of Total	Land Owned	Percentage of Total
Highest	202.6	73	192.0	76
Second	54.2	19	43.8	17
Third	19.6	7	15.6	6
Fourth	1.5	1	1.3	1
Lowest	0	0	0	0
Total	277.9	100	252.7	100
Gini ratio	.7142		.7388	

Source: Fishstein 1985:74.

the farmers owned one-third of the land. This situation was certainly one of the most dramatic instances of a skewed landownership pattern. (The French-owned farms were nationalized in a land reform program initiated in 1962.)

During the 1960s and 1970s, Latin America became notorious for concentration of landownership in the hands of the few. A 1988 study found that, in Colombia, the top 10 percent of owners controlled more than 80 percent of the total farmland (Stevens and Jabara 1988:272–273). Gini coefficients for land concentration in Latin America run very high. A 1975 collection of such coefficients listed Colombia at 0.86 and Peru, the highest, at 0.95 (World Bank 1975:26).

In Figure 18.2, land distribution in Wisconsin is compared to that in Brazil. For the period shown, over half of the farmers (and over half of the farmland) in Wisconsin lived on farms of between 100 and 500 acres. In Brazil, over three-fourths of the farmers lived on holdings of less than 100 acres, whereas almost half of the farmland is in holdings greater than 2,000 acres in size.

In the late 1990s, a major land reform program was instituted in Zimbabwe. In 1997, President Mugabe proposed a plan that would seize 10 million acres of farmland owned by about 1,500 large commercial farmers and redistribute it. The land reform initiative was a response to landownership patterns that were established during colonialism when blacks in Zimbabwe (then called Rhodesia) were legally prohibited from owning some of the best farmland. As a result, "whites made up 2 percent of

Figure 18.2   Agrarian Ownership Structure in Wisconsin and Brazil, 1980

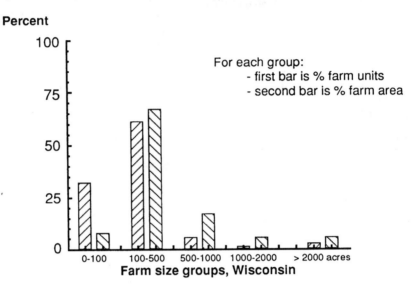

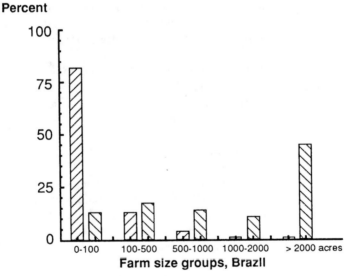

Source: Adapted from Carter 1989:1.

Zimbabwe's population but own[ed] 70 percent of the nation's best land"
(Duke 1998). The land reform has been harshly criticized for the way in
which it has been implemented, with extralegal bands of squatters seizing
farms, and is a contributing factor to the famine conditions in Zimbabwe in
recent years.

Not only is land reform attractive as a means of wealth redistribution, but it has compelling logic for productivity. Remember in Chapter 14 we pointed out that production per unit of land in the third world is typically higher on smaller farms (Figure 14.5). This suggests that dividing up large landholdings should result in increases in productivity.

But we see another compelling productivity argument. Farmers with limited capital typically operate their farms on shares, splitting a share of the harvest (typically around 50 percent) with the landlord. A share tenant who receives only half of the returns from his last hour of labor on the farm is presumably less motivated to work long hours than would an owner. Because tenant farmers normally operate on a short-term lease, often on a year-to-year basis, the insecurity of tenure discourages them from making land-associated capital investments such as fences, irrigation, or fruit trees (Herring 1983:253). These arguments suggest increased productivity from transferring landownership from the landlord to the tiller.

Deininger and Squire (1998) show that rates of growth are higher in countries where land is distributed more equally. Using a similar data set, Deininger and Olinto (2000) examine the experiences of sixty countries over the period 1966 to 1990. Of the thirty-five countries with Gini coefficients on land distribution of less than 72 (remember, a lower Gini means a more equal distribution), twenty-one had growth rates that were higher than average. Of the twenty-five countries with land Gini coefficients higher than 72, only six had growth rates higher than average.

Disillusionment about land reform.   Despite the compelling nature of the equity and productivity arguments for land reform, many oppose the concept. The history of the twentieth century is replete with instances where land reform failed to live up to its promise. The Communist Revolution in China brought with it an agrarian reform that eliminated private ownership of land in the early 1950s (see Box 2.1). The move to communal ownership initially spurred agricultural production; but by the late 1950s agricultural production had stagnated. During the 1980s, laws were changed to permit leasing and sales of agricultural land, thus returning agricultural land to private ownership. A World Bank paper describes the effects: "Gradual reform in rural areas lifted agricultural production and income and controlled poverty. In the early stages of reform inequality also lessened, although it has increased in recent years. (The Gini coefficient . . . increased to 30.7 in 1993, from 27.4 in 1978 and 21.5 in 1984)" (Ying 1996).

But not only the grand socialist experiments with collectivized agriculture have experienced major disappointments. Various other types of reform have produced unforeseen consequences, some of which made the supposed beneficiaries worse off than they might have been without the reform. A few examples will illustrate some of the common difficulties.

One of the most pressing goals of the 1962 Algerian land reform was to provide employment for as many workers as possible. Yet it did not take the self-management committees on the newly nationalized large estates long to realize that fewer workers on their farms meant more returns per worker, and an early study of the situation showed employment on the farms actually decreasing after reform (Foster and Steiner 1964). A later study of the ongoing land reforms in Algeria (Pfeifer 1985:81) concluded that the reform "promoted, rather than curtailed, the class differentiation of agricultural producers into successful commercial farmers and propertyless wage workers." Pfeifer goes on to observe rather caustically that "in this, the 'agrarian revolution' in Algeria in the 1970s seems to have completed the historic task begun by the French intruders in 1830."

An agrarian reform law passed in Peru in 1969 was intended to do something about the skewed landownership in that country. An important principle of the reform legislation was "land to the tiller." By late 1978 ownership of 8.6 million hectares had been transferred, and some 370,000 families had benefited from the reform (Alberts 1983). But the benefits went largely to the rich. Reforms carried out on the sugar estates, for instance, mainly benefited the permanent workers. The families living outside the sugar plantations received no benefits at all. In a detailed study of the reform, Alberts (pp. 47, 49, 141–142, 175, 226) concluded that "the poor majority of Peruvian peasants has only received land, credit and technical assistance to a minor extent." According to him, "the agrarian reform did not accomplish a radical and lasting improvement in the degree of equity within the agricultural sector. The economic policies implemented by the military government were not conducive to agricultural growth nor did they accomplish anything toward reducing the urban-rural income gap."

In the early 1950s Burma undertook an economic development program that included a land reform component also designed to provide land to the tiller. All agricultural landholdings in excess of 50 acres were subject to confiscation, and those up to 50 acres were also subject to confiscation unless the entire 50 acres were worked by the owner and his family. To retain their lands, absentee owners began working the land themselves, forcing their former tenant farmers off the land and making landless laborers of them. The former tenants usually stayed on as laborers, but they no longer enjoyed some of the benefits that had been theirs as tenants (Walinsky 1962:137, 294).

This same Burmese economic development program undertook to protect farmers from losing their land to banks and moneylenders when they defaulted on their loans by making it illegal to foreclose on mortgages on agricultural land. This not only denied landowners the opportunity to use their land as collateral to raise capital for farm investments, but the diminished security for the lender meant that the farmer-borrower had to pay higher interest rates for his money. Thus the protection afforded the cultivator came at a high cost (pp. 504–505).

In 1972 a land reform law in the Philippines gave permanent tenure rights to those who had sharecropped a piece of land for three or more years. Sharecropping had traditionally been a way for the young landless worker to get started in farming, but after passage of this law it became next to impossible for a landless worker to gain access to land through sharecropping. Landowners were too worried about becoming disenfranchised again.

The disillusionment with land reform comes not only from the multiplicity of disappointments in real-world attempts to implement it, but from a growing realization that who owns a piece of land is only one, and sometimes only a minor one, of the variables that affect the productivity of the workers and of the land they work. After all, some form of tenant farming (renting, share-renting, sharecropping) in the highly productive U.S. corn belt is, in places, the predominant pattern. As was noted by Bromley (1981), availability of low-cost purchased inputs, attractive farm-gate prices for farm produce (prices the farmer receives at the farm gate, before paying transport costs to market), appropriate technical assistance, paved farm-to-market roads, and so on often turn out to be more important in determining farm productivity than who owns the land.

With so many botched cases of land reform on the record, people are asking whether land reform can even be expected to do a creditable job of redistribution. De Janvry (1981:389) makes this observation: "With agriculture well advanced on the road to modernization . . . any drastic land redistribution is likely to nullify past technological achievements and imply shortfalls in production, at least in the short run. Where the population is increasingly landless and urbanized, the social cost of higher food prices [because of the inefficiencies resulting from land reform] may be more widespread than the welfare gains of land redistribution."

Critics of land reform ask if the inequality in the ownership of land is any greater than the inequality in the ownership of oil wells, or ships, or factories, or radio stations, or automobile plants. And if concentration in these sources of wealth turns out to be greater than that in land, they ask, why should these sorts of concentration not be shared among the people along with the land?

An important problem associated with land reform, or even the threat of land reform, is the chilling effect it may have on investment in agriculture relative to investment in other productive activities. Landowners who fear that land reform may be in the offing are understandably hesitant to invest heavily in productive improvements for their farms. In this view, land reform is part of a number of antiagricultural policies collectively referred to as *urban bias,* about which we will have more to say in Chapter 22.

■ Economic Growth

There is no doubt that broad-based economic growth is one of the most effective antipoverty programs (Dollar and Kraay 2002). Economic growth creates jobs and raises the incomes of the poor. Figure 10.1 provides some evidence of the benefits of economic growth. To a limited degree, government projects can contribute directly to economic growth; but in general governments do not create jobs very efficiently. Developing countries must rely on growth in the private sector for their economic prosperity.

The history of the past forty years frames the debate over what kinds of policies best promote economic growth. A couple things are obvious:

• *Economic growth is possible.* For example per capita income in Taiwan grew from $1,256 in 1960 to $12,181 in 1998 (in constant, or "inflation-adjusted" dollars). South Korean incomes grew from $904 to $9,454 over the same period. Of a comprehensive sample of fifty-eight countries with low incomes (per capita incomes of less than $1,500) in 1960, per capita incomes doubled in twenty of them.

• *Economic growth is not inevitable.* In these fifty-eight low-income countries, per capita incomes declined in twelve countries, and grew by less than 1 percent per year in nineteen other countries. Per capita income in the Democratic Republic of Congo fell from $489 in 1960 to $197 in 1998. Per capita income in Madagascar fell from $1,191 (above where South Korea was) in 1960 to $581 (about 5 percent of the South Korean level) in 1998.

A comprehensive literature deals with prerequisites and policies concerning economic growth. See the World Bank website on economic growth—http://econ.worldbank.org/programs/macroeconomics/topic/22009—for a review of the issues and a guide to the literature.

In 1990, John Williamson published a paper that laid out the general consensus about what policies Latin American countries should adopt at that time to promote growth. This set of recommendations became known as the "Washington consensus" because it reflected the thinking of economists at the World Bank and the International Monetary Fund. The Washington consensus is based on the observation that economic growth comes from three main sources:

• High savings leading to increased capital stock
• High labor productivity
• Adoption of new technology

This translates into three broad sets of policy recommendations:

- Promotion of savings and investment through good macroeconomic policy
- Promotion of labor productivity through education, health, and antipoverty programs
- Market orientation to promote appropriate incentives to economic decisionmakers

Macroeconomic Policy

Good macroeconomic policy, based on the experience of East Asia, where growth was extremely rapid in a number of countries for a long period up to the 1997 "Asian crash," should have the following three objectives: (1) low inflation, (2) low budget deficits, and (3) stable exchange rates.

Low inflation contributes to growth by encouraging savings. Suppose you could earn 5 percent a year interest by leaving your money in a savings account, but that during the year, all prices increase by 20 percent. At the end of the year, you have $1.05 for every dollar saved, but the $1.05 does not buy as much at the year's end as the $1 bought at the year's beginning. In this way, high inflation discourages savings. As inflation becomes lower, individuals are more confident that their savings are not going to be eaten up by inflation, and therefore saving increases. This makes more money available for lending to businesses and entrepreneurs who can buy new equipment (which increases economic production) and start new businesses (creating new jobs). The principal cause of high inflation is rapid growth of the money supply. In many countries the size of the money supply (the amount of currency in circulation) is under the control of a central bank. Experiences in different countries show that inflation is lower in countries where the central bank is independent of the political process. In the United States, for example, the Federal Reserve determines the size of the money supply. The chairman (and other policymaking officers) of the Federal Reserve are appointed for seven-year terms and are subject to confirmation by the Senate. The length of the term, and the checks and balances of Senate confirmation, make the Federal Reserve, to a large extent, independent from the political process.

A government budget deficit occurs when the amount of spending by the government exceeds the government's income from taxes and fees. Low budget deficits contribute to growth in the following ways: First, one way governments finance the budget deficit is through printing extra money to pay their bills. This increases the money supply and causes inflation, creating problems discussed in the previous paragraph. A second way to finance budget deficits is to borrow the money to pay the bills. This uses savings that would otherwise be invested in private businesses. For example, think of a number of people who have some savings and are considering whether to buy government bonds or bonds from a private company. If they buy government bonds (lending their money to the government), the money will be used to finance the budget deficit. If they buy bonds from a private company (lending their money to the private company), the money will be used to buy capital equipment for the business. In this way, high government deficits discourage economic growth. (It should be noted that not all government expenditures are nonproductive. If the government is investing in projects that yield a higher return than the projects of the private company, the running of deficits would actually improve economic growth.)

Finally, stable exchange rates contribute to economic growth by attracting foreigners to invest in the country. Exchange rates are also determined largely by money supplies in each country, and therefore are in the hands of the central banks.

Investments in Human Capital: Education, Health, Improved Nutrition, Antipoverty

The second general policy recommendation is the improvement of labor productivity through programs aimed at education, healthcare, and nutrition. Education improves labor productivity in an obvious way—by making workers better able to do their jobs. In addition to training directly related to job performance, general education gives workers a better ability to learn new jobs, and therefore improves average labor productivity as workers are able to move from industry to industry with relative ease. Improved healthcare and nutrition lead to improved labor productivity by making workers healthier, giving them additional physical strength and endurance, and improving their mental capacities.

Market Orientation and Appropriate Economic Incentives

A third general policy for growth, market orientation, allows prices determined in free markets to be used as a means of organizing the production, distribution, and consumption within an economy. Relative prices provide incentives to producers and consumers: A high price sends the message "produce more, consume less"; a relatively low price sends the message "produce less, consume more." In economies where market prices are severely distorted by government programs and interventions, the signals being sent are distorted as well, and the activities undertaken in response to those signals are likely to be suboptimal.

Market-determined prices provide reasonably good indicators of desirability and scarcity of goods. The kinds of policies that promote market orientation include: openness to free trade and world markets; assignment of property rights to give individuals the right to buy and sell goods, resources, and services; the discouragement of price setting by administrative fiat; and the encouragement of government regulation that operates through the price system rather than by command and control.

One easily overlooked aspect of a market-oriented policy is the assignment and enforcement of property rights. Suppose a farmer works a plot of land that he does not own; perhaps the land is owned communally and the community leaders decide who farms each plot of land each year. That farmer has little incentive to improve the land—to build irrigation ditches, or to protect soil from erosion—because he is not guaranteed to gain the benefit of any such improvement. The community leaders may reassign the plot to another farmer next year. The failure to have a clearly identified and enforceable right to the land discourages investment and retards economic growth. A recent example of assignment of property rights occurred in Peru, where the government issued property titles to over a million people who had been "squatting"— living on land that was ownerless.

One element of a policy to guarantee property rights is the elimination of corruption in legal and administrative processes. This requires honest police and judges, and an institutional framework that allows quick resolution of competing claims to ownership. See Box 18.1 for a description of what happens when the rule of law fails.

Agricultural Development

In addition to the recommendations above, some economists would add a fourth recommendation for growth: promoting growth of the agricultural sector (Department for International Development 2002). The economies of almost all developing countries are dominated by the agricultural sector. One of the most important stimulants to economic growth and increased employment in these economies is increased agricultural production. This is important not only because increased agricultural production increases farm employment but because increasing the quantity of food supplied lowers its price.

Food is a wage good (Mellor and Johnston 1984). That is, the cost of food can substantially affect the wage rate. Consider two developing countries that are competing in the international marketplace to sell a labor-intensive product such as shoes. In country A the price of food is high, and in country B it is low. Even though a shoe manufacturer in country B pays lower wages than his competitor in country A, the workers in the shoe factory in country B can live as well as those in country A because they can buy food more cheaply. Low food prices stimulate employment.

As low food prices make possible low wage rates, employment is stimulated not only in the export sector but in the domestic sector of the economy. Local manufacturers can compete more successfully with importers to manufacture goods. Low food prices reduce the proportion of the household budget that all people, middle- and upper-income people as well as

---

Box 18.1   Property Rights and the Rule of Law in Mexico

Roldolfo Montiel is a farmer in El Mameyal, Mexico, a poor village about 40 miles from the Pacific Ocean. In 1998, poachers began to steal trees from his land. He appealed to the local police, only to discover that they were part of the gang of thieves, controlled by local political bosses.

Montiel formed a group of fellow farmers to protest against the deforestation, but this only marked him as a troublemaker. Soon he was arrested on trumped-up charges and sent to jail.

A *New York Times* reporter (Weiner 2000) collected these opinions from Montiel and his fellow farmers:

"Here there's no justice. The strongest one, the one who can kill someone else, is the one who makes the law." (Jesús Sánchez)

"People are afraid of [the thieves]. They have a lot of power. Because they have made money from the wood, they can hire gunmen and pay off the government." (Rodolfo Montiel)

"There's been no investigation, there's been no justice, there's been no consequences—there's been nothing, nothing." (Hermalinda Sanchez)

"We live in fear of the law here. They can accuse us of anything." (Senso Figueroa)

"This is a place were people can kill without fear. . . . We're losing our land. We're losing our lives, and we don't even have anyone to complain to. We go to the local authorities, and they say it's not their problem. And when we go to the governor, we have even less chance of an answer. We sure won't get it from the president. Maybe it's better for us to be quiet now." (Albertano Peñaloza)

---

low-income people, must allocate to food, thus release purchasing power for nonfood items. This raises the demand for nonfood goods and services and further increases employment.

Stimulating third world agricultural production will involve making policy shifts away from the large number of production disincentives now in place and toward production incentives. There are other avenues to stimulating increased agricultural production, such as government sponsorship of agricultural research and educational services. The main policy alternatives available in that direction are outlined in Chapter 23.

■ **Globalization**

In the past decade, the issue of "globalization" has become widely debated. Though the term may mean different things to different people, it refers generally to a policy of increasing integration of countries in the world economy. For developing countries, a policy that embraced globalization would entail:

- Opening borders to trade by reducing impediments to imports and exports, and subjecting these regulations to restrictions imposed by the World Trade Organization
- Adopting macroeconomic policies required as conditions for loans from the International Monetary Fund (IMF)
- Adopting market-oriented industrial, agricultural, and sectoral policies, as a condition of obtaining IMF loans
- Reducing restrictions or regulations that discourage foreign investment
- Adopting labor and/or environmental policies that will attract foreign investment

As this list makes clear, globalization promotes the same kinds of policies that make up the Washington consensus. Critics of globalization raise the following objections:

- Policies that attract investment are policies that encourage or permit low wages, poor working conditions, and poor environmental quality.
- Fiscal policies imposed by the IMF require countries to reduce or eliminate health, education, and poverty alleviation programs.
- Policies imposed by the IMF and the WTO are antidemocratic, since these international organizations may countermand decisions made by democratically elected leaders and legislatures.
- There is also a suspicion on the part of globalization critics that the international organizations are controlled by multinational corporations, and that the entire globalization effort is intended to harm ordinary people in order to enrich these corporations.

The comparative experiences of Asia (which experienced dramatic economic growth from the early 1980s to the late 1990s) and Africa (which had stagnant growth over the same period) suggest that integration into the global economy can be good for growth.

Per capita income in Southeast Asia and sub-Saharan Africa were nearly identical from 1970 to the mid-1980s. Then per capita income in Southeast Asia shot up, while incomes in Africa regressed. By 1997, the Asian incomes were more than three times higher than those in Africa. Court and Yanagihara (n.d.) provide evidence that this was related to the fact that Asian governments adopted policies that embraced world markets. Exports from Southeast Asian countries grew at over 12 percent per year from 1985 to 1995; exports from sub-Saharan African countries grew at only 3 percent over this period. In the mid-1970s, exports were about 30 percent of GNP in both regions; by 1997, exports were over 50 percent of

Asian GDP, but were still at 30 percent in sub-Saharan Africa. In the early 1970s, foreign direct investment was nearly zero in Malaysia, Indonesia, Ghana, and Kenya. By the late 1990s, it was still nearly zero in the African countries, but had grown to $4–6 million a year in the Asian countries.

A more recent assessment of the impact of globalization on poverty in developing countries was undertaken by the World Bank (2003).

The financial crisis in many Asian economies in the late 1990s reveals some of the weaknesses of the globalization strategy. Nobel Prize–winning economist Joseph Stiglitz (2002) points out that policies imposed by international bodies do not always take into account the special circumstances of each country. Private-sector solutions require the existence of an institutional and cultural infrastructure that may not exist in every case. The best macroeconomic policy is not the same for all countries at all times. The pace of globalization can influence its effectiveness. Stiglitz calls for the globalization process to be reformed so that it can help poor countries grow.

19

Policies Aimed at Demographic Causes of Undernutrition

> One result of [population/resource] projections and their use in public discussion of population policy has been a shift in concern toward future generations. In China, as in most traditional societies, childbearing decisions were shaped by a desire by parents to be looked after in old age. By emphasizing future population/resource relationships in shaping family planning programs, government officials have shifted the focus of childbearing from the well-being of parents to the well-being of children.
> —Brown 1983:38–39

Chapter 18 discussed policies that increase the incomes of the poor. Chapters 19 through 23, in one way or another, discuss policies that might address undernutrition by reducing the price of food.

It may at first appear that population policy has little to do with food price. But Figure 19.1 illustrates how a policy that reduces population growth relaxes the upward pressure on price and increases food availability per person. A successful policy to reduce population growth will result in an aggregate demand curve for food that is closer to the origin. The resulting equilibrium is at a lower price and a lower quantity than the equilibrium that would exist if the population growth stayed high. But although the quantity of food drops, it drops by less than the decline in population; therefore, the food availability per person increases.

In addition to the upward pressure a growing population puts on price, rapid population growth makes the task of education more difficult, thins out the supply of capital per person, and tends to decrease equity, all of which exacerbate undernutrition. In addition, as we saw in Chapter 6, undernutrition tends to be concentrated among the youngest children of large families. Thus, we have both indirect and direct ways through which reducing the tendency toward large family size will improve nutrition.

The theme of this chapter is the examination of policy alternatives for lowering the fertility rate. We should note at the outset that, worldwide, fertility rates are already falling. The demographic policy problem for the nutrition planner in countries with high fertility and high undernutrition

Figure 19.1   If Population Grows More Slowly, Food Price Drops and Food Available per Person Increases

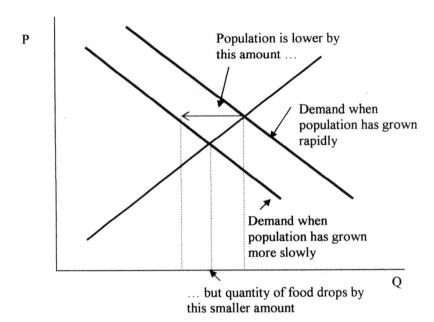

rates, then, is how to accelerate the downtrend or, in other words, how to hasten the demographic transition.

We begin with a review of the causes for the downtrend in fertility rates, which has proceeded furthest, of course, in those countries that have completed or almost completed the demographic transition. Those variables that have contributed to the slow but substantial fertility decline in the high-income, industrialized countries provide a road map to possible policies to reduce fertility in developing countries.

■ Ongoing Reasons for the Fall in Fertility Rates

Over the years, research has produced increasingly reliable and convenient methods of contraception, thus making it easier to limit fertility. But at the same time many other things have been happening that have lowered human fertility rates (Caldwell 1983; Pullum 1983). It is a widely observed phenomenon, for example, that high income yields lower fertility, at least after the initial stages of extreme poverty are overcome. This relationship is illustrated in Figure 19.2 and Table 19.1. (In some European countries, fertility rates have dropped so low that policies to *increase* fertility are being considered. See Box 19.1.)

Figure 19.2   Relationship Between Fertility and per Capita Income

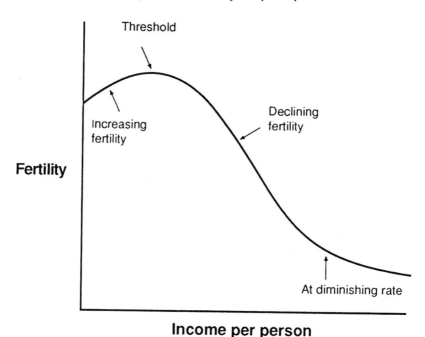

Source: Adapted from Chandra 1980.

When very poor families experience an increase in income, their initial reaction is often to have more children. (The increased income, for instance, may enable a marriage that otherwise might have been postponed for want of adequate dowry. Or the increased income might motivate the substitution of bottle-feeding for breast-feeding, with its consequent increase in the mother's fertility.) But as incomes rise, other factors mitigate to reduce fertility. Higher income is usually associated with better education, and with more education parents tend to trade child quantity for child quality. They spend a greater proportion of their child-rearing resources on their children's health and education, with correspondingly smaller resources left over for raising more children. As income continues to rise, alternative uses of family resources open up: travel, more education, more leisure-time activities, for example. These, in turn, further compete with child-rearing resources in family decisionmaking, putting more downward pressure on fertility.

As education, income, and health improve, a decline in infant and child mortality rates normally occurs. After one or two generations of low infant and child mortality rates, people are less inclined to produce large numbers

Table 19.1 Population Growth, Birth Rates, and Death Rates for Selected Country Groups, 2001

Region	GNI per capita (PPP)	Population growth, 1991–2001	Total fertility rate (births/woman)	Births per thousand population	Deaths per thousand population	Rate of natural increase	Life expectancy at birth	Infant mortality per thousand
World	7,376	14.8	2.7	20.9	8.8	0.1	63.8	53.1
Less-Developed Countries	3,850	17.8	2.97	23.2	8.5	-0.4	62.3	58.3
More-Developed Countries	26,989	4.0	1.58	11.2	10.1	1.8	75.9	8.8
Sub-Saharan Africa	1,831	28.6	5.42	39.1	16.1	-0.5	47.6	91.7
Asia	3,581	14.9	2.46	19.7	7.6	-0.1	66	50.4
Latin America & Caribbean	7,050	17.4	2.56	21.3	6	-1.6	71.2	30.2

Sources: GNI per capita, UNDP, *Human Development Report 2003*, table 1. Groups are: "Developing countries," "High-Income countries," "Sub-Saharan Africa developing countries," "Latin America and Caribbean developing countries," and a population weighted average of "East Asia and Pacific developing countries" and "South Asia developing countries." Available online at: http://www.undp.org/hdr2003/indicator/index_indicators.html. Remaining population data from U.S. Census, International DataBase.

Box 19.1 Fertility and Population Policy in Russia

Russian population is shrinking. Why are Russians deciding to have fewer and fewer children? Mariya Kakturskaya (2003) thinks that it is because the health system discourages childbearing.

The cost of pregnancy and child birth is high. Prenatal care in Moscow costs 10–20 percent of average annual income; the birth itself costs another 10–20 percent.

The quality of maternal healthcare is low. Kakturskaya reports unheated birthing rooms, botched Caesarean births, babies discharged from the hospital while suffering from infections. One expectant mother arrived at a clinic and was told: "Why do you think you're going to have a baby? Look at yourself—bags under your eyes, scrawny. You'll have a miscarriage for sure."

Low-income families receive additional government assistance for each child, but the increment is only about $2 a month.

Maternity leave is not guaranteed and some women report losing their jobs after taking a three-month leave.

Kakturskaya concludes: "Politicians . . . speak of a demographic crisis in the country. They're saying that Russian women must be forced by any means to have not just one child but two or more."

This raises an interesting question for students of constitutional law in the United States. If there is no "right to privacy" in the Constitution, as some scholars claim, could a state pass a law requiring all married women of childbearing age to have three children? On what basis (other than the right to privacy) could such a law be declared unconstitutional?

of children to ensure that at least some offspring will survive to maturity. Very high levels of income lead to a proliferation of private pension programs, or even government-sponsored social security programs, all of which lessen the pressure to have children to provide someone to take care of you in your old age.

The education of women is particularly significant in reducing fertility. Educated women are more likely to postpone marriage in order to enter the work force, more likely to delay having children in order to remain in the work force, and are more likely to know about and use contraception than are uneducated women (Anonymous 1988). The relationship between education and fertility for selected countries is shown in Figure 19.3.

Increased employment of women outside the home lessens their dependence on men (who sometimes are less motivated to limit family size than are women) and increases their tendency to make decisions in favor of using contraception; at the same time, it is inclined to change women's images of themselves. As women gain more and more equality with men in the work force and elsewhere in society (gaining the right to vote, to inherit property, to own land, to participate in the choice of a husband, etc.), they

Figure 19.3   Total Fertility Rate by Education of Wife, Selected Countries

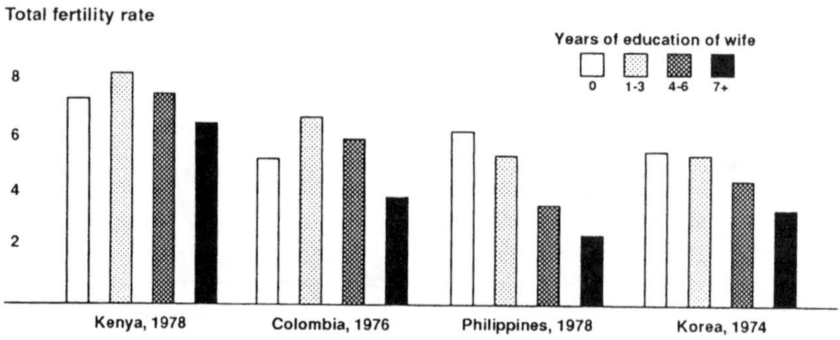

Source: Adapted from World Bank 1984:110.

move away from thinking of themselves primarily as wives and mothers and toward thinking of themselves as playing multiple roles in life. And as they do this, they tend to have fewer children.

■   Public Measures to Accelerate the Demographic Transition

The phenomena we have been discussing will continue to put downward pressure on worldwide fertility rates. But in some regions of the world the advantages of lower fertility rates are so great that governments want to accelerate the downward movement.

Most countries have a set of pronatalist public policies left over from the days when wars, famines, and high mortality rates from uncontrolled infectious diseases, such as smallpox and the bubonic plague, regularly decimated their populations. Pronatalist policies include tax deductions in proportion to the number of children in the family (common throughout much of the world), unlimited subsidized maternity leaves sponsored by government or private industry (again, common throughout the world), and child care subsidies during the first several years of a child's life (found only in certain high-income countries, e.g., Canada, France, and Australia). For countries with such policies, a first task in the direction of reducing fertility is to modify these policies so that they favor small families.

Economic Incentives and Disincentives

Economic incentives to reward low fertility and economic disincentives to discourage high fertility can both be used to motivate lower fertility.

One of the more imaginative incentive schemes was set up on three tea estates in India. By law, the tea estates are required to provide substantial maternity and child care benefits for their workers (tea pickers are usually women). The benefits include hospitalization and medical care for the mother and infant as well as long-term food, clothing, schooling, and medical care for the child. The tea estates set up a "savings account for family planning." Each woman employee of childbearing age is offered a savings account, the proceeds of which are available to her on retirement, and into which the firm will pay the equivalent of one day's wages for each month that she is not pregnant. If a woman becomes pregnant, the company suspends payments for one year. For third and more pregnancies, the company not only suspends payment for a year, but also reclaims part of its past payments into her account to help pay for its legally mandated maternal and child care expenses. Women thus have a choice: maternity and child care benefits for more children, or a better retirement program. Many women are opting for fewer children and more retirement benefits (Brown 1974:169; World Bank, *World Development Report 1984*:126).

Economic incentives for lower fertility are attractive, but they are expensive. In Bangladesh a program was proposed that would provide a twelve-year bond with a maturity value of around $350 for women of childbearing age who had only two or three children and who underwent sterilization. Attached to the proposal was a scheme whereby couples who signed certificates to delay their first birth for three years after marriage, or who delayed their second and third births for at least five years, would be given $20 on presentation of their certificates after the agreed time, provided they had kept their pledge. It was estimated that to cover the entire population with both schemes would require about 10 percent of the annual government budget (World Bank, *World Development Report 1984*:126).

Not only are incentive payments for low fertility expensive, but they waste a certain amount of public resources, as people who would have had fewer children despite the program go ahead and claim its benefits.

While economic incentives involve payments provided to delay or limit childbearing, economic disincentives usually involve the withholding of social benefits from those couples who produce more than some targeted number of children.

In the early 1980s a series of economic disincentives to large families was in use in Singapore. The system (which was dropped subsequent to a decline in birth rates) included incentives to have two children but disincentives for more than two. The system was summarized by a Draper Fund report (Salaff and Wong 1983:16) as follows:

- Paid maternity leave for the first two children, but not for third and subsequent children
- Preference in the choice of primary school given only to the first

two children, with highest preference to the two children of a parent who has undergone sterilization before age forty

- Removal of the large-family priority in the allocation of subsidized housing; only families with three or fewer children are allowed to rent rooms in public housing units
- Escalating delivery fees in public hospitals for higher-order births, as well as fees for prenatal care (fees are remitted if sterilization follows delivery)
- Full tax relief only for the first two children, and none for fourth or subsequent children

During this same period a somewhat more draconian set of rewards and punishments, using "Glory Certificates" to promote the one-child family, was in place in China (see Box 19.2).

The government can also influence infertility indirectly by adopting policies that reduce benefits to parents having more children, and raise the

---

Box 19.2   The Chinese Glory Certificate System

Lynn Landman

To stimulate acceptance of the one-child family, the Chinese have instituted a system of incentives. Those who contract to limit their families to one child receive "Glory Certificates." Such couples are widely publicized and held up as models for their countrymen, as are the rewards they earn. In general, these may include free and priority medical care for the child; priority admission to nurseries, kindergartens, and primary schools; allotment of larger housing accommodations; and bonuses for city workers and increased work points, as well as large private plots and larger housing, for peasants. All these benefits remain in effect until the child reaches fourteen.

If holders of Glory Certificates renege on their commitment, they must return all the benefits and, in addition, their annual income may be reduced by 5 to 15 percent for varying lengths of time. Those who already have two children and go on to have a third must pay all the expenses associated with childbearing, and will not be entitled to paid maternity leave. Salaries are reduced and the usual subsidized grain allotment is not provided for the third child, obliging parents to purchase it on the open market at higher prices. Job promotions may be withheld for a time and mothers sometimes are fired from their jobs.

In a country where per capita annual income is only about $235, where housing is in short supply, and schooling and jobs are not guaranteed, these incentives and disincentives may be presumed to carry considerable clout.

Source: Landman 1983:9.
Note: In 2000, the fertility rate in China was estimated to be 1.83 children per woman.

costs of child rearing. For example, policies described by the catch-phrase "empowering women" work to reduce fertility in a variety of ways. First, as women feel that society and culture give them greater permission to participate in childbearing decisions, the costs to women of childbearing and child rearing are more fully taken into account. Second, as women become better educated, they become more aware of birth control techniques. Third, as women become better educated, their value as workers increases; thus they see higher costs of foregone earnings or production as they devote time and attention to childbearing and child rearing. Fourth, as women become more socially accepted in the labor market, their value as workers increases. Fifth, better education of women is likely to lead to reduced infant and child mortality rates, so that fewer births are necessary to achieve the desired number of surviving children. Sixth, better-educated women are more likely to want a good education for their children. This reduces children's availability to the labor force and therefore reduces the economic benefits and raises the costs of having children.

Moral Suasion and Regulation

The average age at marriage for women in Bangladesh is sixteen. Half the women in South Asia and sub-Saharan Africa are or have been married by the time they are nineteen. The younger a woman is when she marries, the longer she is exposed to the risk of conception. So, to reduce fertility it seems reasonable to try to persuade people to postpone marriage. Minimum marriageable age legislation is commonly used to attempt to encourage support for later marriage. Of those countries that have tried it, China seems to have been most successful. In 1980 the government of China raised the legal minimum age at marriage to twenty for women and twenty-two for men.

India has long promoted a vigorous advertising campaign to encourage the small family, with government-sponsored advertisements appearing on billboards, buses, at movie theaters, in magazines and newspapers, and on radio and television. (India's total fertility rate in 1986 was 4.4. By 2000, it had fallen to 3.1.)

Some countries have tried intense community pressure on couples of childbearing age to limit their family size. Examples of such efforts in Indonesia and China are described briefly in Box 19.3.

Subsidizing Family-Planning Services

Use of contraceptives among married women of childbearing age varies widely in the Third World, from less than 10 percent in sub-Saharan Africa to around 40 percent in Latin America to as high as 70 percent or more in China and Singapore (World Bank, *World Development Report 1984*:128). Controlled experiments conducted in Mexico, India, Bangladesh, Korea,

Box 19.3   Community Pressures to Lower Fertility
Rodolfo A. Bulatao

Pressures can be exerted by the community, or by major sections of it, to promote lowered fertility. Two cases will illustrate group pressures: *banjars* in Bali and production teams in China.

Banjars—traditional units of local self-government, which serve as centers for mutual aid and cooperative work—consist of all the male household heads in a hamlet or subvillage. The form is centuries old. The traditional head of a banjar is democratically elected but has no official standing. Instead, the banjar also has a second, official head, who may be appointed and may have charge of more than one banjar (Hull 1978).

Banjar meetings may be held every month (or thirty-five days), usually with perfect attendance (there is a system of fines for absence or lateness), and typically discuss development of the community and religious affairs (Astawa 1979).

Since 1974 these meetings have also included discussion of the family-planning status of each family. Each member is asked what he and his wife are doing about family planning. A register is kept, and a color-coded map of the community indicating eligible couples and their contraceptive status is prominently displayed in the banjar hall (Meier 1979).

The decline in marital fertility in Bali of about 30 percent in less than a decade has been dramatic enough to be labeled a "demographic miracle" (Hull et al. 1977). How much of the change has been due to the community pressures exerted through the 3,700 banjars is a difficult and probably unanswerable question. Other elements of the Balinese situation, such as acute pressures on the land, the penetration of modern influences (through such means as consumer goods, communication, and transportation systems, and Western-style schooling and tourism), and cultural factors such as the relative independence of young couples—which may facilitate contraceptive decisions—may encourage the decline in fertility. Furthermore, the effective logistical system of the family-planning program and creative uses of native art forms to communicate family-planning messages, and a stable, supportive government, may be influential.

Production teams in China, which are usually the effective unit in rural areas for production and income sharing, consist of thirty to forty households in a small village, within which kinship ties may be strong. Production teams assume important responsibility for the fertility of their members. As part of the national *wan xi shao* campaign (named for the reproductive norms of later marriage, longer birth spacing, and fewer births), the production teams were responsible for deciding which couples could have births, in line with the reproductive norms and with team quotas set from above (Chen and Kols 1982). The team birth-planning leadership group (the leaders all being local residents) might call all eligible couples to a meeting, at which their individual birth plans could be scrutinized and allocations made. Under the one-child campaign, which replaced the wan xi shao campaign in 1979, community birth planning still takes place, although allocation of birth quotas follows different norms. As couples become familiar with the system, the time-

(continues)

Continued

consuming meeting to adjust birth plans may be dispensed with, and the leaders may simply notify couples of their decisions. Adherence is in theory voluntary, resting on persuasion and education. Such elements as adult study groups and visits from birth-planning delegations maintain the peer pressure (Chen 1981).

As with the Balinese banjars, it is not possible to determine the specific impact of the social pressures exerted through production teams, which are only one element in the Chinese population program.

Source: Bulatao 1984a. For greater detail on local control of fertility, see Bulatao 1984a.

and the Philippines have all demonstrated that the provision of family-planning advice, technology, and materials significantly reduces fertility.

In a thirty-one-country study, Bongaarts (1982) looked at determinants of fertility decline as it proceeds from rates well above six to rates close to two. The difference in total fertility was almost five children. He found that, in the countries studied, higher age at marriage reduced total fertility by 1.4 children. Increased use of contraception reduced fertility by 4.5 children. More induced abortion accounted for a reduction of 0.5 children, for a total reduction of 6.4 children. Reduced breast-feeding, of course, works the other way around, and accounted for an increase in fertility of about 1.5 children. On the bottom line of Table 19.2, these data are expressed as percentage contribution to reduction in fertility decline. Data for selected individual countries are also shown in Table 19.2.

In most third world countries a substantial gap exists between women who would like to limit their fertility, and their access to modern contraceptive methods (Table 19.3). In the conclusion to a major National Research Council survey of how specific program elements contribute to the effectiveness of third world family-planning programs, Simmons and Lapham (1987) note that family-planning programs increase the availability of contraception and the level of contraceptive use and that they lower fertility, but that their impact varies with programmatic and environmental factors. For instance, the availability of multiple public and private channels for the delivery of services increases the effectiveness of national programs. A wide choice of methods is more effective than a narrow choice, because diverse groups of clients have different needs. Good leadership and positive political support also increase the effectiveness of such programs.

Table 19.2   Accounting for Fertility Decline in Selected Third World Countries

Selected Countries and Years	Total Fertility Rate			Percentage of Reduction by Contributing Factor				
	Initial	Final	Difference	Higher Age at Marriage	Reduced Breast-feeding	More Use of Contraception	More Induced Abortion	All Other Factors
India (1972–78)	5.6	5.2	.5	41	−58	114	—	3
Indonesia (1970–80)	5.5	4.6	.9	41	−77	134	—	2
Korea (1960–70)	6.1	4.0	2.2	50	−38	53	30	4
Thailand (1968–78)	6.1	3.4	2.7	11	−17	86	16	4
Composite of 31 countries (long term)	>6	<3	5	28	−29	90	10	1

Sources: Composite of 31 countries: Bongaarts 1982; all other data: Bulatao 1984b:38.

Note: — = not available. The composite of 31 countries' data account for the decline in total fertility typical of countries that started their fertility decline with rates around six (the predecline phase of fertility rates) and ended rates below three (the postdecline countries). The difference in pre- to postdecline rates among these countries amounts to almost five children.

Table 19.3   Percentage of Married Women, Age 15–44, Who Do Not Want to Become Pregnant and Who Use Contraception

Region, Country, and Year of Survey	Percentage Who Do Not Want a Birth During the Next Year	Percentage Who Do Not Want Any More Births	Percentage Who Use a Modern Contraceptive Method
Africa			
Benin 1981–82	70*	8	1
Botswana 1984	76	31	19
Cameroon 1978	—	—	1
Ghana 1979–80	65*	11	6
Ivory Coast 1980–81	41*	4	1
Kenya 1984	77*	35	10
Lesotho 1977	—	14	3
Mauritania 1981	54*	14	0
Nigeria 1981–82	33*	4	1
Senegal (rural) 1982	78	7	0
Sudan (north) 1978–79	—	18	4
Zimbabwe 1984	76	22	28
Near East			
Egypt 1980	74*	53	23
Jordan 1983	86	42	21
Morocco 1983–84	—	41	22

(continues)

Table 19.3 Continued

Region, Country, and Year of Survey	Percentage Who Do Not Want a Birth During the Next Year	Percentage Who Do Not Want Any More Births	Percentage Who Use a Modern Contraceptive Method
Syria 1978	—	36	15
Tunisia 1983	86	67	35
Yemen, Arab Republic 1979	27[a]	19	1
Asia			
Bangladesh 1979–80	71[a]	48	9
Fiji 1974	84[a]	51	36
Java and Bali 1976	—	42	24
Republic of Korea 1979	81[a]	76	43
Malaysia 1974	90[a]	43	26
Nepal 1981	55	42	7
Pakistan 1975	—	42	4
Philippines 1978	—	58	17
Sri Lanka 1982	91	65	32
Thailand 1981	89	66	56
Latin America and Caribbean			
Barbados 1980–81	—	52	45
Bolivia 1983	89	74	11
Brazil (northeast) 1980	90	58	29
Brazil (south) 1981	87	49	52
Colombia 1980	84	69	43
Costa Rica 1981	84	53	57
Dominican Republic 1983	88	72	43
Ecuador 1979	91	59	27
El Salvador 1978	93	53	32
Guatemala 1983	79	40	21
Guyana 1975	—	62	32
Honduras 1981	92	76	24
Jamaica 1983	97	54	49
Mexico 1979	88	65	34
Panama 1979–80	90	63	57
Paraguay 1979	84*	31	25
Peru 1981	92*	74	18
Trinidad and Tobago 1977	—	56	49
Venezuela 1977	—	57	38

Source: Galway et al. 1987:43.

Notes: Percentages not wanting a birth are adjusted to exclude the percentage undecided or not stated. Modern methods of contraception include voluntary sterilization, oral contraceptives, intrauterine devices (IUD), condoms, injectables, and vaginal methods (spermicides, diaphragms, and caps).

a. Only fecund married women are included.

■ The Complementarity of Fertility Reduction Policies

Fertility reduction policies often complement each other. For instance, providing subsidized family-planning services not only makes the technology available for reducing fertility but sends a message to the community that government supports the idea of fertility regulation. Joel Cohen (1996b) recommends, as part of any population control policy, "doing everything at once."

However, fertility reduction policies are often also complementary with other programs that help to reduce undernutrition. For instance, successful promotion of prolonged breast-feeding not only reduces fertility but improves childhood nutrition and health. Persuading couples to marry later in life not only reduces fertility but, as women remain in the work force longer as a result, raises per capita income, improving nutrition. Increasing the educational level of women not only decreases fertility but increases their future productivity and undoubtedly improves the quality of the child care they deliver. Cohen (1996b) quotes economist Robert Cassen as saying, "Virtually everything that needs doing from a population point of view needs doing anyway."

20

Policies Aimed at Lowering the Price of Food Through Subsidized Consumption

> In developing countries . . . direct government intervention in the production, pricing, and distribution of foods on a massive scale is common. There is a profound distrust of the ability of the market to value and allocate resources. . . . Government intervention gives rise to price distortions in the domestic economy that have serious allocative and efficiency effects. In order to defend domestic controls, it becomes necessary for governments also to control border trade. This type of policymaking, thus, has a lock-step nature to it where the implementation of certain policies necessarily requires further controls on other parts of the economy. . . .
>
> The policies of intervention are rooted in a model of development where it is thought desirable, in the interests of growth and development, to skim excess resources from agriculture and direct them toward industrialization; the assumption being that such a diversion of agricultural surpluses does not reduce agricultural output. . . . Only recently have the self-defeating nature of these interventions, in the longer run, and the extent of their generally negative effect on agricultural output been fully understood.
>
> —Bale 1985:abstract and 10–11

In Chapter 8 we argued that lack of purchasing power is one of the leading causes of undernutrition. Purchasing power is a function of both income and the price of the goods and services purchased. In Chapter 18 we surveyed policies designed to increase the income of the poor. Food is a major component in the budget of the low-income people most at risk for undernutrition, so in this chapter we survey policies aimed at lowering the food prices paid by consumers.

■ Rationale for Explicit Food Subsidies

There are a number of reasons why food consumption subsidies have been so popular. Developed countries have generally followed farm production policies that have led to burdensome agricultural surpluses. Furthermore, large numbers of people are hungry now and it is tempting for policymakers to feed people today rather than to sponsor programs, such as enhanced agricultural production research, that may take months or years to produce obvious benefits. And as we saw in Chapter 2, donors of famine relief are more charitable when their donations are directed to the most needy.

There are other reasons for the popularity of food consumption subsidies. By and large, rich people prefer to give hungry people food rather than cash (see the discussion of "basic needs" in Chapter 16). Further, particular groups of rich people derive benefits from food distribution programs: these groups include food processors and input suppliers in food-exporting countries; farmers, who see the demand increased for their products; grain elevators, which hope to store the food before shipment; the sea-freight shippers; and finally, the private voluntary agencies such as CARE and Catholic Relief Services that assist in distributing surplus food.

Box 20.1   The Increasing Cost of Increasing Food Consumption Through a Subsidy

Shlomo Reutlinger

If households allocate only an increasingly smaller share of additional income to the augmentation of their energy intake, then the marginal cost of inducing energy augmentation through public intervention rises sharply as higher levels of intake are sought.

As an illustration, consider a nation in which 5 million people have average daily energy intakes of 1,500 calories, 15 million of 1,600 calories, 10 million of 1,700 calories, and the remainder of 1,800 calories and more. Let us further assume that, with declining income elasticity of demand as income rises, the additional (annual) income required to increase daily energy intake by 100 calories is $10, $15, and $25, respectively, at the level of intake of 1,500, 1,600, and 1,700 calories. If the goal of the public intervention is to assure the entire population a minimum energy intake of 1,600 calories, 5 million people at very low levels of intake would have to get a total cash transfer of $50 million. If the goal were to assure a minimum of 1,700 calories in the population, an additional $15 per capita would have to be provided to the 5 million people with the lowest energy intake as well as to 15 million more people. The additional cost would be $300 million more. If a minimum energy intake of 1,800 calories were to be assured, the additional cost would be $1 billion. The marginal cost of raising minimum energy intakes from 1,700 to 1,800 calories is twenty times the marginal cost of raising minimum intakes from 1,500 to 1,600 calories.

The above calculations are illustrative, but not unrealistic, given what we know about the declining marginal propensities of households, at different levels of energy intake and income, to allocate additional income to energy intake. The marginal cost of public interventions to increase energy intake rises sharply as higher levels of intake are sought.

Source: Extracted from Reutlinger 1985: pp. 10–11.

In developing countries, political leaders are interested in creating or continuing such programs. The groups most likely to influence political power are the military, civil servants, urban labor, and industrial interests. All of these groups are happy to be the recipients of cheap food, and political leaders are generally happy to curry favor among them, even at the expense of the country's rural sector (Hopkins 1988). (See Box 20.1.)

Proof of the political popularity of food price subsidies can be found in the morning newspaper. In several countries people have responded to the elimination of these programs by rioting in the streets. For example, in 1996, the IMF pressured Jordan to cut food price subsidies, with the result that bread prices doubled. In response, angry demonstrators in several Jordanian cities demanded that the prime minister be removed from office (Reuters Information Service 1996). In Zimbabwe, an economic crisis lead the government to increase prices for food staples by 30 percent in 2000. Riots began in the capital city of Harare, and 160 people were arrested (Shaw 2000).

■ Marketwide Explicit Subsidies

In an attempt to reduce food prices, some countries have adopted marketwide food subsidies—that is, subsidies that are available to all, not just to the needy. Some developing countries (for example, China and Brazil) have borne most of the costs of their food subsidies themselves. Other countries (for example, India and Egypt) have shared the costs with foreign donor countries who donate food for the purpose. (Food aid is discussed later in this chapter.)

We will look at experiences with marketwide food subsidies in several countries:

- Brazil, an upper-middle-income country that bore most of the costs itself
- Egypt, a middle-income country that shared the costs with foreign donors
- Sri Lanka, a low-income country that shared a small part of the costs with foreign donors and eventually decided to shift from a marketwide food subsidy to a subsidy targeted at the needy
- Kenya, Zambia, Zimbabwe, and Mozambique subsidized maize meal consumption and production by distributing it through government parastatal companies

Brazil

During the period 1966–1982 the government of Brazil attempted to achieve self-sufficiency in wheat production and at the same time provide cheap wheat to its consumers. As part of its attempt to achieve these goals, the government became the sole seller and buyer of both domestically produced and imported wheat. The prices of wheat and wheat products were rigidly controlled throughout the economy. Farmers were encouraged to increase wheat production through a price-support subsidy, and millers were provided with wheat at a price substantially below that paid to the producer, with the government making up the difference out of the general tax till.

In their study of the Brazilian wheat policy, Calegar and Schuh (1988:9–10, 43–45) determined that 86 percent of the subsidy went to consumers. That means only 14 percent of the subsidy costs went to administration or were lost through slippages such as manipulations by the millers. Even so, only 19 percent of the total subsidy went to the true target group, the low-income consumers. Furthermore, gains in consumer welfare were slightly biased toward the high-income population groups (they bought more bread per capita than did the low-income groups). Calegar and Schuh conclude that the marketwide wheat consumption subsidy was not an effective policy for redistributing income and suggest that a preferred policy would be to target the food subsidy specifically at low-income groups.

Egypt

The Egyptian government has a history of intervening in the food-marketing system that dates back to Biblical times when Joseph, interpreting the pharaoh's dream, recommended storing grain during seven fat years to prepare for the seven lean years that he prophesied were to come (Genesis 41). Since the mid-1970s, the Egyptian government has taken on a substantial burden of public expenditures for food subsidies, with the share of the government expenditures for this purpose running as high as 17 percent (Alderman and von Braun 1984:12).

Additional costs of the Egyptian food subsidy have been borne by North American and European governments, which have provided substantial quantities of food at below-market prices. Indeed, the availability of such programs may be one of the reasons that Egyptians embarked on such an ambitious market-wide food subsidy.

As of the late 1980s, the Egyptian government was handling the major share of the sales of bread, flour, pulses, sugar, tea, and cooking oil in the country, making these commodities available to householders at prices significantly below world prices. Farm-gate prices (prices the farmer receives at the farm gate, before paying transportation costs to market) deviated less from world prices than did retail prices (Table 20.1), but both sets of prices demonstrated a priority goal of Egyptian policy: cheap food for all.

Table 20.1   Farm-Gate and Retail Price of Selected Agricultural Commodities, Egypt, 1982

	Price as Percentage of World Price	
	Farm-Gate	Retail
Wheat	64.5	36.8
Rice	26.6	17.7
Sugar	46.0	27.3
Beans	75.4	49.0
Cotton	27.2	41.3

Source: Rountree 1985.

The policy is widely credited with keeping the Egyptian rate of undernutrition to a minimum. Average calorie consumption was above standard even among the poorest 12 percent of the population as a whole (U.S. Dept. of Agriculture 1984:9), although significant numbers of urban households in the lowest-income quartile were found to be calorie-deficient (Alderman and von Braun 1984).

Despite the apparent success of the Egyptian food subsidy, it has been criticized as inefficient. Sources of inefficiency include:

• *Waste.* With bread as cheap as it is in Egypt, farmers purchase significant quantities of it for livestock feed. The resources spent processing the wheat into bread are a dead loss to society when the bread is fed to livestock.

• *Underinvestment in industry.* The more foreign exchange that is spent on a food subsidy the less is available for industrial investment. One study estimated that a 10 percent increase in available foreign exchange would increase industrial investment by 6 percent and industrial output by 4 percent (Scobie 1983). High rates of government spending on imported food could adversely affect industrial employment among the poor.

• *Consumption inefficiencies.* Because of the depressed price of wheat, Egyptians eat more wheat than they would if they were paying the world price. A loss to Egyptian society associated with this overconsumption results because government paid more for the last tons of wheat it bought at world market prices than Egyptian citizens would have been willing to pay for them. The amount of this cost above worth is represented by triangle 1 of Figure 20.1, which illustrates the case where the government uses subsidies to keep both the consumer price and the producer price below equilibrium, and makes up the difference in quantity demanded minus quantity supplied with (donated) imports from abroad.

**Figure 20.1   Cost Above Worth and Producer's Surplus Lost Due to a
Marketwide Explicit Subsidy**

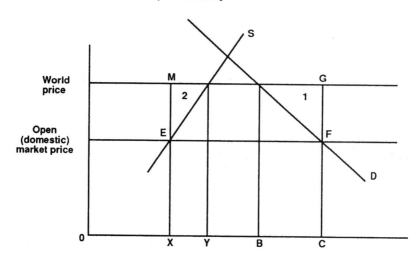

Cost above worth: Suppose that D represents the demand curve for wheat, and that amount OC represents the wheat consumed, given the domestic market price. If BC quantity of wheat is imported, then the area of the triangle 1 is a loss to society since government paid more for this wheat than it was worth to consumers.

Producer's surplus lost: Now suppose that S represents the supply curve for wheat, assuming no concessionary sales were available. Quantity OX represents wheat produced in Egypt given a depressed, domestic market price. Quantity XY represents wheat imported that would have been produced locally had the local price of wheat been equal to the world price. The area of triangle 2 is a loss to the Egyptian farmer because it is a producer's surplus he could capture were he getting the world price, but which he now misses out on. Notice that the consumer would not care whether he paid the world price to the farmer or to a foreigner. But the Egyptian farmer cares because he can produce that quantity of wheat with fewer resources than can the foreigner. And the economy cares, too. Triangle 2 is a loss to the Egyptian economy.

Sri Lanka

When a general food subsidy is substantial, the costs of the program become so high that it becomes necessary to limit access through a system of rationing. This is illustrated by the experience of Sri Lanka. During World War II, when rice supplies were limited, the government instituted a program under which rice was sold at a subsidized price, but the quantity to each consumer was rationed (Edirisinghe and Poleman 1983).

In 1953, the costs of the rice program became too high, and price increases of nearly 300 percent were announced. A massive protest stopped the price increases and forced the resignation of the prime minister. From 1954 to 1966, Sri Lankans could buy rice at prices substantially below the market price, but, through rationing, access was restricted to 4 pounds per week (equivalent to about 1,000 calories per person per day) (Edirisinghe 1987:12–13). In 1966, the basic weekly ration was cut in half, but issued at no charge. Two things were significant here: (1) because government did not need to purchase as much rice overseas, substantial foreign exchange savings accrued, and (2) there were no food riots.

In 1978, the ration system was targeted to the lower end of the income range through a means test. A year and a half later, food stamps were substituted for the ration cards. Food stamps carry a fixed rupee value; therefore their purchasing power declines with inflation, resulting in an automatic reduction of the costs of the food subsidy with no further government action. In 1985, targeting was restricted further, so that only the poorest quarter of the population was eligible for food stamps (Sahn and Edirisinghe 1993). The policy reforms reduced government costs: food subsidies amounted to 23 percent of government expenditures in 1970, 19 percent in 1978, and 4 percent in 1984.

Maize Subsidies in Southern Africa

Maize is the staple food crop in many countries of southern Africa. For example, in Zambia, maize makes up about two-thirds of the calories consumed. During the 1980s, countries in the region experimented with government monopolies in the marketing of maize. Farmers could only sell to the government and consumers could only buy from the government. By operating these monopolies at a loss, the government effectively subsidized both consumption and production as illustrated in Figure 20.2.

(Notice the difference between Figure 20.1 and Figure 20.2. Figure 20.1 describes a policy that sets domestic price lower than the world price, but domestic consumers and producers face the same low price. The quantity consumed at this price is higher than the quantity produced; this difference must be made up with imports. Figure 20.2 describes a policy that allows the price farmers receive to be higher than the price consumers pay. But the quantity consumed is equal to the quantity produced.)

However, the costs of the subsidy program were enormous (Mwanaumo, Preckel, and Farris 1994). For example, in 1990 in Zambia the cost of the maize subsidy program accounted for over 10 percent of the total government budget. The food subsidy programs contributed to overall government budget deficits (the Zambian government ran a deficit equal to 20 percent of their expenditures in 1986). As the countries sought help to finance these budget deficits, the IMF made eliminating the subsidies and privatizing the parastatals a condition of the loan. Between 1990 and 1996—before and after the elimination of the maize subsidy programs—the percentage of population suffering from undernutrition *declined* in three of the four countries involved, and increased slightly in Zambia. Jayne et al. (1995) conclude:

Figure 20.2   The Impact of a Government Subsidy on Consumption: Lower Consumer Price, Higher Producer Price, Higher Quantity Consumed

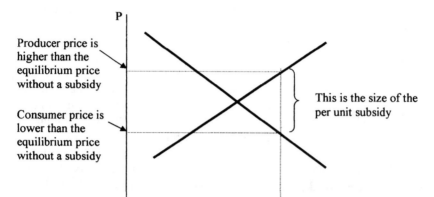

Producer price is higher than the equilibrium price without a subsidy

Consumer price is lower than the equilibrium price without a subsidy

This is the size of the per unit subsidy

Quantity is higher than the equilibrium quantity without a subsidy

Consumer subsidies on refined maize meal in [the four countries] have not necessarily promoted food security, because they have entrenched a relatively high-cost marketing system and impeded the development of lower-cost channels from developing. The negative effects of eliminating subsidies . . . have been partially or wholly compensated by relaxing controls on private grain trade, which has raised consumers' access to less expensive whole maize meal distributed through the emerging informal markets. A 53 percent rise in the price of refined meal in Kenya (due to subsidy removal) has been estimated to raise household expenditures by less than 1 percent of total income for low income groups, due to the widespread availability of cheaper whole meal.

■ Subsidies Targeted to the Chronically Needy

The Sri Lankan experience (as it had evolved by the 1980s) illustrates a second category of food price subsidies: those targeted to the poor or chronically undernourished. *Targeting* means that a person receives the food subsidy only if he or she meets certain criteria. Common criteria involve some measures of undernutrition and economic status. For example, a study of the Philippines advised a two-step procedure for targeting: (1) identify target villages with high concentrations of underweight preschoolers; (2) within the selected villages, identify households containing preschoolers whose anthropometric measurements indicate they are at high risk for undernutrition (Garcia and Pinstrup-Andersen 1987:78). In other cases, a maximum income or wealth level is established, and individuals must fall below that level to participate in the subsidy. It is difficult to enforce these targets. For example, the Sri Lankan program in 1978 restricted participation to households with annual incomes below Rs 3,600 (about $240). A survey of household income indicated that only 7.1 percent of the population lived in households below this eligible income level. Yet almost half the population managed to qualify for the program (World Bank, *World Development Report 1986*: 93).

Targeted subsidies can be administered in a number of ways. For example, they can be targeted geographically: limit the programs to regions where large numbers of the undernourished live. To some degree, donors of food aid choose recipient countries based on this criterion. Other methods of targeting include self-targeting, direct distribution, rationing, food stamps, and food-for-work.

Self-Targeting

The easiest way to target a food subsidy is to subsidize foods with negative income elasticities of demand: the inferior goods, to use the economists' jargon that we introduced in Chapter 7. Inferior foods vary from culture to culture but are typically starchy staples such as cassava, yams, maize, sorghum, or millet. As income increases, people usually eat less of these foods (review Figures 7.7c and d).

The government of Bangladesh experimented with this idea in one area by subsidizing sorghum consumption, but the experiment, although supposedly successful, was not implemented countrywide (Karim, Majid, and Levinson 1984; Ahmed 1988:226).

The review cited above (Jayne et al. 1995) of maize meal subsidies in four countries in Southern Africa concluded that a distinction should be made between programs that subsidized refined maize meal and programs that subsidized whole maize meal. As Table 20.2 shows, a majority of households in the poorest 20 percent of the income distribution in Kenya consume whole maize meal, a less expensive type of meal produced by small hammer mills. The richest households in the income distribution predominantly consume refined maize meal produced by large-scale roller mills.

Direct Distribution

Affluent countries are familiar with direct food distribution programs carried out through school lunch programs or by soup kitchens set up in low-income urban areas. In the third world, direct distribution of food is more likely to take the form of supplemental feeding programs targeted at the groups most vulnerable to undernutrition: pregnant and lactating women, infants, and preschoolers. Despite the popularity of such programs, the results have been disappointing (Kennedy and Knudsen 1985).

**Table 20.2   Targeting Food Subsidies for Maize Meal in Kenya:
Percentage of Households in Each Income Group That
Consume Refined and Whole Maize Meal**

	% of households in this income group consuming:	
Income group	Refined maize meal	Whole maize meal
Poorest 20 percent	38	59
20th–40th percentile	53	44
40th–60th percentile	74	25
60th–80th percentile	76	22
Richest 20 percent	80	18

Source: Jayne et al. 1995.

Beaton and Ghassemi (1982) found that in the eight supervised feeding programs and thirteen take-home food programs for which they had data, the net increase in food intake by the target recipients ranged from 45 to 70 percent of the food distributed, with one program showing a net effect of only 10 to 15 percent. Some of the reasons for these disappointing results are discussed in Box 20.2.

Rationing
A subsidized food-rationing system allows a consumer who holds a ration card to purchase a specific amount of some food or foods in a given time at a price lower than the market value.

A subsidized food-rationing system requires either that the government set up a marketing system of its own, which it operates or licenses to operate parallel to the regular market (which may be declared illegal and is then called a black market), or that the government set up a system for reimbursing commercial retail outlets for the discounts that they give for the rationed food. In either case government must employ auditors to monitor the system to minimize cheating.

A 1983–1984 experiment in the Philippines provides a case study of costs and benefits from a real-world, subsidized food-ration scheme. The experiment was set up so that all households in seven villages, known for a high incidence of undernutrition and poverty, were provided subsidized food. These villages were matched with seven control villages. The program did increase food consumption among the target villages. Although distribution of the extra food within the household favored adults, preschool children also consumed more and showed improvements in their nutritional status. If only weight gains among the undernourished were counted as benefits, the cost of adding 1 kilogram to the weight of an undernourished preschooler was estimated at $101 per year. (Edirisinghe

Box 20.2 Supplementary Feeding

Eileen T. Kennedy and Per Pinstrup-Andersen

Supplementary feeding programs distribute foods through noncommercial channels to pregnant and lactating women, infants, and preschoolers. These programs are the most common form of nutrition intervention in developing countries.

There are three common forms of delivery: (1) on-site feeding, (2) take-home feeding, and (3) nutrition rehabilitation centers (NRCs). NRCs include both residential facilities and programs in which children are cared for during the day but return home at night.

Data from more than 200 supplementary feeding projects indicate that many supplementary feeding programs have had a significant and positive effect on prenatal and child participants (Anderson et al. 1981; Beaton and Ghassemi 1982). Despite the significant, positive effect, however, the benefits are usually small. Increments in birth weights attributed to the supplementary feeding programs are typically in the range of 40–60 grams. Similarly, the increases in growth seen in preschoolers, although significant, are small.

Several reasons are given for these small but significant effects. First, it appears that only a part of the food given is actually consumed by the target population. "Leakages" occur when the food is shared by nontarget family members or when the food is substituted for other food that normally would be consumed. Other factors, such as the timing of supplementation, duration of participation, nutritional status of recipients, and related services available, all influence the effectiveness of supplemental feeding.

Timing of supplement. Pregnancy and the period from six months to three years of age are the most nutritionally vulnerable times. Studies indicate that it is the last trimester of pregnancy that is the most critical for supplementation. Preschoolers below the age of three are also at special risk. Inappropriate weaning practices, delayed introduction of solid foods, food taboos, and infection all contribute to a higher prevalence of second- and third-degree malnutrition in this group.

Duration. For prenatal women, there appears to be a minimum participation of 13–15 weeks needed to produce significant changes in birth weight. For infants and children, the minimum level of participation needed to affect growth depends heavily on the type of delivery system used.

Nutritional status of participants. Children with second- or third-degree malnutrition exhibit greater benefits from supplemental feeding than do marginally undernourished children. The same is true for pregnant women.

Other services. Inadequate intake of food is only one of several factors that contribute to undernutrition. Undernutrition and infection often occur simultaneously. It is not surprising, therefore, that the most successful supplementation activities have been those with strong ties to primary healthcare programs.

Source: Extracted from Kennedy and Pinstrup-Andersen et al. 1983:35–40.

[1987:70], in his study of food subsidies in Sri Lanka, found that discrimination against younger family members diminished when the more productive members of the household had at least 80 percent of their energy requirements met.)

The researchers in the Philippine experiment estimated that the cost-effectiveness of the program compared favorably with other programs. Costs were kept low through careful targeting, the cooperation of the local bureaucratic structure in administering the program, and by using existing retail outlets instead of a parallel, government-operated marketing system (Garcia and Pinstrup-Andersen 1987:9, 78–79).

Although the Philippine effort was targeted at rural villages, it has been found that nationwide subsidized ration schemes generally show an urban bias. For instance, the subsidized wheat ration system in use in Pakistan was found to contribute about 11 percent of household income for urban households with incomes below the median. Rural households gained less than 1 percent of their income from the system. The reasons for the difference are that rural households are less likely to participate in the program, smaller quantities of rationed food are available there, and wheat is not sold in many rural areas (Rogers 1988c:247).

For an example of corruption in a food rationing system see Box 20.3

Box 20.3   Corruption in Food Distribution Programs

In earlier parts of the book, we have seen how government programs sometimes have unintended consequences because they create incentives for individuals to pursue objectives other than those intended by the program. A good example of this general rule was uncovered in a investigation of India's food ration-card system.

Under this system, the poorest people of India receive ration cards that they can use to buy wheat from government run "ration shops" at very low prices. But in the village of Kelwara, ration shopkeepers turned card holders away, saying the shops had received no wheat supplies from the government.

In fact, the ration shops had received government wheat, but had sold it at higher market prices to people who did not qualify for ration cards. The shop keepers covered their tracks by keeping a fraudulent set of books, that showed sales to ration card holders, when in fact those sales had not occurred.

When a grass-roots advocacy group obtained the shopkeepers records, they discovered the fraud by tracking down the ration card holders and asking whether or not they had purchased the quantities shown in the records. The group was able to obtain the records because of a recently passed law guaranteeing public access to government information (Lakshmi, 2004).

Food Stamps

Food stamps are somewhat different from ration coupons for purchasing subsidized food. Food stamps have a face value that can be used in any food store to purchase food at the market value. In addition, people are usually expected to purchase their food stamps. Since a food stamp plan does not require government to set up a parallel marketing system for the subsidized food, the system may be cheaper than rationing.

The first food stamp plan ever was introduced in the United States just before World War II, but it is the 1961 revision of the plan that economists like to talk about. In this version, eligible families got stamps with a cash value depending on household needs for food. They paid varying amounts for the stamps depending on their income level. This arrangement made it possible to vary the food-linked income transfer according to need and therefore extend the limited government food welfare expenditures to a broader segment of the population.

In his study of the food stamp program in Sri Lanka, Edirisinghe (1987:55) found that the caloric intake response to an additional rupee from food stamps was exactly the same as from an additional rupee of income. Because of decreasing income elasticity of demand as income rises, the cost of providing 100 additional calories through food stamps increases as income increases. Despite this finding, food stamp programs will probably stay around simply because they are more acceptable politically than straight cash transfers.

Food-for-Work

Adding the requirement that recipients of food aid work in exchange for the food-linked income transfer is an interesting twist. Food-for-work (FFW) has the potential to increase the productivity of the region in which it is applied and, at the same time, provide productive activities for recipients who would otherwise be unemployed or underemployed (Mellor 1988:1004). FFW projects typically improve rural infrastructure through building farm-to-market roads, constructing irrigation canals, and so forth. They have also been used in improving squatter settlements or in erecting community buildings (Jackson and Eade 1982:24).

During the early 1980s an FFW project in the Rift Valley of Kenya employed low-income farmers on local public works projects, particularly for erosion control and water-harvesting devices. The project had two positive economic outcomes: a good deal of farmland was improved and its access to irrigation water enhanced, and the participating farmers used some of their food-linked income transfers for capital investments on their farms and thus increased their own productivity. In fact, during the second year of the program the farmers devoted fewer hours to FFW activities,

apparently in part because of a greater need to tend their own farms (Bezuneh, Deaton, and Norton 1988).

This success story is heartwarming, yet at the same time it introduces one of the problems with FFW: the benefits often go mainly to those who possess land. Typically, the recipients of FFW food are not landowners but the landless unemployed and underemployed. If their projects improve the productivity of land owned by others, the inequality of asset distribution in the area could increase. In one FFW tree-planting project in Ethiopia, the workers became so resentful that their work was enhancing the private property of already powerful landed people that they planted all the trees upside down (Maxwell 1978a:40).

Another problem stems from the growing number of FFW laborers who are women. The extra time they put into FFW programs may detract from the quantity and quality of care that they give their children. Typically they leave their infants and preschoolers to be cared for by older siblings (Kennedy, Pinstrup-Andersen, et al. 1983:28).

■ Food Aid and the Costs of Explicit Food Subsidies

Explicit food subsidization is an expensive way of improving nutritional status. This is especially true of food aid—subsidized food sold (or given away) by food-exporting countries (e.g., the United States, Canada, and Europe). In recent years, the magnitude of food aid to the developing countries has declined, but it still remains significant. Table 20.3 shows country-to-country donations, and also includes donations from the World Food Program—a multilateral agency of the UN that is funded by donations from developed countries.

Oxfam, one of the leading voluntary agencies involved in distributingt-surplus food to third world countries, commissioned a report on food aid for such purposes as disaster relief, food-for-work, mother and child health, and school feeding programs. Jackson and Eade found that the cost of the

Table 20.3   Quantity of Food Aid from All Donors, 1981–2001 (in metric tons)

Year	Cereals	Non-cereals	Totals
1981	9,140,159	736,527	9,876,686
1986	12,557,080	965,967	13,523,047
1991	13,626,220	1,143,480	14,769,700
1996	5,057,775	921,861	5,979,636
2001	7,417,330	1,435,758	8,853,088

Source: FAOSTAT 2004a

sea-freight to the U.S. food aid program came to 53 percent of the value of the food. When the food arrives at a third world port, there are other costs—warehousing, transportation, and administration as the food is distributed to the needy. The Oxfam report's authors found that the sea-freight plus within-country costs of the U.S. food aid program in one country, Guatemala, ran to 89 percent of the original cost of the food (Jackson and Eade 1982:65).

Jackson and Eade cite a number of disturbing studies that suggest that sometimes ways can be found to improve third world nutrition more cheaply than with explicit food subsidies. To cite one example, a study in India found that it cost 1.5 times as much to prevent a child's death through supplementary feeding as it would to provide basic medical services, and that "for children aged 1–3 years, nutrition supplementation was up to 11 times more expensive in terms of lives saved than medical services." The study concluded that "even where it has been nutritionally effective, supplementary feeding has not proved to be cost-effective" (Maxwell 1978b:295 fn. 36, 297).

Despite their expense, these programs can provide a solution to the most immediate of third world nutritional needs, such as famine relief. Note, however, that to be effective, they must be well administered, and this in itself is expensive. Note also that these programs do not become self-sustaining. Long-term, self-sustaining solutions to the hunger problem will have to involve changes in population growth rates, purchasing power of the poor, income distribution, and health.

Effects of Explicit Food Subsidies

Explicit food subsidies succeed in transferring income, but they are expensive. Third world governments seldom own the resources to sponsor explicit food subsidies on their own. Therefore, the direction of income transfer through these programs has been mainly from the developed to the underdeveloped world, chiefly through the U.S. food aid program PL480 and the World Food Programme.

These subsidies increase food consumption. Because of the fungibility of the food transferred (commonly grains or grain products) in the third world setting, the food received is usually treated as the equivalent of cash. Therefore some of the resulting increased purchasing power is spent on nonfood items.

Marketwide subsidies usually benefit urban consumers far more than rural consumers. This is due in part to the difficulty of running a subsidy program in rural areas and in part to the greater political clout of urban special-interest groups. In these untargeted subsidies, the rich enjoy a greater income transfer than the poor because the rich purchase more food. Even so, the poor may well get a greater percentage increase in income from the subsidy.

In very low-income households the lion's share of the increased food consumed may go to the productive adults unless the subsidy is sufficient to approach food adequacy among those adults.

Even with foreign assistance, explicit subsidies can be expensive to third world governments, often claiming more than 10 percent of their annual budget expenditures. The question must be raised whether the same amount spent on other programs would accomplish more for the poor. Careful targeting of the subsidy can save considerably on costs.

Food subsidies put downward pressure on wages, which partially offsets the real-income transfer. Still, lower wages may increase employment among the poor.

If the food for an explicit food subsidy is purchased in the same country where it is dispensed, the demand for food is increased, because the poor are now eating more than they otherwise would. This results in higher food prices, which work as an incentive to agricultural production. The U.S. food stamp and school lunch programs thus provide an incentive to U.S. agriculture.

Conversely, if the subsidized food is purchased in a developed country and dispensed in a third world country, the effect is to raise farm prices in the developed country and lower them in the third world country. The program thus acts as an incentive to agriculture in the developed country but as a disincentive to agriculture in the third world country. In the developed world, special-interest groups who benefit from food surplus disposal programs are likely to insist that their donated food does not depress third world farm prices. We find it hard to see how they can claim the incentives to the developed world's agriculture without recognizing the corresponding disincentives to agriculture in the recipient countries.

If third world farmers bear some of the costs of explicit food subsidies through the price disincentives described above, those costs are small beside the costs they may incur from implicit food-linked income transfer programs.

21

Policies Aimed at Improving Access to Food: It's All About Distribution (Isn't It?)

In Chapter 9, we saw that the world food supply is sufficient to allow every person in the world to consume an adequate number of calories. It seems logical to ask, therefore, "So, it's really all about distribution, right?" Serious students of the world food problem draw similar conclusions: "Enough food is available to provide at least 4.3 pounds of food per person per day worldwide. The problem, therefore, is not of production but clearly of access and distribution" (Mittal 2002:304). The purpose of this chapter is to take seriously this line of argument, and to demonstrate that this conclusion is grossly misleading.

■ There Is Sufficient Food, But . . .

Let us begin by reviewing the numbers. The worldwide requirements for food are about 2,350 calories per person per day. This reflects an average of requirements that are smaller for children (and the elderly) than for adults, and are smaller for women than for men, as shown in Table 3.2. In 2001, food supply was 2,807 calories per person per day (FAO 2004b). The "average food surplus"—the difference between average supply and average requirement—is about 450 calories per person per day.

A more detailed exploration of the world's *Food Balance Sheet* suggests several ways that the average food surplus might be considered to be even larger. Nine hundred and sixty-one calories per capita per day are lost in processing or waste. Of course, it is impossible to eliminate all such losses, but even reducing these losses by one-half would double the average food surplus. Another 1,094 calories per (human) capita per day are fed to animals, but animal products provide the average human with only 460 calories per day. (Recall the discussion in Box 11.1. That reflects an additional 600-plus calories per person that could be obtained without increasing food production.)

■ Diet for a Small Planet:
Redistribution Through Voluntary Restraint

This last fact has led some to conclude that voluntary changes in diet in developed countries might succeed in reducing or eliminating hunger in the developing world. The Hearts and Minds website (2003) on "socially responsible food" states, for example, that "if the USA reduced meat consumption by 10 percent, we would free more than 12 million tons of grain a year—enough to feed 60 million starving people."

We can analyze the assertion as follows. Table 21.1 shows calories per day, per capita and in total, for the United States and for the world in 2001. This provides a basis for understanding the Hearts and Minds claim quoted above. First, assume that the United States reduces all calories from animal products (not just meat, but also dairy, eggs, and fish) by 10 percent. The reduction is 102.9 calories per day per person, or 29.42 billion calories per day for the country as a whole, or 10.77 trillion calories per year. A metric ton of grain has about 3.15 million calories, so 12 million metric tons of grain would provide 37.8 trillion calories per year, enough to provide 60 million people with 1,726 calories per day.

The feed-to-meat ratio used here (37.8/10.769 = 3.5) is larger than the feed/animal products ratio in the last section (1,094/460 = 2.4), but that difference is not the primary reason why the conclusion in wrong. There are two fundamental flaws in the reasoning: First, the world food supply is not a fixed quantity, so that if less is taken by one group, that difference is available to the other group. Farmers produce food because consumers buy it. If one group of consumers were to reduce their food demand, prices would drop, other consumers would increase their consumption, and producers would react by producing less food. Second, the increase in grain available is not automatically allocated to the world's hungry.

Figure 21.1 illustrates the impact of a small backward shift in aggre-

Table 21.1   Food Consumption Patterns in the United States and the World, 2001

	USA (population 285,926,000)		World (population 6,110,437,000)	
	Per capita	Total (billions)	Per capita	Total (billions)
Calories per day	3,764	1,076.225	2,807	17,151.997
Calories per day from animal products	1,029	294.218	460	2,810.381
Calories per day from vegetable products	2,735	782.007	2,347	14,341.616

Source: FAOSTAT food balance sheets.

Figure 21.1   Impact of a Reduction in per Capita Demand for Food in the United States on Consumption in the Rest of the World

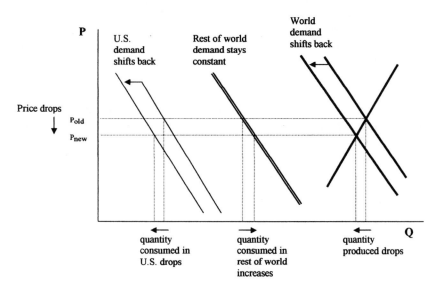

gate demand for calories for animal products in the United States. What is the relative size of these effects? Imagine that U.S. consumers reduce their calories from animal products by 10 percent (by 29.422 billion calories) at the current price levels. This is 1.047 percent of world demand for animal calories. Assuming an elasticity of demand of –0.5, and an elasticity of supply of 0.6, to close the gap of 1.047 percent of quantity supplied, price will drop by .952 percent. Quantity of animal products demanded in the rest of the world will increase by about 11 billion calories per day (from 2,516 to 2,527), quantity demanded in the United States will drop by about 27 billion calories per day (the 10 percent decline is eroded slightly by the price decline), and quantity supplied will drop by about 16 billion calories per day.

This net drop of 16 billion calories per day in production of animal products will shift the supply of grain to the right by 38–56 billion calories per day or 14–20 trillion calories per year (about half of the 37.8 trillion calories projected by Hearts and Minds). (Recall the difference between the FAO *Food Balance Sheet* and the Hearts and Minds assertion about whether the proper conversion rate is 2.4 or 3.5 calories of grain for each calorie of animal products.)

If there were some way to direct this "freed-up grain" into the hands of the most hungry, it is sufficient to feed 20–35 million people a diet of 1,700 calories per day. But the market mechanism for allocating goods relies on price. As a gap appears between aggregate quantity available and aggregate quantity demanded, the price will fall; producers will cut their production and consumers will increase their consumption, as shown in Figure 21.2.

The 38–56 billion calories per day of grain added to the market is .26–.39 percent (less than 1 percent) of the total calories from plant (non-animal) products. In the calculations below we assume that the elasticity of supply for plant calories is 0.4, that elasticity of demand for plant calories is –0.15 in developed countries and –0.35 in developing countries. As an additional .26–.39 percent of plant calories are made available for human consumption, the price will drop by .38–.55 percent. Consumption in developed countries will increase by 15–22 billion calories per day. This would provide each resident of the developing world with 3–4 additional calories per day. See Table 21.2.

To review the logic by which the 37.8 trillion calories per year (or 1,700 calories per day for 60 million starving people) projected by Hearts and Minds has shrunk to 3–4 calories per day:

• The direct impact of a reduced meat consumption by some people is partially offset by increased meat consumption by others, responding to a

Figure 21.2   Impact of Increase in Proportion of Grain Produced That Goes to Human Food Rather Than to Animal Food

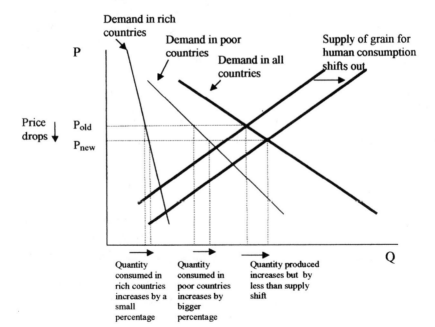

Table 21.2   Food Consumption Patterns in Developed Countries and Developing Countries, 2001

	Developed countries (population 1,317,872,000)		Developing countries (population 4,792,565,000)	
	Per capita	Total (billions)	Per capita	Total (billions)
Calories per day	3,283	4,326.574	2,575	12,820.111
Calories per day from animal products	855	1,126.781	350	1,677.398
Calories per day from vegetable products	2,428	3,199.793	2,325	11,142.714

Source: FAOSTAT food balance sheets

lower meat price. If changes in diet create a direct reduction of 10.739 trillion calories per year in animal products, about half of this is offset, so the net impact is to reduce animal calories consumed by 5.84 trillion calories.

• The calories of feed "freed up" for each calorie of animal products may be 2.4 rather than 3.5, so the 5.84 converts to 14.016–20.44 trillion calories of feed.

• The direct impact of an increase in available plant calories drives down the price and is partially offset by reduction in supply of plant calories that would otherwise have been available. Of the 14–20 trillion calories of animal feed newly available for human consumption, about 60 percent of this is offset, so the net impact is to increase plant calories consumed by humans by 6.0–8.7 trillion calories.

• Some of this increase in plant calories takes place in developed countries: of the 6.0–8.7 trillion calories increase, about 5.4–7.9 trillion calories occurs in the developing world.

• Within the developing world, consumption increases among the adequately nourished as well as the undernourished. Dividing the 5.4–7.9 trillion calories among the 4.7 billion people in the developing world yields 1,150–1,680 additional calories per person *per year*, or 3–4.6 calories per day.

This demonstrates that voluntary restraint in the developed world will do little to improve the world undernutrition problem. Complete elimination of animal products from the diets of all people in the developing world would increase calories per day in the developing world 120–180 calories. This would make substantial inroads into the undernutrition problem, but would not eliminate undernutrition. FAO's estimates of "depth" of undernutrition list many countries in which the average calorie deficiency among the undernourished exceeds 200 calories per day.

■ Policy Approaches

Of course, those who argue that we can solve the world food problem through redistribution are not restricting themselves to purely voluntary measures. What kinds of programs would be a part of a redistribution solution?

- "Overconsumption" in developed countries must be reduced.
- Overall production must be maintained at current (or close to current) levels.
- "Underconsumption" in developing countries must be reversed, and the increased consumption must be targeted to those who are undernourished.

Reducing overconsumption is conceptually quite simple, but impossible in practical, political terms. Food consumption will drop in response to a tax on income, or a sales tax on food. But huge taxes would be needed to achieve a substantial drop in consumption. In the United States, a reduction in average daily calories consumed from the current level of 3,750 to 3,000 (still a little above calories produced per person worldwide) is a 20 percent drop, too large to apply standard elasticity calculations. However, we can make some inferences about the size of the taxes needed by looking at the historical experience in the United States. The U.S. populace last had an average consumption of 3,000 calories per capita per day in 1968. In 1968, real (inflation-adjusted) disposable income per person was $17,266, about half of the current income of $32,350. Food prices have risen more slowly than prices in general since 1968. Therefore a sales tax on food of about 4 percent, combined with an income surtax of about 45 percent, would be needed to return the United States to the consumption patterns of the late 1960s.

The second policy objective of the "redistribution solution" requires that while consumption in developed countries is reduced, overall production remains unchanged. Of course, the tax revenues collected under the programs to reduce overconsumption may well provide government revenues to operate such a program. (Undoubtedly, an income tax surcharge of the size projected here [45 percent] would have substantial incentive effects. Those are ignored here.) A program of government purchases of food could be used to bridge the gap between current levels of production and the reduced levels of consumption attained by the taxes. Assuming that the government purchased 20 percent of farm marketings (current value about $240 billion), the program would cost the U.S. government about $50 billion (about 2.5 times the cost of current commodity programs).

The third part of the "redistribution solution" would be donations of the food purchased by the developed-country governments to countries with undernourished people. The U.S. foreign aid budget is currently about $11 billion and less than half of this goes to low-income countries. Thus, the kind of food distribution envisioned here would mean not only a huge change in the scope of foreign assistance (increasing it by a factor of five), but also a radical change in the targeting of foreign assistance.

A fourth part of the "redistribution solution" would be a set of programs to ensure that the food donated by the developed countries actually reaches the undernourished people in the recipient countries. Here again, it is not difficult to conceive of programs to target the undernourished; but it may be problematic to get these programs adopted and implemented administratively.

Of course, the kinds of policies considered here are policies that would be adopted within a market-oriented system. Two alternatives to a market-oriented economic system might be considered: central planned production and consumption, and household food self-sufficiency or subsistence agriculture. Both of these alternatives have been tried (or are being tried), neither with notable success in eliminating undernutrition.

■ Why Does This Matter?

The main conclusion that we draw from the previous section is that a policy to solve the world's food problem solely through redistribution is politically infeasible. Huge taxes to reduce food consumption and huge increases in government expenditures for foreign assistance are not realistic policy proposals. But does it matter?

A sage once said: "In policy debates, never let the obvious go unstated." The reason that it is worthwhile to examine the "redistribution solution" argument seriously is that the conclusions drawn from the argument may actually impede progress toward solving the world food problem. The "dangerous" conclusions are:

- Protection of natural resources can be achieved by cutting back on (or at least halting the growth of) food production.
- It is unnecessary to develop and adopt new technology to increase food production.

The first of these conclusions is illustrated by a quote from Rosset, Collins, and Lappe (2000): "Where dominant technology destroys the very basis for future production, by degrading the soil and generating pest and weed problems, it becomes increasingly difficult and costly to sustain yields. Under these . . . conditions, mountains of additional food could not eliminate hunger. The alternative is to create a viable and productive small farm agriculture using the principles of agroecology."

The second of these conclusions is also illustrated by Rosset, Collins, and Lappe: "We must be skeptical when Monsanto, DuPont, Novartis and other . . . companies tell us that genetic engineering will boost crop yields and feed the hungry. . . . [A] second Green Revolution they promise is no more likely to end hunger than the first." Or consider "Myth Seven: Biotechnology Will Solve the Problems of Industrial Agriculture," by Kimbrell (2002: 62) in which he concludes: "If biotech corporations really wanted to feed the hungry, they would encourage land reform, which puts farmers back on the land, and push for wealth redistribution, which would allow the poor to buy food."

Underlying these conclusions is a deep-seated suspicion of technology: technology causes problems, it does not solve problems. And if agricultural production cannot be increased substantially without new technology, it is reassuring to believe that increased production is not necessary to solve the world food problem.

A clearer view of what kinds of policy changes would make up a "redistribution solution" suggests that improved technology must be a part of the solution to the world food problem. The enormous improvement in the world food situation in the last forty years (the percentage of people suffering from undernutrition in the developing world has dropped from 35 percent in the early 1960s to less than 20 percent today) is undoubtedly attributable in large part to new technology. In addition to boosting yields, new technology (low-impact tillage, drip irrigation, integrated pest management) can also reduce the impact of food production on resource degradation. Perhaps technology alone will not solve the world food problem, but increased production will be an integral part of any solution.

Finally, we should emphasize that although redistribution alone is unlikely to solve the world food problem, food distribution programs that target the poor and hungry are an absolutely critical part of any strategy to reduce undernutrition. We say in Chapter 16 that providing adequate nutrition to the average undernourished person requires a very small investment—the average hungry person is a peanut-butter sandwich a day away from adequate nutrition. The lack of political will in developed countries and in the world community to undertake the necessary investments can be explained in large part by the belief that the efforts will not in fact put food into the mouths of the needy, but will instead enrich the already well-fed who have learned how to use the programs to their own advantage.

22

Policies That Raise Prices Paid to Farmers: Direct Subsidies and Eliminating Urban Bias

The most important class conflict in the poor countries of the world today
is not between labor and capital. Nor is it between foreign and national
interests. It is between the rural classes and the urban classes.
—Lipton 1977:13

Chapter 21 shows that increasing production is almost certainly a necessary
part of any solution to the world food problem. This conclusion is buttressed further by the findings in Table 22.1. This table shows that at least
26 percent of the populations in the eighty-three countries reported were
undernourished in the period 1979–1981. The countries are split into three
groups according to how fast cereals yields grew in the country between
1979–1981 and 1998–2000. "Low yield growth" is defined as growth of
less than 10 percent; "high yield growth" is defined as growth of greater an
50 percent; and "medium yield growth" is between 10 percent and 50 percent. In 1979–1981, prevalence of undernutrition was virtually identical in
the three groups. But in the 1998–2000 period, the prevalence of undernutrition had declined sharply in the high-yield group; it had declined modestly in the medium-yield group; and prevalence of undernutrition had actually increased in the low-yield group. This suggests that increasing
agricultural yields and output may be an important component in a effort to
reduce undernutrition.

Figure 22.1 illustrates two different ways of increasing the quantity of
food produced. In this chapter we focus on the left hand-side of Figure
22.1. What kinds of policies can increase prices received by farmers? Here
we consider two general approaches: increasing farm prices through subsidies and increasing farm prices through removal of programs that impose
an implicit tax on farm output.

■ Direct Subsidies

We saw an example of a direct subsidy in Chapter 20 (Figure 20.2).
Although the discussion there was couched in terms of a subsidy on consumption, we saw that the per unit subsidy created a wedge between the

Table 22.1   Yield Growth and the Prevalence of Undernutrition

	Growth in cereal yields between 1979–1981 and 1998–2000	Number of countries	Average % of population undernourished in 1979–1981	Average % of population undernourished in 1998–2000
Low Yield Growth	< 10%	29	27.3	29.5
Medium Yield Growth	10–50%	30	26.7	25.3
High Yield Growth	> 50%	24	27.2	18.6

Source: Calculated from FAOSTAT 2004a

Figure 22.1   The Difference Between an Increase in Quantity Supplied and an Increase (or Outward Shift) in the Supply Curve

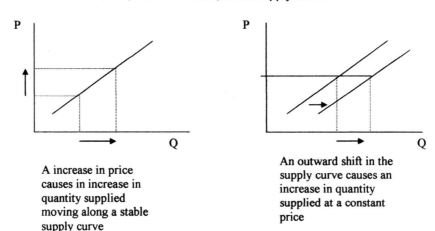

A increase in price causes in increase in quantity supplied moving along a stable supply curve

An outward shift in the supply curve causes an increase in quantity supplied at a constant price

price consumers paid and the price farmers received. Direct price subsidies to farmers have exactly the same effect: the price farmers receive is the price paid by consumers plus the subsidy amount, so the program has the impact of increasing quantity, reducing consumer price paid, and increasing producer price received.

Historically, many agricultural subsidies have been administered as "target price–deficiency payment" programs. Under these programs the government announces the target price that they will guarantee for farmers. Then, once the crop is produced and sold at the market price, the government makes a payment to farmers (a "deficiency payment") that makes up the difference between the market price (the price paid by consumers) and the target price (the price received by farmers). As described in Chapter 20, in some cases these subsidies are implemented by having the government purchase farm output at a specified price and then act as the marketing agent to consumers.

The difficulties with these programs are the same as the difficulties with consumption subsidies: the programs are expensive, and they are economically inefficient (recall the discussion of Figure 16.1). In addition, they often fail to provide farmers with incentives to produce high-quality output. (See Box 22.1 for an example.)

Agricultural Subsidies and the World Trade Organization

As part of the World Trade Organization negotiations to reduce impediments to freer international trade, countries have been negotiating reduc-

---

Box 22.1 Removing Farm Subsidies in Iraq

Under the regime of Saddam Hussein, agriculture was dominated by government bureaucracy. The government provided seeds, fertilizer, chemicals, and machinery to farmers at below-market prices. It leased land to farmers at concessionary rates. It bought all wheat and barley produced at a fixed price, regardless of quality. Then government flour mills distributed flour free to consumers.

When the Saddam government fell, the U.S.-led occupation authority was in charge. They discovered that some of the grain produced by Iraqi farmers was of such low quality that it threatened to gum up the flour-milling equipment. To avoid ruffling the feathers of the Iraqi farmers, the occupation authority continued to buy grain as under the old regime. But they fed much of the crop to cattle, and destroyed some by burning. Wheat was imported from the United States and Australia to provide flour for Iraqi consumers.

One Iraqi official told a *Washington Post* reporter that he blamed the subsidy system.

"People were making so much money that the incentive to work harder, to increase production—it wasn't there," said Salam Iskender, the new head of the agriculture section for the Wasit [provincial] governorate. . . . As a result, the yield in some regions plummeted from one ton of wheat per [unit of land] to a third of that and, particularly in the last two years, a large percentage of the crop came up 'black,' meaning that it couldn't be eaten" (Cha 2004).

Western advisors to the provisional authority are certain that a more market-oriented approach will succeed in increasing output by 20 percent, and the upcoming crop year will see an end to government provision of inputs (though the output price subsidy will remain, and will even increase). Iraqi farmers are not so sure: " 'We are afraid of the free economy. We don't understand it. If we grow crops, who will help us and who will buy it?' " asks one farmer. " 'We are like a child which stage by stage needs to grow up. . . . We need time,' " says another.

tions in their agricultural subsidies. In these negotiations, an important distinction has emerged about the difference between "distortionary" versus "nondistortionary" subsidies.

Distortionary subsidies are subsidies that work through the price mechanism, and give a farmer a subsidy *per unit of production*. This means that the more the farmer produces, the larger the subsidy received. Because of this, the subsidy program influences or "distorts" farmer decisions. (Farmers move up the supply curve as shown in the left-hand side of Figure 22.1.) In the context of international trade, a program that encourages increased production domestically interferes with free trade because it reduces the market for imports, or because it creates additional exports that must compete with other countries. The deficiency payments described above are an example of a distortionary subsidy. Under WTO rules, distortionary subsidies are limited in size, and future negotiations are likely to limit them still further.

However, under WTO rules there are few restrictions on nondistortionary subsidies. Nondistortionary subsidies are subsidies that do not work through the price mechanism and therefore are not tied to the quantity produced by a farmer. During the last two decades, agricultural subsidies in the United States and Europe have evolved from distortionary to nondistortionary subsidies. For example, a farmer in the United States receives a payment based on how many acres he has farmed over a historical period. (Confusingly, these payments are called "deficiency payments," a terminology that harkens back to a period when they were in fact distortionary; but they do not function as the deficiency payments we have described above.) If he increases his acreage, that does not increase his subsidy payment. If he increases his yield per acre, that does not increase his subsidy payment. If he shifts crops from wheat to potatoes, that does not change his subsidy payment. Since the subsidy does not influence the farmer's decisions about how much to produce, they are regarded as nondistortionary, and are not limited by WTO agreements.

A few caveats are in order before leaving this subject. First, the description of U.S. subsidies as nondistortionary applies to the bulk of U.S. farm payments, but there are some exceptions. For example, in May 2004, the WTO determined that payments under the U.S. Cotton Program violated WTO rules. Second, even these lump-sum subsidy payments can be distortionary in the longer run for two reasons: (1) The subsidies can influence (or distort) a farmer's decision about whether to quit or retire from farming. Low incomes from low prices may be compensated for by the government subsidy payment; (2) the subsidy system creates a guaranteed source of liquidity that may make it easier for many farmers to obtain loans and therefore to make investments that increase their future output.

■ Urban Bias

Another way to increase farm prices is to remove policies that have the effect of depressing prices. Figure 20.1 illustrated a policy that reduced both producer and consumer prices in a country by increasing imports. Many developing countries have adopted policies that reduce food prices in the economy as a whole—both the prices paid by consumers and the prices received by farmers.

As pointed out in Box 22.2, one of the surprising anomalies of the world food problem is that developed countries (where agriculture is already highly productive and food supplies are abundant) have generally stimulated farm production by engaging in agricultural policies that result in high farm prices, whereas developing countries (where agricultural pro-

---

Box 22.2   Urban Bias and Agriculture

Michael Lipton's 1976 book, *Why Poor People Stay Poor: Urban Bias in World Development*, laid out a compelling case that the most important "class struggle" in developing countries was the competition between the rural population and the urban population for control of the policymaking apparatus. The urban class, he argued, was winning this competition because they had overwhelming advantages: lower poverty, better education, better capacity to organize and communicate.

The result is that urban-dominated ruling classes directed resources toward low-return projects that helped city dwellers rather than rural investments that had much higher payoffs. "Scarce investment, instead of going into water-pumps to grow rice, is wasted on urban super-highways. Scarce human skills design and administer not village wells and agricultural extension services, but world boxing championships" (p. 13).

Not only is urban bias inefficient, it is inequitable. The people who benefit most from government programs in developing countries are the comparatively rich urbanites, rather than the rural poor. Lipton concludes, "A shift of resources to the rural sector and within it to the efficient rural poor . . . is often, perhaps usually, the *overriding* developmental task" (p. 18).

Anandarup Ray (1986) pointed out that in the 1970s and 1980s, this urban bias could also be seen in agricultural pricing policies of developing countries. Whereas rich countries such as the United States, Canada, Europe, and Japan heavily subsidize their agricultural sectors, "developing countries tend to tax agriculture—even those low-income countries that depend critically on agriculture for their economic growth. Some pay their producers no more than half the world price for grains and then spend scarce foreign exchange to import food. Many subsidize consumption to help the poor, but end up reducing the incomes of farmers who are much poorer than many of the urban consumers who benefit from the subsidies" (p. 2).

duction is often marginal and food supplies are scarce) generally have discouraged farm production by engaging in agricultural policies that result in low farm prices. A central idea underlying developing-country policies that result in these low farm prices is that they represent an easy way to transfer income. Popular as they are, such pricing policies are not an efficient way of transferring income to the poor.

Recall our discussion about policies that lower consumer prices, illustrated in Figure 20.1. When a government policy also reduces producer prices, it gains the additional impact of discouraging domestic production. Because the domestic price of wheat is depressed below the world market price, farmers produce less than they would if they were paid the world market price. This loss of production is represented by triangle 2 in Figure 20.1.

Implicit Subsidies to Consumers, Implicit Taxes on Farmers

Government activities that result in low (that is, below-world-market) farm prices include: noncompetitive procurement of grain from farmers; below-market food prices set by law; foreign trade controls; support of an overvalued domestic currency; and limits on cash cropping. All these activities are carried out in the name of lower food prices, and all of them, in turn, amount to implicit food subsidies to consumers, and implicit taxes on farmers.

Implicit food subsidies are almost always paid for by the farm sector through the below-market food prices. The difference between the depressed price the producer gets for his food (depressed because of an implicit consumer subsidy program in operation) and the international price for that food is a hidden cost to the farmer. The farmer's contribution to the food subsidy represents an income transfer from the farmer to the recipient of the subsidized food.

In this way, farmers have sometimes paid the lion's share of a food subsidy. In Table 22.2 we see data on the distribution of costs of food subsidy systems in three South Asian countries—Sri Lanka, India, and Pakistan—during the 1970s. During the years cited, rationed food in these countries was available at about half the market price. In all three countries, but particularly in India and Pakistan (where producers were picking up the tab on over half the cost of the subsidy), part of the heavy burden of price subsidization was shifted to farmers through the use of forced government procurement at below-market prices. Marketing regulations such as administered prices also helped to keep producer's prices below world levels. India and Pakistan set prices in their fair-price ration shops at a high enough level to cover most of their procurement costs, administrative expenses, and possible losses on imports, leaving the rest of the cost of the subsidy to be borne by the farm population (Scandizzo and Tsakok 1985:60–76).

Table 22.2 Extent and Cost of Food Subsidy Systems for Sri Lanka, India, and Pakistan, 1970s

	Ration Price as Percentage of Open Market Price 1	Quantity Rationed as Percentage of Total Consumption 2	Fiscal Cost of Subsidy to the Economy			
			Per Capita Cost (U.S. dollars) 3	Government's Share of Cost (%) 4	Producer's Share of Cost (%) 5	Budgetary Cost as Percentage of Total Expenditure 6
Sri Lanka						
1974	48	46	15.01	68	32	17
1975	60	54	10.14	87	13	16
1976	65	53	7.02	89	11	—
India						
1974	47	15	7.88	10	90	—
1975	47	18	4.22	20	80	—
1976	60	13	3.54	10	90	—
Pakistan						
1974–75[a]	44	32	7.19	24	76	13
1975–76	55	27	7.34	45	55	11
1976–77	51	33	5.03	36	64	—

Sources: Ration price as percentage of open market price in Sri Lanka: Edirisinghe 1987:12; all other data: Scandizzo & Tsakok 1985:64.
Note: a. For Pakistan the cost estimate refers to the calendar year; for example, the 1974 estimate appears under 1974–75.

Because of their nature, most implicit food-linked income transfers are market-wide, but some can be and are, occasionally, targeted to low-income groups. We now examine several commonly practiced programs that result in implicit, food-linked income transfers from farmers to the recipients of subsidized food.

Noncompetitive procurement.   A number of countries have used compulsory procurement to obtain grain from farmers at below-market prices. In India, for instance, the Food Corporation of India (FCI) is empowered to obtain grain from farmers through compulsory means. State corporations often act as agents for the FCI for both procurement and later distribution through the "fair-price" shops. In 1981 in India there were about 280,000 fair-price shops distributing subsidized grain through a rationing program available to some 660 million people. During the 1980/81 agricultural year, about 35 percent of the rice and 60 percent of the wheat sold in the market in India was procured by government agencies (George 1988).

Compulsory procurement amounts to a tax on the growers of the commodities procured. One problem is that it may motivate some farmers who have the opportunity, because of climate, soil, and topography, to switch from producing grain to producing nontaxed alternative crops, such as vegetables and fruits. Increasing the quantity supplied and thus lowering the price of vegetables and fruits benefits chiefly the high-income consumer. Low-income consumers do not spend much on these types of foods.

Administered prices.   In many third world countries, farm-gate and retail food prices have been set by government regulation. An administered price may be fixed substantially below the international price. This ceiling price becomes the highest price that can legally be offered to farmers. When this price is below the market price, it may be necessary to dissuade farmers from selling their crops on the black market by making it illegal for anyone but government representatives to purchase or transport the commodities covered by the ceiling price. This requires that government enter the marketing system as an active participant or at least license certain firms to do so.

Malcolm Bale (1985:13) describes how such a system of below-market ceiling prices worked in Pakistan in the decade prior to 1981, after which the administered prices were allowed to rise:

> The government sets a price at which it will buy wheat. Farmers may sell to government agents or private traders. The government buyers resell to ration shops at a fixed (low) price, which essentially sets the upper limit of the open market price. Private middlemen typically pay producers less than the government price because they provide extra services such as credit or transportation to growers. Wheat procured by the government is

milled and sold by privately owned ration shops to ration card holders at the same price at which the government sells the flour to them. The ration shop covers costs and profits by selling the gunny bags in which flour is delivered. Until 1981, the government price of wheat was as much as 60 percent below the border price.

Pakistani wheat farmers were implicitly taxed, and Pakistani consumers were implicitly subsidized by the support prices. A similar program kept the price of rice in Pakistan at an average of 35 percent below the border price until the 1980s (Bale 1985).

In Tanzania, where, until the early 1990s, the government controlled most aspects of agricultural marketing, government-controlled farm prices were lowered between 1970 and 1984 so that the average of official producer prices declined 46 percent. Rising export taxes and the costs of the government marketing program reduced the farmers' share of the final sales value of export crops to 41 percent in 1980. Output of some export crops (cashews, cotton, and pyrethrum) fell drastically in the 1970s. By 1984 the tonnage of export crops moving through the government marketing boards was 30 percent less than it had been in 1970 (World Bank, *World Development Report 1986*:74–75). The implicit tax on agriculture was a substantial disincentive to agricultural production.

A common aspect of administered prices has been pan-territorial and pan-seasonal pricing—that is, the practice of maintaining identical prices across time and place within the economy. The policy discourages private traders from storing food just after harvest and shifts the burden of storage, together with its costs, to the government. Jamaica practiced pan-pricing when, for several years prior to 1980, it placed a ceiling price on the retail price of wheat flour, all of which was imported. Most of the flour imported into Jamaica is landed at Kingston, and the administered ceiling price made it just barely profitable for supermarket operators in the city and suburbs to stock flour. But the cost of transporting the flour to remote markets in the mountains some distance from the port was greater than the legally allowed marketing margin. In time, the only flour available in many remote locations was black market flour, which sold at a considerable premium. Thus the rural poor ended up paying more for their flour than they would have paid without the government policy, while the urban rich found flour available at reasonable prices in their supermarkets.

Export taxes. Third world governments have placed taxes on the export of agricultural commodities. This not only generates revenue for the government but lowers the domestic price of the commodity, because exporters can pay farmers only the world price minus the export tax they have to pay to the government. The lower price can be a substantial disincentive to production. The government of Ghana set up its own Cocoa Marketing Board and gave it a monopoly on buying, transporting, and exporting cocoa. Then it undertook to raise significant tax revenue from cocoa exports. This combined with exchange-rate manipulations to raise the effective export duty on cocoa from a high of 54 percent in the last half of the 1960s to 90 percent in the last half of the 1970s. Domestic cocoa prices fell to levels far below those in competing cocoa-exporting countries, and Ghana's share of world cocoa exports fell from 40 percent in 1961–1963 to 18 percent in 1980–1982 (World Bank, *World Development Report 1986*:76).

From 1940 to 1972 the government of Argentina generally maintained a policy to keep agricultural prices low relative to the prices of nonagricultural goods. This was accomplished through a variety of measures that, in general, added up to a high tax on agricultural exports and a tariff on non-agricultural imports. This resulted in an implicit tax on agriculture that is estimated to have amounted to 50 percent of total agricultural output during the period. Among the consequences of this policy were that employment in agriculture declined, agriculture lost resources to nonagriculture, and agricultural productivity grew more slowly. In fact, per capita agricultural production in the 1970s was less than it was before World War II. And this in a country known for its excellent agricultural soils and climate and during a period when per capita world agricultural production was growing (Cavallo and Mundlak 1982:13–14).

Overvalued domestic currency. In additon to skimming resources from the agricultural sector through export taxes on farm products, governments of developing countries have also engaged in activities that further tax agriculture through an overvalued exchange rate (Schuh 1988). Here is what typically happens: as economic development proceeds in a third world country, local demand for attractive foreign goods usually becomes so great that a foreign currency deficit develops. People want lots of foreign currency so they can buy foreign-made goods, which ultimately must be paid for in foreign currency. (To simplify the discussion, we will refer to local currency as rupees, a common third world currency denominator, and to foreign currency as U.S. dollars, the standard currency of world trade.)

As the dollar deficit develops, the value of the rupee falls relative to the dollar. That is, you must spend more and more rupees to buy one dollar. As the value of the rupee falls, the cost (in terms of rupees) of imported goods rises. Government frequently attempts to stop this progression by fixing into local law the price of rupees relative to the dollar. This fixed ratio becomes the official exchange rate. As the free-market value of the rupee continues to fall, government usually defends the exchange rate by discouraging the purchase of foreign goods. It does this by such measures as requiring that approved buyers obtain a license to buy dollars (at the official exchange rate) from the central bank, placing quotas on imports,

and placing high tariffs on imports. The limitations on imports serve to protect domestic industry by cutting back on foreign competition and by raising the local price for industrial products. (For the level of protection
afforded to industry in selected countries, see Table 22.3.) One result of
this, of course, is that prices rise on the inputs that farmers use for increasing their production, such as fertilizers, irrigation pumps, and pesticides,
whether foreign or domestic. But perhaps more important to farm profitability is what it does to the prices of farm products that are exported.

Let us assume that rice costs $0.25 per pound on the world market.
And let us further assume that the official exchange rate is Rs 6 to $1. A
dollar will buy four pounds of rice on the world market, and Rs 6 will buy
four pounds. The local farmer can therefore export his rice at Rs 1.50 a
pound (assuming no export tax).

But let us also assume that, because of the continued deterioration in
the free-market value of the rupee, it now takes Rs 10 to buy a dollar on the
unofficial market. The value of a pound of rice on the international market
is really Rs 2.50 (Rs 10 equals $1, so four pounds of rice are really worth
Rs 2.50 a pound at the market rate). The farmer who exports his rice at Rs
1.50 a pound because he gets only the official exchange rate for his rice is
being taxed Rp 1 per pound for his exports. Since the export price sets the
domestic price, the farmer who sells on the domestic market is also being
taxed Rp 1 per pound for his sales. The domestic consumer receives the
benefit of the tax when he purchases the rice at Rs 1.50 rather than at the
world price of Rs 2.50.

When you combine the implicit tax resulting from the overvalued
domestic currency with an explicit export tax and thus force farm prices

**Table 22.3   Protection of Agriculture Compared with Manufacturing in Selected
Developing Countries**

	Year	Relative Protection Ratio[a]
Philippines	1974	0.76
Colombia	1978	0.49
Mexico	1980	0.88
Nigeria	1980	0.35
Egypt	1981	0.57
Turkey	1981	0.77
Ecuador	1983	0.65

Source: World Bank 1986:62.

Notes: A ratio of 1.00 indicates that effective protection is equal in both sectors; a ratio
less than 1.00 means that protection is in favor of manufacturing.

a. Calculated as $(1 + EPR_a)/(1 + EPR_m)$, where EPR_a and EPR_m are the effective rates of
protection for agriculture and the manufacturing sector, respectively.

well below the international market, and when, in addition to this, you throw in the condition that the farmer is required to pay more than the world price for his modern purchased inputs, you have a recipe for a substantial disincentive to agricultural production.

Bale (1985:24) studied five developing countries from the point of view of the impact of overvalued domestic currency on agricultural production. He found that:

> The extent to which currencies are misaligned in most developing countries is not widely recognized, and certainly its effect on output is not generally appreciated by their policy makers. For example, in the Philippines during most of the 1970s, the exchange rate was overvalued by an estimated 25–30 percent; in Jamaica during the early 1980s by 35 percent; in Colombia in the early 1980s by about 25 percent; and in Nigeria during the past five years by 44 percent. When margins of less than 10 percent determine the outcome of a sale or a profit, the effect of implicit taxes of these dimensions on domestic agriculture can be devastating.
>
> The results of these World Bank studies show that misaligned exchange rates have played the prime role in inhibiting agricultural performance.

In a study of the impact of trade and exchange-rate policies on agricultural production incentives in the Philippines, it was found that a 10 percent rise in the domestic price of imported goods (caused by tariffs, for example) results in a 6.6 percent decline in the domestic price of agricultural export products relative to home goods (Bautista 1987:9).

Thirty-one countries of sub-Saharan Africa, for which data on changes in the degree of overvaluation of domestic currency were available, were examined for the relationship between these changes and agricultural productivity. The countries fell into two groups of approximately equal size: those whose degree of overvaluation was lessening and those whose degree of overvaluation was increasing. Those countries found to be lessening the degree of overvaluation of their domestic currency were found to be increasing their agricultural production, on the average, at 2.4 times the rate of those who were increasing the degree of overvaluation of their currency (Cleaver 1985:18–19).

Limits on cash cropping.   A cash crop is one that is produced for sale. The commercial orientation of the crop (regardless of whether it is a food or a nonfood crop) identifies it as a cash crop. An export crop is, of course, a particular kind of cash crop: one that is ultimately exported from a country (von Braun and Kennedy 1986:1). In contrast to cash crops, those grown by farm families for their own consumption are called subsistence crops.

It is often argued that the growing of cash crops, and in particular, the growing of cash crops for export, limits the local food supply and therefore raises local food prices. So limits on growing cash crops for export from third world countries are often proposed as a means of forcing a shift in cultivation to food crops, thereby lowering the local price of food.

Lappe and Collins (1977), proponents of this point of view, quote a Colombian government economist as estimating that, in Colombia, "one hectare planted with carnations brings in a million pesos a year; planted with wheat or corn, the same hectare would bring only 12,500." In other words, the gross returns from a field of carnations in Colombia are eighty times the gross returns from grain. These authors assume that growing carnations for export will automatically raise local food prices through limiting the local food supply, and observe, rather sarcastically, that "if the local peasants cannot afford chicken or eggs, perhaps they can brighten their shacks with cut flowers" (p. 266).

The argument that growing cut flowers in Colombia deprives the local peasants of their food supply misses a couple of important points: (1) Colombians can purchase a lot more grain from the United States (the recipient of the cut flowers) in exchange for a field of carnations than they can raise on that field themselves, and (2) the cut-flower industry is highly labor-intensive. Regardless of who owns or manages the field of carnations, many more peasants are going to be employed to produce an acre of cut flowers than to produce an acre of grain.

What happens when third world farmers do expand their production of cash crops? Let us look at the evidence from recent studies.

Kennedy and Cogill (1987) studied smallholders in a low-income farming region in southern Kenya. These farmers were reducing their activities in subsistence agriculture and increasing their commercial sugarcane production. As sugarcane acreage expanded it replaced maize acreage. However, the return to labor for sugar was three times the daily agricultural wage rate and significantly higher than the return to maize. Incomes of the farmers who had joined the cane-growing scheme were significantly higher than those of nonsugar farmers, and the increased income positively affected household calorie consumption. For each 1 percent increase in sugarcane income, household energy intake was found to increase by 24 calories (p. 9). The increase in household calorie intake translated into modest increases in calorie intake among the children (Kennedy 1989:54). The expansion of the sugar industry in the area also increased employment. Typically the sugar mill hired laborers and supplied them to the sugar farmer for such tasks as weeding, cutting the cane, and transporting the cut cane to the mill (Kennedy and Cogill 1987:9).

Bouis and Haddad (1990) studied families in an area of Mindanao, in the Philippines, where a sugar mill had been introduced seven years earlier. Among those who had access to land, all households grew corn but some had switched part of their acreage from corn to sugar. Women were found to be more involved in corn production than in sugar production, contributing 23 percent of the total labor going into corn production, but only 11 percent of the total labor going into sugar production. During breast-feeding, wives in households that grew some sugar spent less time away from home, more time at child care, and less time in field work. The youngest children in sugar households grew significantly taller than the same age group in corn households.

In a study that looked at the household-level effects of cash cropping in rural Guatemala, von Braun and his colleagues (1989) surveyed four hundred households, about half of which had recently started raising nontraditional vegetable crops for export. The nontraditional export crops were substantially more profitable than traditional crops and were adopted by even the smallest farmers. Net returns per acre from one of the export crops, snow peas, averaged fifteen times those of maize, the most important traditional crop. Returns per unit of family labor for the new crops in general were about twice as high as for maize and 60 percent higher than those for traditional vegetables.

Because the export-crop producers produced yields for their subsistence food crops some 30 percent higher than the nonexport crop yields of their neighbors, the export crop producers usually had larger amounts of maize and beans available, per capita, for home consumption. Among the reasons for their higher yields was their purchase and use of fertilizer; thus, their increased incomes helped increase yields on their subsistence crops. Nontraditional export crops enhance local employment, not only on the farm (see Figure 22.2) but also, through backward and forward linkages, off the farm. The farmers purchased locally manufactured sticks and ropes for tying snow pea plants, for instance. And the marketing of the vegetables for export is labor-intensive, requiring such tasks as selection, grading, and packing of the produce (von Braun et al. 1989:11–12, 48).

In a statistical analysis of seventy-eight developing countries that devote at least part of their farmland to cash crops, von Braun and Kennedy (1986:2) did not find support for the hypothesis that the expansion of cash cropping happens at the expense of producing staples. To the contrary, growth in areas allocated to cash crops positively correlated with growth in staple food production. Furthermore, growth in the share of cropland allocated to cash crops is generally positively associated with per capita staple food production.

We can reasonably argue that limiting cash crop production may, in fact, limit rural incomes and create adverse affects on nutrition. Unfortunately, the advantages of export crop production in the third world are often neglected by policymakers (see Box 22.3).

Figure 22.2   Labor Inputs for Traditional Crops (Maize and Traditional Vegetables) and Export Vegetables (Broccoli, Cauliflower, and Snow Peas), Guatemala, 1985

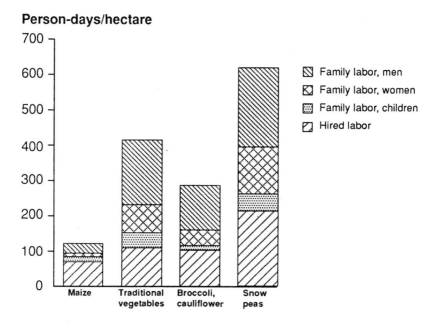

Source: Adapted from Von Braun et al. 1989:49.

Alternatives to Taxing Farm Commodities

Government must be financed. And the taxation system that finances government should not only be fair, it should be economically efficient. For efficiency and fairness, all sectors of the economy must bear a portion of the total tax burden, and the tax incidence should fall proportionally across all sectors. Of course agriculture should be taxed. The problem in the third world is how to avoid *excessive* taxation of agriculture.

We have seen that producers have been taxed as much as 50 percent or more on farm commodities that are involved in implicit food subsidy programs (see India data, columns 1 and 5 of Table 22.2). Rates of export taxation to the order of 50 to 75 percent for farm products have not been unusual (World Bank, *World Development Report 1986*:64).

It is inequitable to place such a heavy tax burden on the agricultural sector when other sectors are taxed at a lower rate or even subsidized with protective import measures. And it is inefficient. Placing an unduly heavy tax burden on agriculture steers productive resources away from this sector

---

Box 22.3   Export Crops and Food Crops

Uma J. Lele

Development debates and government and donor policies have not stressed the critical role of agriculture for the development of the rest of the economy. Instead of promoting policies that support balanced development of the agricultural sector as a whole, they have tended to emphasize the conflict between food and export crop production.

The attainment of food security is of fundamental importance in the farming decisions of small rural households. Assured food crop production releases land and labor for diversification into other higher-value production for domestic use or export. Export crop production, however, helps raise and stabilize household and national income, thereby increasing food security.

Due to labor intensity, export crops tend to generate greater employment than food cropping. Moreover, the production of most export crops tends to be scale-neutral and therefore can be undertaken by farmers with holdings of any size. Despite these features, export crops were neglected by both governments and donors in the 1970s.

Source: Extracted from Lele, n.d.

---

and slows productivity within agriculture. The resources lost to agriculture would have yielded a higher return to society in agriculture than they will at the margin in a protected industrial sector. The growth rate of per capita income slows, and to the extent that such policies exacerbate unemployment, the poor suffer more than the rich.

There are explicit tax alternatives to the implicit taxes on agriculture: taxing agricultural land, taxing agricultural income, and taxing agricultural commodities at the point of consumption rather than lowering farm-gate prices. Because these explicit taxes are readily identifiable, they are more likely to be applied equitably relative to other sectors of the economy than are implicit taxes. And because they are not commodity-specific, they do not favor the production of one agricultural commodity over another. For both of these reasons they are more economically efficient than are implicit taxes.

Complaints about the high administrative costs of taxing agricultural land have been used to explain why this method of taxing agriculture has fallen out of favor. Such complaints are hard to justify. It is, after all, fairly easy to determine who has an economic interest in farming the land; the sort of title search that may be necessary during the transfer of land ownership is unnecessary for tax purposes. Market prices can be a ready guide to the value of the land, and satellite imagery now provides a cheap means of sorting out which regions have access to irrigation water or are growing which crops. Setting up an equitable system of land taxation today is technically feasible and not unduly expensive.

It is possible to tax agricultural income, especially income from the large agricultural holdings. In Latin America, 1 percent of the population controls over 50 percent of the land, and the operations of these landholders account for more than one-sixth of the gross national product for the area (World Bank, *World Development Report 1986*:83). The income of these large landholders would be fairly easy to identify for taxation. For large agricultural corporations, the personal income tax can be used to tax employees and the corporation profits tax can be used to tax the business itself. As the tax collection system improves, it can be extended downward toward the smaller farmers, as appropriate.

Taxing agricultural commodities at the retail level instead of at the farm gate puts a greater burden on the wealthy than on the poor, because the wealthy are more likely to purchase their food at a retail outlet where the tax is collected.

Shifting from implicit taxes on agriculture to explicit taxes does not have to cause the demise of all food-linked income transfer programs. Such programs can be financed by explicit means using money in the public tax till. This type of financing has the advantage of providing considerable motivation to the framers of the food subsidy to target it carefully toward the most needy.

The Costs of Urban Bias
When third world governments adopt policies that lower the price of farm outputs and raise the price of industrial products, they are demonstrating a preference for industrial development over agricultural development. This preference for industry or, more broadly, for the people and resources concentrated in the cities, is sometimes called "urban bias."

Societies pay a heavy price for urban bias. As governments encourage the substitution of locally made industrial goods for imported goods (the policy is sometimes called import substitution, for short), the growth rate of the entire economy is inhibited. In a worldwide study of the effects of such policies, Chenery, Robinson, and Syrquin (1986:356–358) found that "economies which pursued export led growth—as opposed to a strategy of import substitution—grew faster, industrialized sooner, had higher rates of total factor productivity growth, and tended to achieve the input-output structure of an advanced economy faster." These researchers showed that shifting away from a tariff-induced import substitution trade policy to a neutral trade policy can account for an increase of as much as one percentage point in annual rate of growth of the entire economy. They further found that export-led economies are more likely to attract capital inflows. This helps to explain the success of such export-oriented economies as Korea and Taiwan.

A common aspect of third world urban bias is the implicit taxation of grain, which is often the leading agricultural product. Taxing one commodity or set of commodities to the exclusion of others shifts resource use in the direction of the untaxed commodities. When the taxed commodity is grain (the diet of the poor), the tax encourages the production of nongrain foods such as livestock products (livestock can eat the grain before it is taxed), fruits, and vegetables—favorites of the rich. It is hard to make a case that there is any nutritional gain in lowering the price of foods for the rich while limiting the production of the chief foods of the poor.

But perhaps the ultimate problem with urban bias is that, as it slows the growth of the entire economy, it deprives the poorest not only of jobs but of possible income transfers from the rich to programs that would improve the welfare of the poorest.

An End to Urban Bias?

A five-volume World Bank study (Krueger, Schiff, and Valdes 1991) confirmed the policy bias against agriculture in great detail. A synopsis of the findings of that study are found in a 1995 article by Schiff and Valdes. They concluded that (for the eighteen countries in their study), compared to nonagricultural prices, agricultural prices were 43 percent lower than they would have been in the absence of policies biased against the rural sector. Since the mid-1980s, a substantial shift has ocurred in the emphasis of developing-country policies to eliminate much of the urban bias. A paper by Jensen and Robinson (2002) concludes:

> Empirical studies from the 1980s . . . supported the view that policies in many developing countries imparted a major incentive bias against agriculture. Eliminating this bias was one of the goals of policy reform strategies, including structural adjustment programs, supported by the World Bank and others; and many countries undertook such reforms in the 1990s. . . . [Our] analysis indicates that, in the 1990s, the economywide system of indirect taxes, including tariffs and export taxes, significantly discriminated against agriculture in only one country, was largely neutral in five, provided a moderate subsidy to agriculture in four, and strongly favored agriculture in five.

In an article reviewing the literature on agricultural policies in developing countries, Binswanger and Deininger (1997) explore the conditions under which policy reforms are likely to be initiated. They observe that "a fiscal crisis is usually necessary for initiating reform"—the efficiency costs of the urban bias must become high enough to have an impact on the government budgeting process. They argue that the sustainability of the reform effort depends on: (1) whether people who benefit from the reform are organized into groups that can exercise some political clout; (2) whether the central bank and ministry of finance have the will and power to maintain budgetary discipline; (3) whether the reform effort is encouraged by international credit and advice; and (4) whether policy analysts can support the reforms without succumbing to political pressures.

23

Policies Aimed at Lowering the Price of Food by Increasing the Supply

> While the most important reasons for inadequate agricultural output are difficult to ascertain, T. W. Schultz, in the first Elmhurst Memorial Lecture to the International Association of Agricultural Economists, left no doubt as to his ranking of the causes. He stated that the level of agricultural production depends not so much on technical considerations, but in large measure, "on what governments do to agriculture."
>
> —Bale and Lutz 1981:8

In Figure 22.1, we noted the distinction between increasing the supply of food and increasing the quantity of food supplied. An increase in the supply of food—or as economists call it, an outward shift in supply curve—occurs when farmers are willing to produce more food at the same price, or are willing to produce the same amount of food at a lower price. This is the type of change that would permit the quantity of food to increase while the equilibrium price of food declines (see Figure 23.1). What would make a farmer willing to produce more at the same price, or produce the same amount at a lower price? A reduction in the farmer's costs of production. And how can we reduce food production costs? By reducing prices farmers pay for inputs, by encouraging investment, and by developing new technologies that increase farm productivity.

■ Subsidies for Purchased Inputs

The most direct and obvious way to reduce production costs is to subsidize the prices farmers pay for inputs. The government can do this by compensating farmers for each unit of inputs purchased, by subsidizing the production of inputs, or by producing or distributing the inputs themselves. In this section, we will briefly explore programs that subsidize irrigation, fertilizer, and mechanization.

Irrigation

Publicly sponsored irrigation systems date back some six thousand years, to when vast irrigation works were developed for the flood plain of the Tigris

Figure 23.1   Effect of Reduced Costs or Improved Technology on the Supply Curve

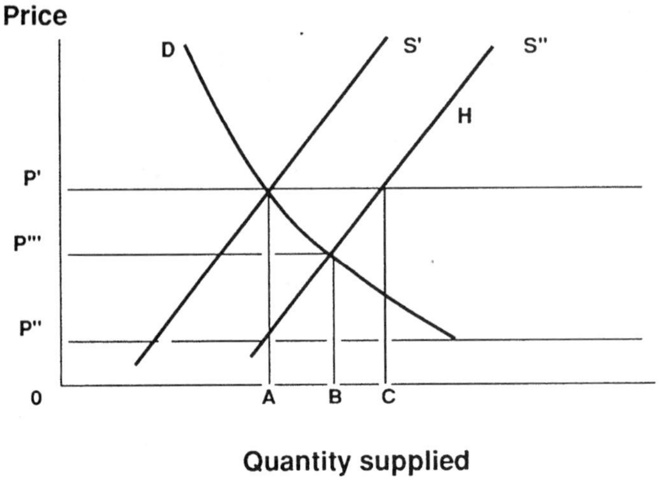

Note: When the supply curve shifts from S' to S", farmers are willing to furnish to the market: (1) an increased quantity (OC rather than OA) at the same old price (P'); (2) the same old quantity (OA) at a new prices (P"); or (3) some other combination of quantity and price—for instance, the quantity and price represented by point H on the diagram.

and Euphrates Rivers in Mesopotamia. In modern times, huge dams thrown across major rivers throughout the world (the Nile, the Indus, and the Colorado, for example) have furnished low-cost irrigation water to millions of farmers. Cost-benefit analysis has shown substantial gains to society from such projects, which usually are promoted for their multiplicity of benefits—flood control, electricity generation, and irrigation water for agriculture.

In most countries, government subsidizes irrigation water. In Egypt it is free. In the Philippines, during 1980–1981, the subsidy amounted to 90 percent of the marginal cost (Bale 1985:17).

Once the dam is built, a couple of conditions may make it illogical to charge for even the marginal costs of water delivery to the farmer: (1) the water supply is so abundant that no allocation problem exists, and (2) monitoring use may be more expensive than the marginal value of the water. In most other situations, economic efficiency would be improved through charging farmers the full cost of irrigation water. For instance, in areas where the underground aquifer is close to the surface and is rapidly recharged, such as on the Ganges plain in India, tube wells give a high payoff. In this situation farmers might as well pay the full cost of the water.

This will make it more likely that resources are being allocated to their highest-valued use for society.

Concerns that the introduction of irrigation and the modern technologies that go with it will lead to increased inequalities in income distribution have proved unfounded. Irrigation was found to increase substantially the income of all sectors of production, although the increases to land, fixed capital, and purchased inputs appear to be higher than those to labor and management. Just the same, poor people benefit substantially from irrigation. Gains in labor income resulting from irrigation ranged from 12 percent in the Philippines to over 400 percent in Thailand (where dry-season irrigation doubles the cropping intensity, and wet-season labor use is higher in irrigated than in nonirrigated areas) (Rosegrant 1986).

For a broad review of agricultural water policies, see Boggess, Lacewell, and Zilberman (1993); Rosegrant, Scheleyer, and Yadav (1995); and Sampath (1992).

Fertilizer and Farm Chemicals

Fertilizer subsidies have been common in the developing world. During the 1980s, for example, urea sold at 56 percent below cost in Sri Lanka and at 60 percent below cost in Gambia. A long list of arguments favoring subsidies to fertilizer include encouraging learning by doing, overcoming risk aversion and credit constraints, helping poor farmers, offsetting disincentives caused by taxing or pricing policies, and maintaining soil fertility (World Bank, *World Development Report 1986*:95). Let us look briefly at each of these arguments.

• When fertilizer was a new idea, it made sense to provide it to farmers at below cost as an incentive to try it. But knowledge of fertilizer is widespread now.

• As we will discuss below, encouraging rural financial markets is the most appropriate way to deal with rural credit constraints.

• Fertilizer subsidies are an inefficient way to help poor farmers. Farmers with large operations, and those on better land, are likely to reap more benefits than the poor farmers. For example, data collected by Leclercq (1988) on size distribution of Brazilian soybean farms showed that the smallest 64 percent of farmers produce only 20 percent of the soybeans, while the largest 2 percent of farms produce over 30 percent of the soybeans.

• The best way to cope with production disincentives caused by anti-farm taxation or pricing policies is to eliminate urban bias (Chapter 22). Subsidizing the price of fertilizer is an inequitable way to transfer income to the farm sector because it provides the greatest subsidy to the biggest farmers.

• Subsidizing fertilizer use to maintain soil fertility is a questionable practice, especially when making fertilizer cheap encourages farmers to substitute it for naturally occurring organic fertilizers that have better moisture-retaining properties.

Similarly, making pesticides cheap through subsidization encourages farmers to use more of the chemicals than they would if they paid the full costs. The subsidies undermine efforts to promote integrated pest management—a method of pest control that stresses biological suppression of insects and weeds and minimal use of chemical pesticides (Repetto 1985; U.S. Dept. of Agriculture 1989a).

As fertilizer use increases, scarcities often develop as the government-subsidized distribution falls behind demand. Furthermore, the cost of the fertilizer subsidy can become a major concern to government. Concern over the budgetary costs of the fertilizer subsidy in Bangladesh prompted a study of the production impact of removing the subsidy. On the one hand, it was found that eliminating the subsidy would result in an increase in the domestic price of fertilizer some 34 percent over what it would have been during 1983–1984, and that this increase in price would result in a decrease in fertilizer use. On the other hand, several factors were found to be of even greater importance than the fertilizer subsidy in stimulating fertilizer use and farm production in Bangladesh. Many of these factors were related (because of the subsidy to fertilizer) to the government's involvement in the distribution of fertilizer, with its attendant bureaucratic inefficiencies. (See Box 23.1.)

Mechanization
Many developing countries have pursued a mix of policies that tend to accelerate mechanization beyond the pace appropriate for their labor force (Binswanger, Donovan et al. 1987:1). They do this in a variety of ways.

Governments often give preferential tariff treatment for machinery, and especially low tariffs for agricultural machinery. Farmers are sometimes given a tax shelter through deductions for farm machinery set at levels greater than the cost of the machinery. Brazil, for instance, has allowed a deduction for farm machinery of six times the value of the machine in the first year of operation. Other farm investments are treated less favorably, and labor costs enjoy no preferential tax treatment at all (World Bank, *World Development Report 1986*:97).

Countries often set the official exchange rate for their domestic currency higher than the market value. The market value for a rupee in India, for example, might be 10 (U.S.) cents, but the Indian government might declare a rupee to be worth more, say 15 cents. The upshot of this artificially inflated exchange rate is that, if you can get dollars from the government at the official rate, you can buy goods, like machinery or food, from abroad

---

Box 23.1   Impact of Eliminating Fertilizer Subsidies in Sub-Saharan Africa

During the 1970s and 1980s, many sub-Saharan African countries began government programs to distribute fertilizer at below-market prices. In the 1990s, responding to pressure from international organizations, these programs were eliminated. The hope was that getting governments out of the fertilizer distribution business would create a vacuum that would be filled by more-efficient privately owned companies.

The early indications of the impact of this policy reform are mildly disappointing. For example in Ethiopia, eliminating the subsidy was estimated to cause an increase in fertilizer prices by 21–39 percent. Derneke, Said, and Jayne (1997) examined fifty-one farms that differed in geography and crop choice; they found that with the subsidy, fertilizer use was profitable in forty-two of these cases. However without the subsidy (assuming no increased efficiency of delivery), fertilizer use would be profitable in only twenty of the fifty-one cases. If cost efficiencies could be realized in the fertilizer delivery system, fertilizer use would be profitable in twenty-eight of the fifty-one cases.

A general review by Reardon et al. (1999: pp. 381–382), concluded:

"African fertilizer use is the lowest in the world and has even decreased over the past decade and a half, i.e., over the same period in which fertilizer and seed subsidies and cheap input financial services programs have been reduced or eliminated. . . . Case study evidence points to a connection between the reduction in fertilizer use and these rising input prices. . . . Moreover, there is growing evidence that private fertilizer and seed merchants have responded much less than was expected to the liberalization of input markets enacted through elimination of fertilizer and seed parastatals. . . . Fertilizer markets in African are plagued by a series of fundamental problems such as risk, seasonal demand, high transport costs, underdeveloped financial services markets, and cash constrained farmers. Small markets add to the problem by limiting economies of scale. . . . Moreover, economies of scale in fertilizer production make domestic production inefficient in most African economies, so domestic fertilizer prices are sensitive to macro trade and exchange rate policies, and to volatile international fertilizer prices. While fertilizer subsidies and domestic fertilizer production schemes have generally proved ineffective in Africa, it appears clear that private market conditions in rural Africa cannot presently support necessary fertilizer deliveries, so some role for government is inevitable in the short-to-medium term. Given the considerable costs of delivering fertilizer to farmers on time and the restricted physical availability of fertilizer to most farmers, investment in improved private marketing infrastructure seems one of the most promising roles for the state."

---

at bargain prices. When this happens, competition immediately arises for these cheap dollars, and the government has to ration them among competing uses. Commonly, agricultural machinery imports receive a substantial allocation. Cheap foreign currency and low tariffs make a substantial subsidy to imported machinery. In addition, subsidized credit (discussed below) makes capital cheaper than it otherwise would be.

The desirability of machinery subsidies has been questioned on several points. First, the benefits of machinery subsidies typically go to large farms. Thus they provide the wealthy farmers with a competitive advantage relative to their poorer neighbors. Second, mechanization does not necessarily increase yields. Binswanger (1978:73), in a careful review of the studies concerning the impact of tractorization on yields in South Asia, found that the surveys failed "to provide evidence that tractors are responsible for substantial increases in intensity, yields, timeliness, and gross returns on farms in India, Pakistan, and Nepal." It seems that, by and large, an acre of land tilled by hand or animal power does not yield less than an acre of land tilled by a tractor (Campbell 1984:47).

From the point of view of improving third world nutrition, there can be no justification for a machinery subsidy. When machinery is profitable, farmers will buy it and society will benefit from it. If the machinery is available only in fairly large units, small farmers can benefit from using rented machinery.

Subsidizing agricultural mechanization denies funding for alternative investments that are at least as productive as the machinery and that do not reduce labor demand as much as the subsidized machinery (Binswanger, Donovan et al. 1987:1).

Stevens and Jabara (1988:272–273) list four undesirable effects from premature acceleration of agricultural mechanization resulting from subsidies: (1) reduced employment; (2) greater income disparities; (3) attempts by those with tractors and other machines to increase farm size; and (4) increased incentives to inventors and manufacturers to develop and produce even more labor-saving agricultural machinery.

■ Credit Subsidies

Rationale for Subsidizing Credit
To the extent that credit can remove existing financial constraints, it can accelerate the use of capital equipment and the adoption of new technology. Third world governments commonly feel that a scarcity of credit is constraining the development of their low-income farm sector and see subsidized credit as a way of transferring income to the poor, who will then benefit by becoming more productive through the use of this cheap credit. Furthermore, as described in Chapter 19, these same governments often engage in policies that result in farm-gate prices below those the market would normally pay, and look to subsidized credit,

with its below-market interest rates, as a way of compensating low-income farmers for their losses from these pricing policies (Adams et al. 1984).

Billions of dollars have been spent on subsidized credit programs in the third world. These programs have arisen because of a number of assumptions about peasant farmers as savers and borrowers and about the credit sources that are commonly available to them. For instance, it is commonly assumed that, despite their ability to repay a loan, small farmers have difficulty obtaining loans because of a lack of collateral or the feeling among rural lenders that small farmers present too great a risk.

Dale Adams and others, having reviewed these assumptions, concluded that many of them are erroneous (see Box 23.2).

As we will see below, subsidized credit is not an effective instrument for transferring income to the poor. Furthermore, subsidized credit may have harmful side effects on financial institutions and other segments of the economy, particularly the poor.

Box 23.2   Common Assumptions About Lenders and Borrowers

Dale Adams and Douglas Graham

Common assumptions about saver-borrower behavior are that the rural poor cannot save and therefore will not respond to incentives or opportunities to save, that most farmers need cheap loans and supervision before they will adopt new technologies and make major farm investments, and that loans in kind are used in the form granted.

Common assumptions about lender behavior are that most informal lenders are exploitative and charge borrowers rates of interest that result in large monopoly profits, that the rural poor do not receive formal loans because formal lenders are overly risk-averse, that nationalized lenders can be forced to ignore their own profits and losses to serve risky customers and the rural poor, and that all formal lenders can be induced to follow government regulations in allocating financial services.

At a national level it is commonly assumed that cheap credit is an efficient way of offsetting production disincentives caused by low farm product prices or high farm input prices, that loan quotas established in the capital city are efficient ways of allocating loans in the countryside, that loans should be a part of a package of inputs, that only production loans should be made, and that rural financial market vitality is not related to projects and policies.

Research is showing that many of these assumptions are either unsubstantiated, weak, or incorrect.

Source: Extracted from Adams and Graham 1981: pp. 347–350.

Methods of Providing Cheap Credit

There are two common ways in which governments provide low-interest loans. One is directly through a government bank or quasi-government bank that loans the money to preferred borrowers at below-market interest rates. For instance, in Jamaica during the 1970s, the parastatal development bank supplied loans at less than half the commercial bank rate.

The other common way of providing low-interest loans is for the government to require commercial banks to supply a given amount of money to preferred borrowers at below-market rates. In Nigeria, for example, banks must devote 8 percent of their loans to the agricultural sector at approximately half the going commercial interest rate (Bale 1985:17).

Beginning in 1965 in Brazil, the law required commercial banks to lend at least 50 percent of their demand deposits to farmers at 17 percent interest per year. At that time the annual inflation rate was ranging from 20 to 40 percent per year; these loans were therefore very profitable for the borrowers. In 1971 the mandated rural interest rate was lowered to 15 percent, even though high rates of inflation continued (Sicat 1983:381).

Problems Associated with Subsidized Credit

When the credit subsidy is paid for directly by government, the costs can run very high, so high that governments often use deficit financing to pay for the programs. The deficit financing, in turn, leads to inflation, which discourages saving, the basis of capital formation. The question must be asked whether the resources devoted to providing cheap credit might better be used in other government programs—more agricultural research, better rural roads, or improved educational services.

When the credit program is paid for implicitly, as happens when you force commercial credit institutions to give low-interest loans to priority borrowers, the costs of this hidden subsidy must be borne by the less preferred borrowers. They get less credit or pay higher interest rates for their loans, both of which are a constraint on development.

Sometimes governments attempt to limit the possibility that someone will make a profit (by obtaining cheap credit and then depositing the money right back in the bank at the [higher] commercial rate) by putting a ceiling on the commercial interest rate. Forcing down the interest rate in this way lessens the rewards from saving, discouraging some people from saving and motivating others to send their savings (and thus their capital) out of the country where they can get a better return.

From the point of view of income distribution, the worst aspect of subsidized credit is that it discriminates against the poor. The subsidized credit almost always goes to those in the community who are better prepared to receive it. In rural areas this means the rural elite: those well connected politically. Seldom does it go to the poorest of the poor.

The impact of a credit subsidy is thus regressive. Loans are seldom all the same size, and the size of the subsidy is directly proportional to the size of the loan. The larger farmers get larger loans and more subsidy. Medium and small farmers get proportionally smaller subsidies. The smallest farmers and landless laborers get no subsidy at all (González-Vega 1983:371).

An Alternative to Subsidized Credit

Evidence shows that the availability of credit in the countryside can be greatly expanded merely by rigging the system to encourage rural financial markets to serve as intermediaries between savers and borrowers. This seems to be the appropriate alternative to subsidized credit.

Contrary to the commonly held assumption, low-income farmers do save. In a review of the available data on savings among rural households in Taiwan, Japan, South Korea, Malaysia, and India, Dale Adams found positive average propensities to save to be the norm. (The propensity to save is the percentage of income that is not spent for consumption or taxes.) Furthermore, rural households' savings are responsive to changes in the real interest rate. (The real interest rate is the difference between the nominal interest rate and the inflation rate.) In 1965 South Korea allowed the interest rate paid on time deposits and applied to loans to almost double. This resulted in real interest rates of over 8 percent per year. During the ensuing four years, total time and savings deposits in all banks increased fourteenfold. The number of savings accounts also increased sharply during this period (Adams 1983:401–405). In Korean farm households, the average propensity to save steadily increased during the ten years following the credit reform (Table 23.1). Interestingly, the rate of increase in propensity to save was greatest among those farm households with the smallest landholdings.

Mere convenience can be a factor in attracting rural savings. In India, when banks were encouraged to open rural branches for the primary purpose of disbursing agricultural loans, but at the same time offered a positive real interest rate on deposits, the response was so substantial that some authorities were concerned about the drain of funds from rural areas (World Bank, *World Development Report 1986*:101).

When rural people are offered convenient, secure savings institutions providing financially attractive real rates of return on savings, they seem to flock to make deposits. This increases the supply of lendable funds, eventually reducing the cost of credit through market mechanisms. Abundant credit at reasonable commercial rates eliminates the need for the capital rationing associated with subsidized credit, with its tendency to favor rural elites, and makes credit more readily available to the rural poor.

Microcredit and group liability. One promising way to make credit available to small farmers is microcredit (see Box 23.3.) The Grameen Bank of

Table 23.1   Average Propensity to Save, South Korean Farm Households, by Farm Size, 1962–1974

Farm Size (in Cheongboa)	1962	1965	1966	1968	1970	1972	1974
0.5 or less	0.05	−0.05	0.01	0.06	0.03	0.02	0.22
0.5–1.0	0.12	0.01	0.09	0.11	0.13	0.21	0.29
1.0–1.5	0.16	0.06	0.10	0.20	0.16	0.34	0.35
1.5–2.0	0.15	0.12	0.13	0.23	0.26	0.30	0.43
2.0 or more	0.22	0.13	0.23	0.24	0.19	0.30	0.40
Average all households	0.15	0.04	0.11	0.16	0.15	0.24	0.33
Total number of households	1,163	1,172	1,180	1,181	1,180	1,182	2,515

Source: Adams 1983:404.
Note: One cheongbo equals 0.992 hectares or 2.45 acres. In this table average propensity to save was calculated as follows: (net income after taxes − consumption)/net income after taxes.

Box 23.3   Microcredit in Practice.

An actual example of microcredit illustrates how it works. A farmer in the Philippines wanted to borrow $52 to buy two piglets. He planned to feed the piglets with table scraps and spoiled food from the family table, so there would be little cost other than the initial investment. He was able to convince his fellow microcredit group members that this was a reasonable investment, and they knew that the farmer had a reputation for honesty and hard work. The farmer received the loan and promised to repay $2.30 a week for twenty-six weeks (a total repayment of about $60). At the end of six months, the farmer was able to sell the fattened pigs for over $200. The money he repaid plus interest was available to finance projects by other group members.

Bangladesh introduced the concept of making small loans to poor families who put up no other collateral than joining and meeting regularly with a support group. The sense of obligation of the borrower to the group was a sufficiently strong incentive so that members do, in fact, pay back their loans (Hossain 1988a:25–26).

The use of small community groups to funnel credit to rural lenders has a number of advantages. The group members know the reputation of the borrowers—who is industrious, who is lazy, who is honest—and can take that into account in making loan decisions. The group members have similar backgrounds and experiences, and so are able to analyze the likelihood that a project will succeed in generating income sufficient to repay the loan. The group members can fairly easily determine whether difficulty in repaying is due to a borrower's bad luck or is due to the borrower's poor performance. Finally, borrowers want to repay the loans in order to preserve their social standing in the community.

One estimate (Global Development Research Center 2003) says that there are currently about 13 million borrowers from microcredit lenders, with the average loan size of about $500. Repayment rates are reported to be above 95 percent.

■ Policies to Encourage Investment:
Rural Infrastructure and Price Stability

Making credit more easily available or reducing the prices of capital goods increases farmers' *ability* to make investments that will lower production costs. In this section, we discuss some policies that can increase farmers' *desire* to make such investments. In particular, we will examine how government investments in rural infrastructure and government programs to stabilize farm prices can reassure farmers about their ability to transport their output to market and sell it.

Subsidizing Farm-to-Market Roads

Building a new road into a region that formerly was reached only by human or animal transport can have an important impact on that region's economy. Because it dramatically reduces the cost of transporting farm products out of the region, it raises the farm-gate price of what farmers sell to country marketing agents who buy and transport food to the city. And because it simultaneously reduces the cost of transporting materials into the region, it reduces the cost of purchased farm inputs such as fertilizer. Higher farm-gate prices and lower input costs increase farm income, stimulate greater farm production, increase the demand for farm labor, and raise local wages.

In a study of the impact of new roads on forty-six Philippine rural communities, Santos-Villanueva (1966) found a decrease in transportation costs of from 17 to 60 percent per kilometer and a substantial increase in the amount of agricultural products sold off the farm (see Table 23.2).

In a study of sixteen villages in rural Bangladesh, it was found that villages with a good infrastructure, including good all-weather, hard-surfaced roads, used 92 percent more fertilizer per hectare than villages with poor infrastructure. They used 4 percent more labor per hectare, and they paid their agricultural laborers 12 percent more per day than did villages with poor infrastructure (Ahmed and Hossain 1990).

Higher local wage rates reduce the pressure for out-migration. In other

Table 23.2   Average Increases in Volume of Sales of Selected Farm Products After the Construction of a Nearby Road from Farm to Market, Philippines

	Percentage Increase
Corn	104
Chicken	69
Swine	47
Coconuts	30
Rice	24
Bananas	12

Source: Santos-Villanueva 1966.

words, good roads help keep people home. Good roads encourage private entrepreneurs to start bus services, often with very small vehicles ranging from large three-wheeled motorcycles to minibuses, and thus make it possible for rural people who live within reasonable commuting distances to work in town but continue to live at home. Good roads enable employment outside the home neighborhood.

As roads lower the cost of transportation to and from the countryside, the annual fluctuation in the price of food is reduced. Remote communities find it cheaper to export food in good crop years and to import food in poor crop years, thus reducing price swings between the bad and the good harvests. Reducing these price swings reduces the probability that low-income families will face undernutrition during the years of bad harvest.

As a good road network reduces the cost of transporting agricultural commodities around the country, increased agricultural specialization by region can take place. For instance, perishable fruits and vegetables can be grown farther from urban markets than previously, making possible a higher-valued use of land far from market and reducing the income disparity between remote areas and the major cities.

The same sorts of advantages that accrue with new roads into a formerly remote territory apply to improvements in old roads. Putting a hard surface on a dirt road, or mending potholes on a worn-out, older, all-weather road, creates benefits similar , albeit less dramatic, to those from putting in a new road.

Other Aspects of Rural Infrastructure

In addition to roads, the parts of rural infrastructure that probably have the most bearing on agricultural production are the electrical system, the communications network, and the marketing system.

Rural electrification makes possible the powering of a host of time-saving and production-enhancing devices. Small irrigation pumps and power tools are efficiently driven by electricity. It also makes communications easier in the countryside, for example by making a modern telephone switching system possible. Access to a telephone (even if there is only one per village) can save lives in a medical emergency. But efficient communications are also important in marketing farm products as well as in gaining access to purchased farm inputs.

An important function of a marketing system is to reflect back to producers the wants and preferences of consumers. As economic development brings changes in food-demand patterns, a good marketing system will efficiently transmit this information to farmers, who can then reallocate their resources to take advantage of the new production opportunities.

And as the sophistication of agricultural production increases with the adoption of new technology and improved management, a good marketing system for agricultural inputs will reflect farmers' preferences back to the farm suppliers. Bureaucratic, government-sponsored fertilizer distribution schemes usually supply only a limited choice of plant nutrient mixes. But if allowed to function in an appropriate institutional framework, a private-enterprise marketing system will make available a wide variety of fertilizers, allowing farmers to choose the most efficient ones for a particular situation.

Government support can supply radio stations and newspapers to pass along price information of interest to farmers. This is especially important for small farmers who, because of lack of information about market prices, might otherwise be at a disadvantage in comparison with the larger farmers who can afford to get such information on their own.

Government-sponsored terminal markets, where buyers can assemble farm products from the countryside and distribute them to retailers in the city, can increase the efficiency of the marketing system. Increasing the efficiency of the marketing system lowers prices to consumers and increases prices to producers, thus improving nutrition and stimulating increases in production. Appropriate government subsidies are important to an efficiently functioning agricultural marketing system. (See Box 23.4.)

Price Stabilization

When farmers make decisions about whether to invest in projects that will improve their long-term productivity, they base their decisions on beliefs about future prices. Economists have found evidence that farmers are *risk-averse*—other things being equal, they would prefer a sure thing or a low-risk investment to a high-risk investment. When output prices are highly variable and unpredictable, farm investments are riskier, and farmers are less likely to make these investments. For this reason, some governments have instituted policies to stabilize prices of agricultural commodities (Newbery and Stiglitz 1981).

Box 23.4   Public Goods and Public Investment

Public investments are usually made because of a failure of the market to provide certain public goods. A small public park, a downtown sidewalk, national defense, and free public education are examples of public goods. Public
goods have two critical properties: (1) it is impossible to exclude individuals
from enjoying the benefits from them, and (2) it is undesirable to exclude
individuals from enjoying the benefits from them, since such enjoyment does
not detract from that of others (Stiglitz 1986:119).

No one wants to produce a public good because, once produced, it is
available to all. The producer cannot sell it and capture his costs.

The distinction between a private good and a public good may be blurred
or fuzzy. For instance, we can think of expenditure on the education of our
children as a private good, since the children benefit directly; but education
also has aspects of a public good because educated children will be more productive later on in life than uneducated children. The fact that education provides benefits (external benefits) to people other than the students themselves
helps explain why governments are involved in paying for public schools.

Likewise, when a consortium of governments pays a public agricultural
experiment station for research to develop high-yielding varieties of rice, we
may want to call it a public investment. All rice farmers can benefit from the
new rice varieties, and of course the public benefits from the lower market
price of rice after the higher-yielding rice varieties are put into use. We could
also call the rice research and the resulting high-yielding varieties a public
good. So it is with many other public expenditures for enhancing agricultural
production, such as research on irrigation machinery or agricultural extension
programs—they are pitched at the farm sector but they benefit the public.

Governments have used four general types of policies to achieve more
stable prices:

1. The most direct policy is that of *administered prices,* under which
the government sets prices, either by administrative fiat, or by acting as the
sole buyer of the commodity. The difficulty with this type of policy is that
the government frequently knows even less than farmers about likely future
price levels. Therefore, the prices established by the government do not
reflect underlying supply-and-demand conditions. Black markets emerge
and either the programs are ineffective or they become an enormous drain
on the government treasury.

2. A second method is a *buffer stock* program under which the government buys the commodity when supplies are plentiful and prices are relatively low, and sells the commodity when supplies are tight and prices are
relatively high. The government storage acts to even out prices over time.
In theory, this program should put a ceiling and a floor on agricultural

prices: when prices threaten to drop below the floor, the government buys the commodity and bids the price back up; when prices threaten to shoot through the ceiling, the government sells the commodity and brings prices back down. In practice, governments have not been particularly adept at establishing the correct range of prices. In addition, the subsidized government storage tends to discourage storage in the private sector.

3. A *buffer fund* accomplishes much the same thing as a buffer stock program, but does so without the government's actually buying and selling the commodity. Under a buffer fund, governments tax sales of the commodity in periods when prices are high (and thereby reduce the price received by farmers), and subsidize sales in periods when prices are low (effectively increasing the farm price). Buffer funds require extensive bookkeeping to verify which farmer sold what quantity at what price.

4. Finally, governments can encourage the development of private market institutions, such as *forward contracting* and *futures markets,* to stabilize prices. These mechanisms allow farmers to lock in a price at the beginning of a growing season, at least for a major proportion of their crop. These types of contracts work well in theory; but farmers have been reluctant to adopt them in the United States and other developed countries.

■ Policies to Promote Technological Improvement

Subsidizing Agricultural Research

Technological change is one of the primary driving forces behind increasing production. Improved technology (e.g., a higher-yielding variety of rice) can increase the productivity of every item of the set of resources that a farmer uses—land, labor, management, and capital. Yet the agricultural researcher intent on developing new technology for agriculture faces an extraordinarily intricate range of scientific challenges. One analysis of technological change (Lele, Kinsey, and Obeya 1989:42) listed these areas as important to researchers in improved crop varieties in third world agriculture:

- Yield potential and responsiveness to available chemical fertilizers and pesticides
- Adaptation to the growing period and drought tolerance
- Disease and pest resistance
- Improvements in quality, palatability, and consumer acceptance
- Storage, transport, and other handling qualities (including processing) with available technology
- Changes in labor requirements in production and processing in rela-

tion to the available mechanical technology, in view of other requirements for household labor and incentives for labor use
• Compatibility with other social, cultural, and economic norms

Not only is the range of challenge complex, but the disciplines brought to bear on agricultural research are varied. Advancing agricultural technology involves research in biology, chemistry, and engineering, as well as in the social sciences, which are crucial to the appropriate integration of the new technology into the production system.

Despite the challenging nature of agricultural research, the payoff has been nothing short of spectacular. As described in Chapter 14, agricultural research has been instrumental in dramatic increases in crop yields per acre as well as in livestock productivity. And when the costs of agricultural research are compared to the benefits to society, agricultural research turns out to be a real bargain.

In Table 23.3, studies of payoffs to research done at agricultural experiment stations around the world are listed. The last column, annual internal rate of return, is of particular interest. The internal rate of return represents the average earning power of the resources used in a project during the project period. For an agricultural research project, this is the equivalent of the interest rate you would have to get from a savings account to receive the same return on your savings as the public got from the agricultural research project.

In one of the earliest studies of this kind, returns to research on hybrid corn (maize) in the United States were calculated by the economist Zvi

Table 23.3   Studies About Rates of Return to Agricultural Research

Commodity	Number of studies	Average over all studies (%)	Lowest rate of return found(%)	Highest rate of return found(%)
Multicommodity	436	80.3	−1	1219
All agriculture	342	75.7	−1	1219
Crops and Livestock	80	106.3	17	562
Unspecified	14	42.1	16.4	69.2
Field crops	916	74.3	−100	1720
Maize	170	134.5	−100	1720
Wheat	155	50.4	−47.5	290
Rice	81	75.0	11.4	466
Livestock	233	120.7	2.5	5645
Tree crops	108	87.6	1.4	1736
All studies	1772	81.2	−100	5645

Source: Alston, J., et al. 2000.

Griliches (1958). (The corn breeding research was carried out by many scientists.) The internal rate of return to hybrid corn research in the United States is calculated to be 35 to 40 percent. That means for every dollar the U.S. public paid for agricultural research on hybrid corn until 1955, it collected from $0.35 to $0.40 every year in benefits (mostly through lower prices for corn). It would be hard to find another set of investments that pay off as well as agricultural research. Swindale (1997) cites an example of research in sub-Saharan Africa into methods of controlling an insect pest—the cassava mealybug. The research cost $27 million, but the benefits from the research exceeded $4 billion.

If agricultural research has such a spectacular payoff, why don't farmers themselves pay for it? Or why don't private companies undertake the research and sell the results to farmers? (See Tables 23.4 and 23.5.) The two reasons why it is not appropriate to ask farmers to pay are (1) most farmers have far too small an operation to sponsor and benefit from agricultural research, and (2) because the elasticity of demand for most farm products is less than one, the majority of the benefits from agricultural research goes to consumers. Farmers generally lose revenue when the new technology is widely adopted because they see their farm-gate prices fall faster than they can increase production. Long-term data from the United States, with a history of public sponsorship of agricultural research dating back to the 1870s, is illustrative:

Table 23.4   Estimated Public and Private Agricultural R&D Investment, 1995

Group	Expenditures in $million			
	Public	Private	Total	% Private
Developing	11,770	609	12,379	4.9
Developed	21,567	10,962	32,530	51.4

Source: Pardey and Beintema 2001.

Table 23.5   Public Exenditures on Agricultural R&D As a Percent of Agricultural GDP

Group	1976	1996
Developing	0.5	0.6
Developed	1.5	2.6

Source: Pardey and Beintema 2001.

The decline in the real price of food has been dramatic. Available data for the period 1888 to 1891 indicate that consumers spent an average of about 40 percent of their income for food. From 1930 to 1960, the food expenditure proportion of consumer incomes ranged from 20 to 24 percent. In the seventies, the proportion of total disposable personal income spent for food dropped to a range of 1–17 percent. By the mid-eighties, that proportion for the average family had dropped to a record low of 15 percent. (Lee and Taylor 1986: 20–21)

Patent laws protect mechanical and chemical innovations more effectively than biological innovations. For this reason, some agroindustrial firms have been able to sponsor research in farm machinery or agricultural chemicals and capture the benefits from that research. Hybrid seeds are protectable by patents and, because they do not breed true, farmers must purchase new supplies each year. So after government-sponsored research led the way, hybrid seed companies set up their own research and are developing their own varieties. But by and large, biological innovations in agriculture have to be paid for by government. Thus, animal breeding, animal nutrition, plant breeding, plant pathology, entomology, agronomy, soil science, and so on are government-sponsored (Judd, Boyce, and Evenson 1987:7).

Some governments are too small to sponsor agricultural research. Their funds are best spent on adaptive agricultural research—finding out which of the innovations discovered elsewhere are most adaptable to their own situations. The Consultative Group on International Agricultural Research stations are helping to fill in the research gap felt by the smaller countries. As of 1998, twelve international agricultural research stations belonged to this group and were sponsored by a variety of sources. The group includes the International Rice Research Institute in the Philippines and the International Maize and Wheat Improvement Center in Mexico, as well as a number of other centers whose activities range from plant and animal breeding to food policy.

Modern-day challenges to agricultural research are legion. The techniques of recombinant DNA and cell fusion are making it possible for biotechnologists to engage in investigations with opportunities for very high rewards, developing highly productive organisms that might not ever have arisen in nature (U.S. Congress, Office of Technology Assessment 1986).

Low-income rural householders could benefit from research on hardy but efficient scavenging animals. High-yielding, disease-resistant breeds of chickens, ducks, goats, pigs, cattle, bees, or fish that can utilize garbage or other food that may be locally available but unfit for human consumption would be of considerable benefit to the third world's poor.

Africa poses a particular challenge to agricultural research. Its soils are more diverse, its climate more varied, its pest and disease hazards more pronounced, and its farming systems more complex than those of monsoon Asia, where the green revolution has been such a success (Lele and Goldsmith 1989; Lipton and Longhurst 1990). African agriculture is characterized by *mixed cropping* (more than one crop at a time is grown in a field), which occupies over 90 percent of the cropped area in most countries on the continent. Mixed cropping falls into three main categories:

1. *Intercropping:* more than one crop on a given area at one time, arranged in a geometric pattern
2. *Relay cropping:* a form of intercropping where not all the crops are planted at the same time
3. *Sequential cropping:* more than one crop (or intercrop) on a given area in the same year, the second crop being planted after the first is harvested

A special challenge for the agricultural research community working in Africa is to intensify agricultural production within this complex farm management system while maintaining its flexibility and its proven sustainability (Dommen 1988). One production innovation that holds promise for sustainability in the semiarid tropics that cover so much of Africa is *agroforestry,* a system of strip-cropping rows of trees between narrow strips of crops. The trees help conserve water, provide a ready source of organic matter, and reduce erosion.

Subsidizing Technology Diffusion and Adoption
Profitable technology will spread from farmer to farmer by itself. But the rate of adoption can be accelerated by government-sponsored educational programs. (See Feder, Just, and Zilberman 1985 for a review of the literature on this.) Such programs are often called *extension* because they were originally conceived to extend the knowledge developed in the U.S. land-grant college system directly to the farmer. Programs that provide education and advice to farmers are now in place in most countries having a significant agricultural economy.

A classic study of Iowa's farmers illustrates the typical growth curve of knowledge that an agricultural community experiences as its farmers gradually become aware of a new technology, then try it out, and finally adopt it as part of their regular farming activities. In this case, a new chemical weed control called 2,4–D had come on the market. It took approximately eleven years between the time only a few farmers (4 percent) had even heard of it and all of them were using it. Notice in Figure 23.2 how awareness precedes trial, which precedes adoption. In 1949, for instance, about midway through the process, 74 percent of the farmers were aware of the existence

Figure 23.2   Cumulative Percentage of Farm Operators at the Awareness, Trial, and Adoption Stages for 2,4–D Weed Spray, by Year, Iowa, 1944–1944

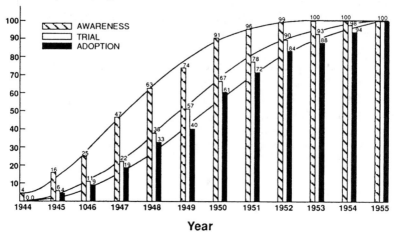

Source: Adapted from Beal & Rogers 1960:8.

of the new weedicide, but only 40 percent had adopted it. By 1955 all farmers in the area were using it. Without the vigorous extension program carried on by Iowa State University, the new technology undoubtedly would have spread, but whether it would have spread as fast is open to question. It is the charge of the extension service to accelerate the adoption of new technology, whether it be new agricultural chemicals, better plant and animal varieties, or better farm management practices.

Accelerating the spread of technology begins with government sponsorship of agricultural training institutions—places where technicians learn the skills necessary for backstopping agriculture in the field: plant and animal sciences, and farm management and finance, for example. Not only do government-sponsored farm advisors need to know agricultural technology, but rural banks need farm appraisers, and rural tax collectors need to know about the economics of farming. Sponsoring the training of these technicians provides an important subsidy to agricultural production. The success of an agricultural extension service depends not only on the quality of training that farm advisors get at their local agricultural colleges but, perhaps more important, on the quality of the technology they have to extend. Building an array of extension agents without providing them with a set of technologies appropriate to the region where they are working does not endear them to farmers and weakens the future effectiveness of their organizations.

■ Policies to Promote Sustainable Farming Methods

Closely related to policies that promote increased productivity in the farm sector through development and adoption of new technologies are policies that promote environmentally friendly (or sustainable) farming. Here too, the government programs are directed at invention—or discovery—of environmentally appropriate practices, and extension—or teaching farmers about those methods. The kinds of policies discussed in the previous section apply here.

The importance of sustainable farming methods was discussed in Chapters 13 and 14. Agricultural production puts a strain on the natural environment. If the strain is too great—if land and water resources become sufficiently degraded—future agricultural production will suffer. Therefore, persuading farmers to adopt sustainable farming methods—methods that by definition do not entail resource degradation, which will in turn lead to future declines in production—will cause future food supply to be greater than it would be in the absence of these methods.

24

World Food Supply and Demand for the Next Half-Century: Some Alternative Scenarios

> And I beheld a black horse; and he that sat on him had a pair of balances in his hand. And I heard a voice . . . say, A measure of wheat for a penny, and three measures of barley for a penny. . . . And power was given unto them over the fourth part of the earth, to kill with the sword, and with hunger, and with death, and with the beast of the earth.
>
> —Revelation 6:5–8

Famine is one of the Four Horsemen of the Apocalypse. And when our visions of the future take an apocalyptic turn, the spectre of widespread hunger is likely to appear. What does the future hold? Will the progress of the last thirty years continue? Or are we on the brink of a slide into catastrophe? Having boldly asked these questions, we less boldly reply, "It all depends . . . " This chapter will briefly review schools of thought about the future of the world food problem and will present a framework for building scenarios about the future.

There are several points on which there is universal agreement. Of course, any prediction is likely to be wrong in certain fundamental ways. But the four Ps identified in Chapter 1—population, prosperity, productivity, and pollution—are almost certain to be the major factors shaping the future. Growth in population and in per capita income will determine, to a considerable extent, demand for food. Growth in yields per hectare and limitations imposed by environmental quality will determine, to a considerable extent, supply of food. The interplay of these factors will ultimately be reflected in the fifth P—the price of food. If demand grows more rapidly than supply, food prices will increase and hunger may become more widespread. If supply grows more rapidly than demand, food prices will drop. The sixth P—policy—is the means by which humankind can hope to influence the future.

■ Two Views of the Future

It is tempting to characterize people's views about the future of world food supply and demand as "optimistic" or "pessimistic." (In fact, at several points in this book, such characterizations are made.) But a more accurate division might be between the *establishment* view and the *antiestablishment* view. The establishment view is reflected in recent reports by the FAO (Alexandratos 1995), the World Bank (Mitchell, Ingco, and Duncan 1997), the International Food Price Research Institute (Pinstrup-Andersen, Pandya-Lorch, and Rosegrant 1998, and other IFPRI 2020 reports), and the U.S. Department of Agriculture (1998). These reports embrace a common vision of the future in which world agricultural production continues to grow (with slight growth in agricultural area and yield growth in the 1 to 1.5 percent per year range), world population continues to grow but ever more slowly than the current 1.14 percent rate, and income per capita continues to grow. Implicit in their vision is an assumption that there will be no catastrophic changes in environmental conditions.

The antiestablishment view is reflected in the works cited in Chapters 12–14 by David Pimentel of Cornell and by Lester Brown and his colleagues at the WorldWatch Institute. See Gilland (2002) for a careful exposition of this view, which puts a much greater emphasis on the possibility of environmental catastrophe. The types of catastrophe that could occur include losses of agricultural land due to erosion or degradation, reductions in availability of usable water for agriculture due to overirrigation, and global warming that could (in the worst cases projected by scientists) cause significant loss of land to rising sea levels, and significant yield reductions from changing climate patterns. The antiestablishment view is also notably less confident about the possibility of a "technological fix" for these future catastrophes if they do occur. As described in Chapter 14, this lack of confidence is based on the slowing of yield growth, and the belief that we are unlikely to see any significant breakthroughs in basic science that would provide a foundation for a new spurt of growth in yields.

Past predictions of global food shortages have been wrong in large part because they underestimated the ability of technological progress to increase food output. The establishment view has confidence that the institutions and processes that generated yield growth in the past will continue to generate yield growth in the future. The antiestablishment view sees the yield growth of the past fifty years as a one-time stroke of good fortune that is unlikely to be repeated.

Both the establishment and antiestablishment views accept the premise that human actions—especially government policies—can influence the future state of the world. The establishment view is more sympathetic to incrementalism—small changes in policies to ensure the world continues to make progress. The antiestablishment view is that major sweeping changes—especially in environmental and population policies—must be made to accommodate and ameliorate future problems.

The antiestablishment view tends to see current prosperity—and the fact that "only" 20 percent of the world's population is currently under-nourished—as coming at the expense of future generations. In effect, they argue, we are "eating the seed"—satisfying our current hunger by guaran-teeing even more severe and widespread problems in the future. The appro-priate response, therefore, is a radical reduction in current levels of con-sumption of food and nonfood alike. At the extreme, it is argued, accomplishing this radical reduction may require radical restructuring of economic and political systems. The establishment view does not accept the vision of inherent conflict between present and future generations: Current prosperity will not cause future poverty; future generations will be on average at least as prosperous as we are today. This attitude leads to a broad endorsement of existing institutions. This is not quite the same thing as saying the establishment view endorses a "business as usual" policy. Rather, the kinds of policies endorsed by the establishment view—market-oriented pricing, increased government funding of research and develop-ment, appropriate macroeconomic policies to promote general economic growth, for example—tend to be policies that can be pursued within the existing institutional framework.

■ Predicting the Future: Principles for Scenario Building

Looking at different scenarios for the future allows us to see how intelli-gent, well-informed people can arrive at such different views about the future. In this section, we present a few alternative scenarios. The main purpose is not to prove that one or the other of these scenarios is "correct," but rather to provide a template from which readers can construct their own scenarios.

These scenarios make projections fifty years into the future. This is further than most projections; but most projections are intended for policy-makers, who recognize that today's projections will be replaced by a new set within a few years. The fifty-year period was chosen to give readers a view of world food supply and demand during their lifetimes.

All scenarios are based on assumptions about annual rates of growth: growth in population, growth in per capita income, growth in area harvest-ed, and growth in yields per hectare. The rates of growth assumed are *aver-age* rates for the entire fifty-year period. Growth may be higher than aver-age for some years, and lower than average for others. As laid out at the end of Chapter 11, projections about world food demand are based on assumptions about growth in population and growth in income per capita. As suggested at the beginning of Chapter 12, projections about world food supply are based on assumptions about growth in agricultural land area and growth in yields.

In developing scenarios, we use a set of assumptions that is internally consistent. The complexity of interconnections among the factors has been illustrated throughout the book. Agricultural productivity, and the concomitant prosperity in the farm sector, contributes to economy-wide prosperity and growth in per capita income. Higher per capita income is associated with better healthcare and sanitation, and therefore lower infant mortality; this in turn leads to reduced fertility and ultimately lower population growth rates. Environmental catastrophes, should they occur, are likely to be associated with lower per capita incomes, and increased mortality—and therefore possibly lower population growth.

An "Establishment View" Scenario

At the end of Chapter 11, we presented some sample scenarios for growth in total food demand. There we saw a number of different assumptions that were consistent with a doubling of demand for food over the next fifty years. Here, we revisit that, and expand it to include the supply side. The assumptions and conclusions are summarized as scenario A in Table 24.1.

Population. Chapter 9 showed us that both the U.S. Census Bureau and the UN medium variant projected average population growth of slightly less than 1 percent per year. Here we use an average growth rate of 0.95 percent per year. At the end of fifty years, population will be 60 percent higher than the current population. (Note that this is slightly higher than the UN and census projections of 50 percent growth between 2000 and 2050.)

Income and calories per capita. Chapter 10 showed that over the last ten years, growth rates in the income per capita worldwide have been about 1 percent per year. Nevertheless, the establishment view studies cited above typically project average growth in the 2–3 percent per year range. However, the studies are for shorter periods than fifty years. For our establishment view projection, we assume an average worldwide income growth of 1.5 percent per year. This means that by the end of the fifty-year period, the average income will be more than twice as high as the current level (210 percent of the current level). As described in Chapter 11, assuming an income elasticity for food of 0.14, this means that calories per capita will increase by about 15 percent over the fifty-year period. In addition, we assume an increase in calories from animal sources will increase the effective demand per person by an additional 13 percent. The cumulative effect is to increase (plant-equivalent) calories per capita by 30 percent.

Total shift in demand. The above allows us to project that at the end of fifty years, food demand (at constant prices) would be (1.60 x 1.30 =) 208.6 percent of its current level—slightly more than twice current demand. Can supply keep pace?

Increase in agricultural land. Chapter 12 discusses the potential for increasing agricultural land. Here we assume that land in agriculture

Table 24.1 Assumptions and Outcomes of Different Scenarios for the Food Supply and Demand Situation: Comparison of the Situation as Projected 50 Years in the Future to the Current Situation

Scenario	Population	Income per Capita	Plant-Equivalent Calories per Capita	Agricultural Land	Yields per Acre	Total Demand for Food	Total Supply of Food	Price of Food	Calories/Capita/Day After 50 Years
A	+60%	+110%	+30%	+13%	+86%	+108.6%	+110%	-2.1%	3,528
A-1	+22%	+110%	+30%	+13%	+86%	+59%	+110%	-72%	3,843
A-2	+60%	+110%	+30%	+13%	+49%	+108.6%	+68%	+57%	3,327
B	+60%	+28%	+6%	-15%	+10%	+70%	-7%	+108%	2,495
B-1	+120%	+0%	0	-15%	+10%	+120%	-7%	+181%	2,256
B-2	+60%	+28%	+6%	-15%	+49%	+70%	+27%	+61%	2,655

Notes: A number such as "+60%" means that the scenario projects that, after 50 years, the level of the variable will be 60% higher than the current levels. The details of the scenarios are described in the text.

increases by 2.5 percent per decade (not per year), or 13 percent over the fifty-year period.

Increases in agricultural yields. As mentioned above, the establishment view projects increases of from 1.0 to 1.5 percent per year in yields. The graphs in Chapter 14 show that this range is consistent with historical trends and experience. Here we take the midpoint of that range (1.25 percent per year) as our assumption. Under this assumption, yields grow to 186 percent of current levels over the next fifty years.

Total increase in supply. Under these assumptions, total food supply (at constant prices) would increase to (1.13 x 1.86 =) 210 percent of current levels.

Effect on price. If food demand grows to 208 percent of current levels while supply grows to 210 percent of current levels, we see a slight downward pressure on prices. Assuming a demand elasticity of 0.2 and a supply elasticity of 0.5, food price would decline by about 2 percent from current levels.

Extent of undernutrition. Of course, we cannot estimate what happens to the extent of undernutrition with any precision by using only these worldwide aggregate numbers. But ample evidence shows that the extent of undernutrition will decline substantially under this scenario. The projected calories per capita per day increase from the current 2,700 to 3,500 (about the level in the United States during the mid-1980s). In addition, notice that while the price of food (in this scenario) is essentially unchanged at the end of fifty years, average income per capita has doubled. This should lead to a substantial reduction in the extent of undernutrition. In fact, this is the prediction of the establishment view. For example, the FAO projects that the number of food-insecure people should drop from 840 million (about 20 percent of the developing world's population) in the early 1990s to 680 million in 2010 (about 12 percent of the population). The International Food Policy Research Institute projects that by 2020, the number of malnourished children will have dropped 20 percent from 1993 levels; during the same period, total population will increase by more than 30 percent.

"Sensitivity Analysis": What Happens If We Change Assumptions? The base scenario permits us to modify assumptions one at a time and see how sensitive the results are to changes in the assumptions.

Scenario A-1: lower population growth. If population grows at the UN low-variant, population at the end of fifty years is higher by only 22 percent. If we hold all other assumptions constant, this would mean supply growing much faster than demand, and huge price decreases (72 percent declines). Although the supply curve shifts out by 110 percent, the price decline causes a movement along the supply curve of 36 percent (based on a 0.5 supply elasticity). Thus the total increase in quantity of food supplied is 74 percent.

Scenario A-2: lower yield growth. If average yield growth is 0.8 percent per year, rather than 1.25 percent in the base scenario, yields at the end of fifty years will have increased by 49 percent above current levels. Food supply increases less rapidly than food demand; therefore prices rise substantially, although less rapidly than the increase in incomes. Per capita calorie intake increases modestly. A scenario of higher population growth (at the UN high-variant of 1.3 percent annual growth) yields results that are qualitatively similar: demand grows faster than supply; quantity supplied per capita increases slightly; food prices increase but less than the increase in average incomes.

The reader is invited to create other alternative scenarios. Again, let us stress the importance of consistency. For example, if we construct a high-income-growth scenario, but maintain our initial assumption about yield growth, we will conclude that demand growth outstrips supply growth and prices rise. But economy-wide prosperity is likely to be linked to increased agricultural productivity: if the economy is prosperous, more money can be invested in agricultural productivity; in developing countries where agriculture is a large sector of the economy, agricultural productivity is a prerequisite for high rates of economic growth.

An "Antiestablishment View" Scenario

A scenario (scenario B in Table 24.1) that is consistent with the antiestablishment view is likely to reflect the following assumptions.

Population. The antiestablishment view does not take a strong stand on population projections. At least at the outset, population growth is assumed to be the same as in the establishment-view scenario—average annual growth of 0.95 percent per year. If the base-case scenario (with the UN medium-variant and U.S. Census population growth) appears to entail widespread undernutrition, we can revisit the scenario with lower population growth.

Income and calories per capita. The antiestablishment view is similarly silent on explicit projections about growth in income per capita. However, the view does predict a considerable degree of stagnation or depression in the agricultural economy. Therefore, to be consistent with the antiestablishment view, we will assume that income per capita grows much more slowly—at a rate of 0.5 percent per year. This translates into an increase in income of 28 percent over the fifty-year period, and an increase in calories demanded per capita of about 4 percent. We will assume that the impact of dietary diversification is an additional 2 percent. The cumulative effect is to increase plant-equivalent demand per capita by 6 percent. (It is important to note here that this is an increase in demand—holding prices constant. If prices increase—as is likely under the antiestablishment scenario—actual food intake per capita may decline.)

Total shift in demand. Given the above assumptions, total demand for food will be higher by a factor of (1.60 x 1.06 =) 170 percent—70 percent higher than current demand.

Increase in agricultural land. As noted in Chapter 11, the antiestablishment view believes there may be declines in agricultural land due to degradation and a rise in sea level from global warming. In this scenario, we assume that agricultural area decreases by 15 percent over the fifty-year period.

Increases in agricultural yields. The antiestablishment view is doubtful that historical rates of growth can be continued. It may be reasonable (from the standpoint of this view) to assume that yields do not increase at all, or even that they decline as irrigation and land quality decline. Here we assume that yields do continue to grow, but at only a 0.2 percent rate for the next fifty years. Under this assumption, yields grow by 10 percent over the next fifty years.

Total increase in supply. Under these assumptions, total food supply (at constant prices) would decrease to (0.85 x 1.10 =) 93.5 percent of current levels.

Effect on price. If demand grows by 70 percent and supply declines by 7 percent, price must increase. Using the 0.2 demand elasticity and 0.5 supply elasticity, this 77 percent difference between quantity demanded and quantity supplied at current prices means that the price must rise by 110 percent to return supply and demand to equilibrium.

Extent of undernutrition. The antiestablishment conclusion is that the extent of undernutrition increases substantially. The decline in average purchasing power supports this conclusion—average incomes increase by 28 percent while prices increase by 110 percent. Additional evidence of food shortage is found in food available per capita. In terms of calories per capita per day, with the current level being 2,700, this scenario implies that at the end of fifty years, there would be available about 2,230 calories per capita per day. (Although the supply curve declines under this scenario, we see an increase in quantity supplied in response to the much higher prices. See appendix to this chapter for details.)

Under this scenario, worldwide calories per capita per day have fallen to levels seen in the mid-1960s. During this period, population was growing at a faster rate than currently and incomes were lower than they are currently. So we might want to investigate what happens under this scenario when population grows more rapidly and income is stagnant. This is shown in scenario B-1. Here, we assume that the population at the end of fifty years has more than doubled—growing by 120 percent. (This rate of population growth is even higher than the UN high-growth variant, but is not as high as growth rates experienced during the 1960s.) Income growth, and growth in demand per capita, is assumed to be zero. The outcome of this scenario is catastrophic: food prices increase by 181 percent and worldwide calories per capita per day decline to 2,256. This is less than the current level of food availability in Africa. At this level, there would undoubtedly be much more widespread undernutrition and large increases in infant and child mortality. The large population results from high fertility and includes therefore many children who die before the age of five.

Scenario B-2 shows that if yields grow a little more strongly (0.8 percent per year rather than 0.2 percent per year as in scenarios B and B-1) major catastrophe is avoided. Maintaining the other assumptions of scenario B, we see that demand grows by 70 percent while supply grows by 27 percent. This leads to a food price increase of 16 percent. The scenario also predicts a slight decline in average food availability per capita from the current 2,700 calories per capita per day to 2,655.

■ Policies

Scenarios such as those presented here may be useful in evaluating the likely impacts of various policies. Policy action or inaction will influence the future course of events and the severity of the worldwide hunger problem. Experts do not agree on all details about what comprises a "best policy," nor do they agree on the likely impacts of any policy option. However, there is widespread agreement that policy initiatives should focus on the following objectives:

- *Reduce the rate of population growth.* In addition to economic incentives to promote small families, general economic prosperity and improved health and education systems can be an important part of these policies.
- *Invest in improved agricultural productivity.* Direct government investment in agricultural research and extension, and improved access to rural credit and markets will play an important role here.
- *Protect soil and water resources.* Agricultural research can assist in this. In addition, clearly assigned and enforceable property rights will give resource owners a personal stake in environmental protection.
- *Encourage economic growth among the poorest.* Appropriate macroeconomic policies, reliance on competitive markets, and investment in human capital are likely to be important elements of this policy.

It is for us, the living, to be dedicated to the unfinished task.
—Abraham Lincoln, The Gettysburg Address

■ Appendix: Mathematics Used In Making Projections

Using Growth Rates to Project the Future

To understand the calculations behind the scenarios presented in this chapter, it is necessary to know some elementary mathematics of growth. A simple example explains the basic point. Suppose a city starts the year with a population of 100,000, and suppose the population grows by 10 percent during the year. At the end of the year (year 1), the city's population will be 110,000. We get this by multiplying the population at the beginning of the year (100,000) by 1 plus the annual growth rate (10 percent or 0.10):

110,000 = 100,000 x (1 + 0.10)

end of year value = beginning of year value times 1 plus growth rate

To conserve verbiage, we assign symbols to these words with V_1 being the value at the end of year 1, V_0 being the value at the beginning of year 1 (or at the end of year zero), and r being the growth rate.

$$V_1 = V_0 (1 + r) \qquad\qquad (1)$$

Now suppose the population grows by 10 percent for the second year. We can use equation (1) to calculate the population at the end of year 2. The population at the end of year 2 will be

110,000 x (1 + 0.10) = 121,000

Notice that we can also write this as:

(100,000 x [1 + 0.10]) x (1 + 0.10) = 121,000

Similarly, at the end of year 3 (if growth continues at 10 percent) the population would be

([100,000 x (1 + 0.10)] x (1 + 0.10)) x (1 + 0.10) = 121,000 x (1 + 0.10) = 133,100

The last two calculations show us a pattern:

$$V_1 = V_0 (1 + r)^1$$
$$V_2 = V_0 (1 + r)^2$$
$$V_3 = V_0 (1 + r)^3$$

The general rule used to calculate values at the end of T periods is

$$V_T = V_0 (1 + r)^T \qquad\qquad (2)$$

To return to Chapter 24, and see how equation (2) is applied, look at the assumption about population growth in scenario A. Population is assumed to grow at an average rate of 0.95 percent (or 0.0095) over the fifty-year period. Applying equation (2) gives us

$$V_{50} = V_0 (1 + .0095)^{50} = V_0 \times 1.6044$$

This means that population at the end of fifty years is "160 percent of current levels" or "60.44 percent higher than population at the beginning of the fifty-year period." This information is entered in Table 24.1 as "+60 percent" in the population column of scenario A. Similarly, yield growth of 1.25 percent (0.0125) per year for fifty years gives us a yield at the end of the period that is $(1.0125)^{50}$ or 1.86 times the level at the beginning of the fifty years. This information is entered in Table 24.1 as "+86 percent" in the yield column of scenario A.

Calculating the Total Impact When Two Multiplicative Factors Are Growing

Total Demand is demand per capita times the number of people. In our scenarios, both of these factors (demand per capita and population) grow. As explained in Chapter 10, when this happens, growth rate for total demand is calculated as follows. Following scenario A for an example, if population grows by 60 percent over the fifty-year period, and if (plant-equivalent) calories per capita grows by 30 percent over the period, growth in total demand is calculated as follows:

$$(1 + .60) \text{ x } (1 + .30) = 2.08$$

Total demand at the end of the fifty-year period is 2.08 times (or 208 percent of) demand at the beginning of the period; or demand has increased by 108 percent. Likewise, total supply is number of hectares (area) times yield per hectare; so growth in total supply is calculated in a similar fashion.

Calculating the Price Change

The changes in demand and supply in our scenarios assume constant prices—we are projecting the degree to which demand and supply curves shift in the future. (Those with more training in economics will notice that our demand factors—population and income—are traditional demand shifters in economic theory; however, our supply factors—area and yield—are not consistent with theoretical economics of supply. We analyze growth in supply using these supply factors because they make the supply side of the equation easier to understand. It is also interesting to note that historical trends in these variables are observed for a period in which real agricultural prices were declining slightly—see Chapter 6.) If demand grows faster than supply, equilibrium price will increase from current levels. If supply grows faster than demand, equilibrium price will decrease.

How do we calculate the size of the price change? Scenario A illustrates the calculation. In scenario A, supply is projected to grow by 110 percent and demand is projected to grow by 108 percent. Thus, at constant prices, quantity supplied would exceed quantity demanded by 2 percent. We expect the price to fall. If the price fell by 1 percent, quantity supplied would drop by 0.5 percent (the elasticity of supply is assumed to be 0.5) and the quantity demanded would increase by 0.2 percent (the elasticity of demand is assumed to be 0.2). To erase the 2 percent difference in supply and demand, the price would need to drop by 2.86 percent. This would create a drop in quantity supplied of 1.43 percent, and an increase in quantity demanded of 0.57 percent.

The general calculation uses the following:

$$\text{Price Increase} = \frac{\text{\% growth in demand} - \text{\% growth in supply}}{\text{elasticity of supply} + \text{elasticity of demand}}$$

(where elasticities are expressed as absolute values). If growth in demand is less than growth in supply, the "price increase" is negative—that is, the price declines. Given the assumptions about elasticities, this becomes

$$\text{Price Increase} = \frac{\text{\% growth in demand} - \text{\% growth in supply}}{0.7}$$

For the scenario we are discussing this is:

$$\text{Price Increase} = \frac{2.08 - 2.10}{0.7} = -.02876$$

This is the calculation that leads us to say that the price would drop by 3 percent (or the price would increase by -2.876 percent, if you prefer).

Calculating the Calories per Capita per Day

To calculate the total quantity supplied, we adjust the growth in supply by movement along the supply curve implied by the projected price change. So the total quantity supplied increases by supply growth plus 0.5 times the price change. If population remained constant, calories per capita per day would increase from the current level of about 2,700 by this amount. But population does not remain constant in our scenarios. Therefore, we divide the growth in quantity supplied by the growth in population and multiply this by the current level (2,700 calories per capita per day) to calculate future food intake.

$$\text{Calories per capita per day in 50 years} = \frac{2700 \times ([1 + \text{growth in supply}] + [0.5 \times \text{price increase}])}{1 + \text{growth in population}}$$

REFERENCES

Abbott, Patrick. 2003. Ireland's great famine, 1845–1849. Online at http://www.ire-landstory.com/past/famine/, accessed June 2003.

Adams, Dale W. 1983. Mobilizing household savings through rural financial markets. In *Rural financial markets in developing countries: Their use and abuse*, ed. J. D. Von Pischke et al., 399–407. Baltimore: Johns Hopkins University Press.

Adams, Dale W., and Douglas H. Graham. 1981. A critique of traditional agricultural credit projects and policies. *Journal of Development Economics* 8:347–366.

Adams, Dale W., et al., eds. 1984. *Undermining rural development with cheap credit*. Boulder, Colo.: Westview Press.

Adamu, H. 2000. We'll feed our people as we see fit. *Washington Post*, September 11, 2000, p. A-23.

Adelman, I., and C. T. Morris. 1973. *Economic growth and social equity in developing countries*. Stanford, CA: Stanford University Press.

Ahluwalia, Montek S. 1976a. Income distribution and development: Some sytlized facts. *American Economic Review* 66 (May):128–135.

———. 1976b. Inequality, poverty and development. *Journal of Development Economics* 3 (September):307–342.

Ahluwalia, Montek S., N. Carter, and H. Chenery. 1979. Growth and poverty in developing countries. Chapter 11 in *Structural change and development policy*, ed. H. Chenery. Oxford: Oxford University Press. Also available in *Journal of Development Economics* 6 (September):299–341.

Ahmed, Raisuddin. 1988. Structure, costs, and benefits of food subsidies in Bangladesh. In *Food subsidies in developing countries,* ed. Per Pinstrup-Andersen, 219–228. Baltimore: Johns Hopkins University Press.

———. 1989. Making rural infrastructure a priority. Washington, D.C.: International Food Policy Research Institute. *IFPRI Report*. Vol. 11, No. 1, pp. 1, 4.

Ahmed, Raisuddin, and Mahabub Hossain. 1990. *Developmental impact of rural infrastructures: Bangladesh*. Washington, D.C.: International Food Policy Research Institute. IFPRI Research Report 83.

Alberts, Tom. 1983. *Agrarian reform and rural poverty: A case study of Peru*. Boulder, Colo.: Westview Press.

Alderman, Harold. 1986. *The effect of food price and income changes on the acquisition of food by low-income households*. Washington, D.C.: International Food Policy Research Institute.

Alderman, Harold, and Joachim von Braun. 1984. *The effects of the Egyptian food ration and subsidy system on income distribution and consumption.*

Washington, D.C.: International Food Policy Research Institute. IFPRI Research Report No. 45.

Alderman, H., J. Hoddinott, and B. Kinsey. 2003. Long-term consequences of early childhood malnutrition. Presented to the International Conference on Chronic Poverty and Development Policy, April 7–9, 2003, IDPM, University of Manchester. Online at http://idpm.man.ac.uk/cprc/Conference/conferencepapers/Alderman.22.01.pdf.

Alexandratos, N., ed. 1995. *World agriculture: Towards 2010, an FAO study.* London: John Wiley.

Allison, Graham T. 1971. *Essence of decision: Explaining the Cuban missile crisis.* Boston: Little, Brown, and Company.

Alston, J., et al. 2000. *A meta-analysis of rates of return to agricultural r&d: Ex pede herculem.* Washington, D.C.: IFPRI. Research Report No. 113.

Alston, Philip. 1997. Recognition of the right to food. *UN/FAO world food summit fact sheet.* Rome: UN/FAO. Online at http://www.fao.org./wfs/fs/e/img/right-e.pdf.

Anderson, J. R., and J. A. Roumasset. 1985. Microeconomics of food insecurity: The stochastic side of poverty. Unpublished paper available through the Department of Economics, University of Hawaii, Manoa.

Anderson, Jock, et al. 1985. *International agricultural research centers: A study of achievements and potential; Summary.* Washington, D.C.: World Bank, Consultative Group on International Agricultural Research.

Anderson, Mary Ann, et al. 1981. *Nutrition intervention in developing countries, study I: Supplementary feeding.* Cambridge, Mass.: Oelgeschlager, Gunn, and Hain.

Angé, A. L. 1993. *Trends of plant nutrient management in developing countries.* Rome: FAO.

Angel, J. Lawrence. 1975. Paleoecology, paleodemography, and health. In *Population, ecology, and social evolution*, ed. S. Polgar, 167–190. The Hague: Mouton.

———. 1984. Health as a crucial factor in the changes from hunting to developed farming in the Eastern Mediterranean. In *Paleopathology at the origins of agriculture,* ed. M. N. Cohen and G. J. Armelagos, 51–73. New York: Academic Press.

Anonymous. 1974. How hunger kills. *Time*, November 11, p. 68.

Anonymous. 1988. Women and development: Education and fertility. *Finance and Development* 43 (September).

Arnold, Jesse C., R. W. Engel, D. B. Aguillon, and M. Caedo. 1981. Utilization of family characteristics in nutritional classification of preschool children. *American Journal of Clinical Nutrition* 34 (November):2546–2550.

Aron, Robert, et al. 1962. *Les origines de la guerre d'Algerie.* Paris: Fayard.

Askari, Hossein, and John T. Cummings. 1976. *Agricultural supply response: A survey of the econometric evidence.* New York: Praeger.

Associated Press. 2000. UN: Nutrition improving in North Korea. November 4.

Astawa, I. B. 1979. Using the local community: Bali, Indonesia. In *Birth control: An international assessment,* ed. M. Potts and P. Bhiwandiwala, 55–70. Baltimore: University Park Press.

Baden, John. 2003. Move over culture war: Here's the aquaculture war. Tech Central Station, August 29. Online at http://www.techcentralstation.com/082903D.html; accessed August 2003.

Bale, Malcolm D. 1984. Opening of the discussion on plenary paper 5. In

Proceedings of the fourth congress of the E.A.A.E., agricultural markets and prices. In *European Review of Agricultural Economics* 12:82–83.

———. 1985. *Agricultural trade and food policy: The experience of five developing countries.* Washington, D.C.: World Bank Staff Working Paper No. 724.

Bale, Malcolm D., and Ernst Lutz. 1981. Price distortions in agriculture and their effects: An international comparison. *American Journal of Agricultural Economics* 63 (February):8–22.

Baliunas, Sallie. 1999. Why so hot? Don't blame man, blame the sun. *Wall Street Journal*, August 5.

Bautista, Romeo M. 1987. *Production incentives in Philippine agriculture: Effects of trade and exchange rate policies* Washington, D.C.: International Food Policy Research Institute. IFPRI Research Report 59.

Bayliss, K., and D. Hall. 2001. A PSIRU response to the World Bank's 'Private sector development strategy': Issues and options. University of Greenwich, Public Services International Research Unit. Online at http://www.psiru.org/reports/ 2001-10-U-wb-psd.doc.

Baylor, K. 1996. Biochemical studies on the toxicity of isocyanates. Abstract from a Ph.D. thesis submitted to University College Cork (Ireland), May. Online at http://www.connect.net/dreggie/Methyl%20I.htm.

Beal, George M., and D. J. Hobbs. 1969. *Social action: The process in community and area development.* Ames: Iowa State University Cooperative Extension Service, Soc-16. August.

Beal, George M., and Everett M. Rogers. 1960. *The adoption of two farm practices in a central Iowa community.* Ames: Iowa State University Agricultural and Home Economics Experiment Station Special Report No. 26.

Bearak, B. 2003. Why people still starve. *New York Times Sunday Magazine*, August 10, p. 33.

Beaton, George H., and Hossein Ghassemi. 1982. Supplementary feeding programs for young children in developing countries. *American Journal of Clinical Nutrition* 35 (April):864–916.

Becker, Gary. 1975. *Human capital.* New York: Columbia University Press.

Becker, K., Chief, Basic Data Unit, Statistics Division, FAO, Rome. 1989. Letter to author. January 16.

Belmont, Lillian, and Francis A. Marolla. 1973. Birth order, family size, and intelligence—A study of a total population of 19-year-old men born in the Netherlands. *Science* 182, no. 4117 (December):1096–1101.

Bengoa, J. M. 1972. Nutritional significance of mortality statistics. In *Proceedings of the third western hemisphere nutrition congress.* New York: Futura.

Berg, Alan. 1973. *The nutrition factor—Its role in national development.* Washington, D.C.: Brookings Institution.

———. 1987. *Malnutrition—What can be done?* Baltimore: Johns Hopkins University Press.

Berry, A. R., and W. R. Cline. 1979. *Agrarian structure and productivity in developing countires.* Baltimore: Johns Hopkins University Press.

Bettany, G. T. 1890. Introduction. An essay published with the 1890 Ward edition of the *Essay on population*, by T. R. Malthus.

Bezuneh, Mesfin, Brady J. Deaton, and George W. Norton. 1988. Food aid impacts in rural Kenya. *American Journal of Agricultural Economics* 70 (February):181–191.

Bhargava, Alok. 1996. Econometric analysis of psychometric data: A model for Kenyan schools. Washington, D.C.: World Bank, Policy Research.

Binswanger, Hans. 1978. *The economics of tractors in South Asia: An analytical review.* New York: Agricultural Development Council; and Hyderabad, India: International Crops Research Institute for the Semi-Arid Tropics.

Binswanger, Hans, and Klaus Deininger. 1997. Explaining agricultural and agrarian policies in developing countries. *Journal of Economic Literature* 35 (December):1958–2005.

Binswanger, Hans, Graeme Donovan, et al. 1987. *Agricultural mechanization, issues and options.* Washington, D.C.: World Bank Policy Study.

Birdsall, Nancy. 1984. Population growth: Its magnitude and implications for development. *Finance and Development* 21 (September):10–13.

Blake, Judith. 1989. *Family size and achievement.* Berkeley: University of California Press.

Bleichrodt, Nico, and Marise P. H. Born. 1994. A metaanalysis of reseearch on iodine and its relationship to cognitive development. In *The damaged brain of iodine deficiency: Cognitive, behavioral, neuromotor, educative aspects,* ed. John Stanbury. Port Washington, N.Y.: Cognizant Communication Corp., 1994.

Bliss, C. J., and N. Y. Stern. 1982. *Palanpur: The economy of an Indian village.* Oxford: Clarendon Press.

Blow, L., A. Leicester, and Z. Smith. 2003. London's congestion charge. Institute for Fiscal Studies, Briefing Note No. 31. Online at http://www.ifs.org.uk/consume/bn31.pdf.

Boediono. 1978. Elastisitas permintaan untuk berbagai barang di Indonesia; Penerapan metode Frisch. *Ekonomi dan Keuangan Indonesia* 26 (September):362.

Boggess, W., R. Lacewell, and D. Zilberman. 1993. Economics of water use in agriculture. In *Agricultural and environmental resource economics,* ed. G. Carlson, D. Zilberman, and J. Miranowski, 319–392. Oxford: Oxford University Press.

Bongaarts, John. 1982. The fertility-inhibiting effects of the intermediate fertility variables. *Studies in Family Planning* 13:179–189.

Boserup, Ester. 1981. *Population and technological change: A study of long-term trends.* Chicago: University of Chicago Press.

Bouis, Howarth E. 1991. The changing focus of economic research on nutrition. Washington, D.C.: International Food Policy Research Institute, *IFPRI Report* vol. 13, no. 2, pp. 1, 4.

Bouis, Howarth E., and Lawrence Haddad. 1990. *The effects of agricultural commercialization on land tenure, household resource allocation, and nutrition in the Philippines.* Washington, D.C.: International Food Policy Research Institute, IFPRI Research Report 79.

———. 1992. Are estimates of colorie-income elasticities too high? *Journal of Development Economics* 39:333–364.

Boulding, Kenneth. 1964. *The meaning of the 20th century.* New York: Harper & Row.

Bread for the World. 1997. *Hunger in the global economy: Hunger 1998.* Silver Spring, Md.: Bread for the World Institute.

Briscoe, J. 1979. The qualitative effect of infection of the use of food by young children in poor countries. *American Journal of Clinical Nutrition* 32 (March):648–676.

Bromley, Daniel. 1981. The role of land reform in economic development, policies and politics: Discussion. *American Journal of Agricultural Economics* 63 (May):399–400.

Brown, Lester R. 1970. *Seeds of change: The green revolution and development in the 1970s.* New York: Praegar.

————. 1974. *In the human interest—A strategy to stabilize world population.* New York: Norton.

————. 1983. *Population policies for a new economic era.* Washington, D.C.: Worldwatch Paper 53.

————. 1988. *The changing world food prospect: The nineties and beyond.* Washington, D.C.: Worldwatch Paper 85.

Brown, Lester, and Hal Kane. 1994. *Full house: Reassessing the earth's population carrying capacity.* Washington, D.C.: Worldwatch Institute.

Brown, Lynn. 1997. The potential impact of AIDS on population and economic growth rates. *2020 Brief* 43 (June). Washington D.C.: IFPRI. Online at http://www.cgiar.org/ifpri/2020/briefs/2br43.htm

Bulatao, Rodolfo A. 1984a. Fertility control at the community level: A review of research and community programs. In *Rural Development and Human Fertility*, ed. W. Schutjer and C. Stokes, 269–290. New York: MacMillan.

————. 1984b. *Reducing fertility in developing countries: A review of determinants and policy servers.* Washington, D.C.: World Bank Staff Working Paper No. 680, Population and Development Series No. 5.

Bumb, Balu L., and Carlos A. Baanante. 1996. World trends in fertilizer use and projections to 2020. *2020 Brief* 38 (October), Washington D.C.: IFPRI.

Burki S., and Robert Ayres. 1986. A fresh look at development aid. *Finance and Development* 23 (March):6.

Byerlee, D., and P. Moya. 1993. *Impacts of international wheat breeding research in the developing world, 1966–90.* Mexico, D.F.: CIMMYT.

Caldwell, John C. 1983. Direct economic costs and benefits of children. In *Determinants of fertility in developing countries,* vol. 1, *Supply and demand for children.* ed. Rudolfo A. Bulatao et al., 458–493. New York: Academic Press.

Calegar, Geraldo M., and G. Edward Schuh. 1988. *The Brazilian wheat policy: Its costs, benefits, and effects on food consumption.* Washington, D.C.: International Food Policy Research Institute. IFPRI Research Report 66.

Campbell, Joseph K. 1984. Machines and food production. In *World food issues,* ed. Matthew Drosdoff, 47–50. Ithaca, N.Y.: Cornell University College of Agriculture.

Carner, George. 1984. Survival, interdependence, and competition among the Philippine rural poor. In *People-centered development*, ed. David Korten and Rudi Klauss, 133–145. West Hartford, Conn.: Kumarian Press.

Carson, Rachel. 1962. *Silent spring.* Greenwich, Conn.: Fawcett.

Carter, Michael. 1989. *U.S. farm exports and third-world agricultural development.* Madison: Department of Agricultural Economics, University of Wisconsin Economic Issues, No. 111.

Cassidy, Claire. 1980. Benign neglect and toddler malnutrition. In *Social and biological predictors of nutritional status, physical growth, and neurological development*, ed. Lawrence S. Greene, 109–139. New York: Academic Press.

————. 1987. World-view conflict and toddler malnutrition: Change agent dilemmas. In *Child survival: Anthropological perspectives on the treatment and maltreatment of children*, ed. Nancy Scheper-Hughes, 293–324. Norwell, Mass.: Reidel.

CAST (Council on Agricultural Science and Technology). 2002. Comparative environmental impacts of biotechnology-derived and traditional soybean, corn, and cotton crops. Washington, D.C.: CAST. Online at http://www.cast-science.org/cast/biotech/pubs/biotechcropsbenefit.pdf.

————. 2003. *Biotechnology in animal agriculture.* Washington, D.C.: CAST.

Cavallo, Domingo, and Yair Mundlak. 1982. *Agriculture and economic growth in an open economy: The case of Argentina*. Washington, D.C.: International Food Policy Research Institute. IFPRI Research Report 36.

Centers for Disease Control (CDC). 2002. Investigation of human health affects associated with potential exposure to genetically modified corn. Atlanta: CDC. Online at http://www.cdc.gov/nceh/ehhe/Cry9cReport/complete.htm.

CGIAR (Consultative Group on International Agricultural Research). 1995. Wheat is doing well in Syria. *CGIAR Newsletter* (October). Washington, D.C.: World Bank. Online at http://www.worldbank.org/html/cgiar/newsletter/Oct95/3syria.htm.

———. 1997. *25 years of food and agriculture improvement in developing countries*. Washington D.C.: World Bank. Online at http://www.worldbank.org/html/cgiar/25years/25cover.html.

Cha, A. 2004. Iraqis face tough transition to market-based agriculture. *Washington Post*, January 22, p. A-1.

Chambers, Robert, Richard Longhurst, David Bradley, and Richard Feacham. 1979. *Seasonal dimensions to rural poverty: Analysis and practical implications*. Brighton, England: University of Sussex, Institute of Development Studies. Discussion Paper 142.

Champakam, S., S. C. Srikantia, and C. Gopalan. 1968. Kwashiorkor and mental development. *American Journal of Clinical Nutrition* 21 (August):844–852.

Chandra, Ranjit K. 1980. Immunocompetence in undernutrition and overnutrition. *Nutrition Review* 39:225–231.

———. 1988. Nutritional regulation of immunity: An introduction. In *Nutrition and immunology*, ed. Ranjit Chandra, 1–7. New York: Alan R. Liss.

Chang, Andrew. 2001. Bitter pill: Is the chocolate that you eat the product of child slavery? May 4. Online at http://abcnews.go.com/sections/world/DailyNews/cotedivoire010504_choco.html; accessed 2003.

Chavez, Adolfo, and Celia Martinez. 1982. Growing up in a developing community—A bio-ecological study of the development of children from poor peasant families in Mexico. Mexico: Instituto Nacional de la Nutricion. (Translated from the Spanish.)

Chen, P. C. 1981. China's birth planning program. In *National research council committee on population and demography: Research on the population in China, proceedings of a workshop*, 78–90. Washington, D.C.: National Academy Press.

Chen, P. C., and A. Kols. 1982. Population and birth planning in the People's Republic of China. *Population Reports*, Series J, No. 25, January-February, vol, X, no. 1:577–618.

Chen, R. S. 1990. Global agriculture, environment, and hunger: Past, present, and future links. *Environmental Impact Assesment Review* 10, no. 4:335–358.

Chenery, Hollis B. 1971. Growth and structural change. *Finance and Development Quarterly* 3:16–27.

Chenery, Hollis, Sherman Robinson, and Moshe Syrquin. 1986. *Industrialization and growth: A comparative study*. New York: Oxford University Press.

Chevalier, P. 1995. Zinc and duration of treatment of severe malnutrition [letter; comment]. *Lancet* 345, no. 8956 (April 22):1046–1047.

Chhibber, Ajay. 1988. Raising agricultural output: Price and nonprice factors. *Finance and Development* (June):44–47.

Chidambaram, G. 1989. *Tamil Nadu integrated nutrition project: Terminal evaluation*. Madras, India: State Planning Commission.

Chisholm, Anthony H., and Rodney Tyers, eds. 1982. *Food security: Theory, policy, and perspectives from Asia and the Pacific rim.* Lexington, Mass.: Lexington Books.

Chu, Yung-Peng. 1982. Growth and distribution in a small, open economy. Ph.D. dissertation, University of Maryland.

CIMMYT. 1989. *Towards the 21st century: CIMMYT's strategy.* Mexico, D.F.: CIMMYT.

———. 2003. Innovation for development: Annual report 2002-2003. Mexico, D.F.: CIMMYT. Online at http://www.cimmyt.org/english/docs/ann_report/recent/pdf/ar03_Reducing.pdf.

Clarendon Press. 1959. *The shorter Oxford economic atlas of the world.* 2d ed. Oxford: Oxford University Press, 1959.

Clark, Colin G. 1973. More people, more dynamism. *CERES* Rome: FAO (November-December).

Clay, Jason W., and Bonnie K. Holcomb. 1986. *Politics and the Ethiopian famine 1984–1985.* Cambridge, Mass.: Cultural Survival.

Cleaver, Kevin M. 1985. *The impact of price and exchange rate policies on agriculture in sub-Saharan Africa.* Washington, D.C.: World Bank. Staff Working Paper No. 728.

Coale, Ansley J., and Edgar M. Hoover. 1958. *Population growth and economic development in low-income countries: A case study of India's prospects.* Princeton, N.J.: Princeton University Press.

Cogill, B. 2003. *Anthropometric indicators measurement guide, 2003 revision.* Washington, D.C.: Food and Nutrition Technical Assistance (FANTA).

Cohen, Joel. 1996a. *How many can the earth support?* New York: W. W. Norton.

———. 1996b. Maximum occupancy. *American Demographics* (February).

Cohen, Mark N. 1984. An introduction to the symposium. In *Paleopathology at the origins of agriculture,* ed. Mark Cohen and George Armelagos, 1–11. New York: Academic Press.

Cohen, Mark N., and George Armelagos, eds. 1984. *Paleopathology at the origins of agriculture.* New York: Academic Press.

Conquest, Robert. 1986. *The harvest of sorrow: Soviet collectivization and the terror-famine.* New York: Oxford University Press.

Cook, Robert C., 1962. How many people have ever lived on earth? *Population Bulletin* 18 (February).

Cooke, G. W. 1967. *The control of soil fertility.* London: Crosby Lockwood.

Court, J., and T. Yanagihara. No date. Asia and Africa into the global economy. Online at http://www.unu.edu/HQ/academic/Pg_area4/August-intro.html.

Coutsoudis, A., and N. Rollins. 2003. Breast-feeding and HIV transmission: The jury is still out. *Journal of Pediatrics, Gastroenterology, and Nutrition* 36:434–442.

Cowell, F. A. 1977. *Measuring inequality: Techniques for the social sciences.* New York: John Wiley.

Craig, B. J., P. Pardey, and J. Roseboom. 1994. International agricultural productivity patterns. Working Paper WP 94-1, St. Paul: Center for International Food and Agricultural Policy, University of Minnesota. Online at http://agecon.lib.umn.edu/cgi-bin/pdf_view.pl?paperid=1746&ftype=.pdf.

Craig, B.J., Pardey, P.G., and Roseboom, J. 1997. "International Productivity Patterns: Accounting for Input Quality, Infrastructure, and Research," *American Journal of Agricultural Economics* 79, no. 4 (November): 1064–1076.

Crosson, Pierre. 1996a. Who will feed China? *Perspectives on the long-term global food situation* 2 (spring). Online at http://www.fas.org/food/issue2.html.

———. 1996b. Resource degradation? *Perspectives on the long-term global food situation* (summer). Online at http://www.fas.org/food/issue2.html

Cunningham, A. S., D. B. Jelliffe, and E.F.P. Jelliffe. 1991. Breastfeeding and health in the 1980s: A global epidemiological review. *Journal of Pediatrics* 15:659–668.

Daberkow, S., K. Isherwood, J. Poulisse, and H. Vroomen. 1999. Fertilizer requirements in 2015 and 2030. IFA Agricultural Conference, Barcelona.

Dagum, Camilo. 1987. Gini ratio. In *The new Palgrave: A dictionary of economics*, vol. 2, ed. John Eatwell et al., 529–532. New York: Stockton Press.

Dalrymple, Dana G. 1964. The Soviet famine of 1932–1934. *Soviet Studies* 15 (January):250–284.

———. 1979. The adoption of high-yielding grain varieties in developing countries. *Agricultural History* 53 (October):704–726.

———. 1985. The development and adoption of high-yielding varieties of wheat and rice in developing countries. *American Journal of Agricultural Economics* 67 (December):1067–1073.

———. 1986a. See U.S. Department of State 1986a.

———. 1986b. See U.S. Department of State 1986b.

Dam, Marjory. 1989. *Report of world health*. Geneva: WHO (September).

Dao, James. 2003. U.S. to resume food aid to North Korea after 2-month halt. *New York Times*, February 25.

Das Gupta, Monica. 1988. Selective discrimination against female children in rural Punjab, India. *Population and Development Review* 13:77–100.

Datta, S. K., S. H. Ghosh, and C. N. Bairagya. 1988. Growth and yield of wet season rice with tilapia fish. *International Rice Research Newsletter* 13 (August):46.

Dawkins, K. 2003. *Gene wars: The politics of biotechnology*. New York: Seven Stories Press.

De Janvry, Alain. 1981. The role of land reform in economic development: Policies and politics. *American Journal of Agricultural Economics* 63:384–392.

De Zoysa, Isabelle, et al., 1985. *Focus on diarrhoea*. London: Ross Institute, London School of Hygiene and Tropical Medicine, Keppel St., WC1E 7HT. For the Save the Children Fund (U.K.).

Deaton, Angus, and John Muellbauer. 1980. *Economics and consumer behavior*. Cambridge: Cambridge University Press.

Deininger, K., and L. Squire. 1998. New ways of looking at old issues: Inequality and growth. *Journal of Development Economics* 52, no. 2:259–287.

Deininger, K., and P. Olinto. 2000. Asset distribution, inequality, and growth. World Bank Working Paper 2375. Washington, D.C.: World Bank.

Deininger, Klaus, and Lyn Squire. 1997. Economic growth and income inequality: Reexamining the links. *Finance and Development* (March):38–41.

DeLong, G. R., et al. 1996. Effect of iodination of irrigation water on crop and animal production in Long Ru, Hotien County, Xinjiang. In *Mineral problems in sheep in northern China and other regions of Asia: Proceedings of a workshop held in Beijing, People's Republic of China, 25–30 September 1995*. Canberra: Australian Centre for International Agricultural Research, 49–51.

Department for International Development (DFID). 2002. Better livelihoods for poor people: The role of agriculture. Glasgow: DFID. Online at http://www.tradeobservatory.org/library/uploadedfiles/Better_Livelihoods_for_Poor_People_The_Role_of.htm.

Derneke, M., A. Said, and T. Jayne. 1997. Relationships between fertilizer use and grain sector performance. Working Paper No. 5, Grain Market Research Project, Ministry of Economic Development and Cooperation, Addis Ababa.

Dever, James R. 1983. Determinants of nutritional status in a North Indian village: An economic analysis. Master's thesis, University of Maryland.

Diamond, Jared. 1987. The worst mistake in the history of the human race. *Discover* (May):64–66.

Dickens, Charles. 1958. *A tale of two cities.* London: Oxford University Press.

Diro Pusat Statik. 1981. Statistik harga yan diterima dan yan dibayar pentani untuk biaya produksi pertanian dan Kebutuhan Rumah Tangga Tani. Jawa: Madura dan beberapa Propinsi Luar Jawa. Jakarta, Indonesia (December).

Dixon, John A. 1982. *Food consumption patterns and related demand parameters in Indonesia: A review of available evidence.* Washington D.C.: International Food Policy Research Institute, International Fertilizer Development Center, and the International Rice Research Institute. Working Paper No. 6.

Dollar, D., and A. Kraay. 2002. Growth is good for the poor. *Journal of economic growth* 7, no. 3:195–225.

Dolot, Miron. 1985. *Execution by hunger: The hidden holocaust.* New York: W. W. Norton.

Dommen, Arthur J. 1988. *Innovation in African agriculture.* Boulder, Colo.: Westview Press.

Donnelly, James. 2001. *The great Irish potato famine.* Phoenix Mill, Gloucestershire: Sutton Publishing.

Dover, Michael, and Lee M. Talbot. 1987. *To feed the earth: Agro-ecology for sustainable development.* Washington, D.C.: World Resources Institute.

Dreze, Jean, and Amartya Sen, eds. 1990. *The political economy of hunger,* 3 vols. Oxford: Oxford University Press.

Dreze, Jean, and Amartya Sen. 1989. *Hunger and public action.* Oxford: Oxford University Press.

Duke, Lynne. 1998. Land reform plan divides Zimbabweans. *Washington Post,* February 15, 1998, p. A-27.

Durand, C. H., and J. P. Pigney. 1963. Revue de 410 cas de diarrhees aqueuses infectieuses chez le nourisson et l'enfant de moins de deux ans, traites pendant quatre ans dan les meme service hospitalier. *Annals of Pediatrics* 39:1386.

Edirisinghe, Neville. 1987. *The food stamp scheme in Sri Lanka: Costs, benefits, and options for modification.* Washington, D.C.: International Food Policy Research Institute.

Edirisinghe, Neville, and Thomas T. Poleman. 1983. *Behavioral thresholds as indicators of perceived dietary adequacy or inadequacy.* Ithaca, N.Y.: Cornell University Press, International Agricultural Economics Study 17 (July).

Edwards, Clark. 1988. Real prices received by farmers keep falling. *Choices* (fourth quarter):22–23.

Elias, Victor J. 1985. *Government expenditures on agriculture and agricultural growth in Latin America.* Washington, D.C.: International Food Policy Research Institute. IFPRI Research Report 50.

Elliott, Kathleen. 1978. Editorial. *Lancet* ii:300.

Erlich, P., and A. Erlich. 1991. *Healing the planet.* Reading, Mass.: Addison-Wesley.

Evelth, P. G., and J. M. Tanner. 1967. *Worldwide variation in human growth.* Cambridge: Cambridge University Press.

Evenson, Robert E. 1981. Benefits and obstacles to appropriate agricultural technology. *Annals of the American Academy of Political and Social Science*

458:54–67, as quoted in *Agricultural development in the third world*, ed. Carl K. Eicher and John M. Staatz, 348–361. Baltimore: Johns Hopkins University Press, 1984.

Evenson, R. E., and P. M. Flores. 1978. Social returns to rice research. In *Economic consequences of the new rice technology*, ed. R. Barker and Y. Hayami, 243–265. Los Banos, Philippines: International Rice Research Institute.

Ewen, S., and A. Pusztai. 1999. Effects of diets containing genetically modified potatoes expressing Galanthus nivalis lectin on rat small intestine. *Lancet* 354, no. 9187.

Falconer, J. 1990. Hungry season food from forests, unasylva 41. Online at http://www.fao.org/docrep/t7750e/t7750e00.htm#Contents.

Family Health International. 1997. Online at http://www.fhi.org/fp/fpfaq/index.html.

FAO (Food and Agriculture Organization of the United Nations). 1974. *FAO/WHO handbook on human nutritional requirements*. Rome: FAO Nutritional Studies No. 28.

———. 1989. *Food outlook* (May).

———. 1991. *Food balance sheets, 1984–86 average*. Rome: FAO.

———. 1994. *Body mass index: A measure of chronic energy deficiency in adults*. Rome: FAO.

———. 1996a. World Food Summit (WFS) Technical Background Papers, nos. 1–15. Rome: FAO, UN. Online at http://www.fao.org/wfs/final/e/list-e.htm.

———. 1996b. *Fact sheet on water and food security*. Rome: FAO. Online at http://www.fao.org/wfs/fs/e/WatIrr-e.htm.

———. 1996c. *Sixth world food survey*. Rome: FAO.

———. 1996d. Special feature: The cereals sector outlook to 2010 seen from mid-1996. *Food Outlook* 5-6 (May-June):8. Online at http://www.fao.org/WAI-CENT/faoinfo/economic/giews/english/fo/fo9606/fo960607.htm.

———. 1997a. Factfile. *Contribution of greenhouse gases to global warming*. Online at http://www.fao.org/news/factfile/ff9715–e.htm.

———. 1997b. Famine Early Warning System (FEWS) special report: Hungry season in the Sahel. FEWS Special Report 97-5. Rome: FAO. Online at http://www.fews.org/fb970825/fb97sr5.html#Hungry.

———. 2000a. *State of food insecurity in the world (SOFI 2000)*. Rome: FAO.

———. 2000b. World agriculture: Towards 2015/2030. Rome: FAO. Online at http://www.fao.org/docrep/004/y3557e/y3557e00.htm#TopOfPage.

———. 2004a. FAOSTAT website. www.fao.org/waicent/portal/statistics_en.asp

———. 2004b. Food Balance Sheets. www.fao.org/waicent/portal/statistics_en.asp

———. No date. Programme Against African Trypanosomiasis website. Online at http://www.fao.org/ag/againfo/programmes/en/paat/home.html.

———. No date. World Food Summit background technical documents. Online at http://www.fao.org/wfs/index_en.htm.

———. various years. *State of Food Insecurity in the World* (SOFI). http://www.fao.org/SOF/sofi/index_en.htm

Fass, Simon M. 1982. Water and politics: The process of meeting a basic need in Haiti. *Development and Change* 13:347–364. London and Beverly Hills: Sage.

Feacham, R. G., and M. A. Koblinsky. 1983. Interventions for the control of diarrhoeal diseases among young children: Measles immunization. *Bulletin of the World Health Organization* 61(4):641–652.

———. 1984. Interventions for the control of diarrhoeal diseases among young children: Promotion of breast-feeding. *Bulletin of the World Health Organization* 62(2):271–291.

Feder, G., R. Just, and D. Zilberman. 1985. Adoption of agricultural innovations in developing countries: A survey. *Economic Development And Cultural Change* 33:255–294.

Fei, John C. H., and Gustav Ranis. 1964. *Development of the labor surplus economy: Theory and policy*. New Haven, Conn.: Yale University Press.

FIAN (FoodFirst Information and Action Network). 1997. *Twelve misconceptions about the right to food*. Online at http://www.fian.org/miscon.htm.

Finch, V. C., and O. E. Baker. 1917. See U.S. Department of Agriculture, 1917.

Fishstein, Paul. 1985. Pre and post green revolution income distribution in a North Indian village. Master's thesis, University of Maryland.

Fitzhugh, H. 1998. Competition between livestock and mankind for nutrients: Let ruminants eat grass. In *Feeding a world population of more than eight billion people: A challenge to science*, ed. J. C. Waterlow et al., 223–231. Oxford: Oxford University Press.

Fogel, Robert W. 1994. Economic growth, population theory, and physiology: The bearing of long-term processes on the making of economic policy. *American Economic Review* 84, no. 3 (June):369–395.

Food for the Hungry Homepage. 1998. Online at http://www.fh.org/.

Foster, Phillips. 1972. *Introduction to environmental science*. Homewood, Ill.: Richard D. Irwin.

———. 1978. See U.S. Department of State, 1978.

———. 1991. Malnutrition, starvation, and death. In *Horrendous death, health and well-being*, ed. Dan Leviton, 205–218. New York: Hemisphere.

Foster, Phillips, and Herbert Steiner. 1964. *The structure of Algerian socialized agriculture*. College Park: University of Maryland. Agricultural Experimental Station MP No. 527.

Frejka, Thomas. 1973. The prospects for a stationary world population. *Scientific American* 228 (March):15.

Frisancho, A. Roberto. 1981. New norms of upper limb fat and muscle areas for the assessment of nutritional status. *American Journal of Clinical Nutrition* 34:2540–2545.

———. 1989. *Anthropometric standards for the evaluation of nutritional status of children and adults*. Ann Arbor: University of Michigan Press.

Gabbert, S., and H. P. Weikard. 2001. How widespread is undernourishment? A critique of measurement methods and new empirical methods. *Food Policy* 26, no. 3:209–228.

Galler, Janina R. 1986. Malnutrition—A neglected cause of learning failure. *Journal of Postgraduate Medicine* 80 (October):225–230.

Galway, Katrina, et. al. 1987. *Child survival: Risks and the road to health*. Columbia, Md.: Westinghouse Institute for Resource Development. Demographic Data for Development Project.

Garcia, Marito, and Per Pinstrup-Andersen. 1987. *The pilot food price subsidy scheme in the Philippines: Its impact on income, food consumption, and nutritional status*. Washington, D.C.: International Food Policy Research Institute. IFPRI Research Report 61.

Gardner, Bruce L. 1979. *Optimal stockpiling of grain*. Lexington, Mass.: Heath.

———. 1987. *The economics of agricultural policies*. New York: Macmillan.

Gardner, Gary. 1996. *Shrinking fields: Cropland loss in a world of eight billion*. Washington, D.C.: WorldWatch Institute.

George, P. S. 1988. Costs and benefits of food subsidies in India. In *Food subsidies in developing countries*, ed. Per Pinstrup-Andersen, 229–241. Baltimore: Johns Hopkins University Press.

Gershwin, M. Eric, et al. 1985. *Nutrition and immunity.* New York: Academic Press.

Gifford, R. C. 1992. Agricultural engineering in development: Mechanization strategy formulation. Vol. I: Concepts and principles. FAO Agricultural Services Bulletin 99/1. Rome: FAO, 74.

Gilland, B. 2002. World population and food supply: Can food production keep pact with population growth in the next half century? *Food Policy* 27:47–63.

Gillis, J. 2003. Debate grows over biotech food; Efforts to ease famine in Africa hurt by U.S., European dispute. *Washington Post*, November 30, 2003, p. A-1.

Gilmore, Richard, and Barbara Huddleston. 1983. The food security challenge. *Food Policy* 8 (February):31–45.

Glewwe, Paul, Hanan Jacoby, and Elizabeth King. 1996. An economic model of nutrition and learning: Evidence from longitudinal data. Washington, D.C.: World Bank, Policy Research Department.

Global Development Research Center. 2003. Microfacts: Data snapshots on microfinance. Online at http://www.gdrc.org/icm/data/d-snapshot.html.

Godwin, William. 1793. Political justice. In *A reprint of the essay on "Property,"* ed. H. S. Salt. London: Allen & Unwin. 1949.

Goldenberg, R. L., et al. 1995. The effect of zinc supplementation on pregnancy outcome. *Journal of the American Medical Association* 274, no. 6 (August 9):463–468.

Gómez, F., R. Galvan, S. Frank, R. Chavez, and J. Vazquez. 1956. Mortality in third degree malnutrition. *Journal of Tropical Pediatrics* 2:77.

González-Vega, Claudio. 1983. Arguments for interest rate reform. In *Rural financial markets in developing countries: Their use and abuse*, ed. J. D. von Pischke, et al., 365–372. Baltimore: Johns Hopkins University Press.

Goodall, Roger M. 1984. CDD Information Papers No. 1 and 2, New York: UNICEF (United Nations Children's Fund) (June).

Gopalan, C. 1970. Some recent studies in the nutrition research laboratories: Hyderabad. *Journal of Clinical Nutrition* (January):35–53.

———. 1986. Vitamin A deficiency and child mortality. *Nutrition Foundation of India Bulletin (NFI Bulletin)*, vol. 7, no. 3.

Gopalan, C., and K. S. Rao. 1979. Nutrient needs. In *Human nutrition: A comprehensive treatise.* Vol. 2: *Nutrition and growth.*, ed. D. Jelliffe and E. Jelliffe. New York: Plenum Press.

Graham, K. K., et al. 1994. Pharmacologic evaluation of megestrol acetate oral suspension in cachectic AIDS patient. *Journal of Acquired Immune Deficiency Syndromes* 7, no. 6:580–585.

Grantham-McGregor, S., L. Fernald, and K. Sethuraman. 1999a. Effects of health and nutrition on cognitive and behavioural development in children in the first 3 years of life. Part 1: Low birthweight, breastfeeding, and protein-energy malnutrition. *Food and Nutrition Bulletin* 20:53–75.

———. 1999b. Effects of health and nutrition on cognitive and behavioural development in children in the first 3 years of life. Part 2: Infections and micronutrient deficiencies: iodine, iron, and zinc. *Food and Nutrition Bulletin* 20:76–99.

Grapentine, Liz. 1998. The official page of breastfeeding propaganda. Online at http://members.aol.com/cgrapentin/brstfeed.html.

Gray, Cheryl W. 1982. *Food consumption parameters for Brazil and their application to food policy.* Washington, D.C.: International Food Policy Research Institute. IFPRI Research Report 32.

Greenland, D. J., P. J. Gregory, and P. H. Nye. 1998. Land resources and constraints to crop production. In *Feeding a world population of more than eight billion people: A challenge to science*, ed. J. C. Waterlow et al. Oxford: Oxford University Press.

Griffiths, Marcia. 1985. *Growth monitoring of preschool children: Practical considerations for primary health care projects*. Geneva: World Federation of Public Health Associations.

Grigg, D. 1993. The world food problem, 2nd ed. Cambridge, Mass.: Blackwell.

Griliches, Zvi. 1958. Research costs and social returns: Hybrid corn and related innovations. *Journal of Political Economy* 66:419–431.

Guggenheim, Karl Y. 1981. *Nutrition and nutritional diseases, The evolution of concepts*. Lexington, Mass.: Heath.

Gupta, Arun, and Jon E. Rohide. 1993. Economic value of breast-feeding in India. *Economic and Political Weekly* 28, no. 26:1390.

Haggblade, Steven, and Peter Hazell. 1989. Agricultural technology and farm-non-farm growth linkages. *Agricultural Economics: The Journal of the International Association of Agricultural Economists* 3:345–364.

Hancock, G. 1985. *Ethiopia: The challenge of hunger*. London: Victor Gollancz.

Harberger, Arnold. 1983. Basic needs versus distributional weights in social cost-benefit analysis. *Economic Development and Cultural Change* 32, no. 3:455–474.

Harlan, Jack R. 1975. *Crops and man*. Madison, Wis.: American Society of Agronomy.

Harris, M. 1974. Cows, pigs, wars, and witches: The riddles of culture. New York: Vintage Books.

———. 1977. Cannibals and kings: The origin of cultures. New York: Random House.

Hartini, T., A. Winkvist, L. Lindholm, H. Stenlund, V. Persson, D. Nurdiati, and A. Surjono. 2003. Nutrient intake and iron status of urban poor and rural poor without access to rice fields are affected by the emerging economic crisis: The case of pregnant Indonesian women. *European Journal of Clinical Nutrition* 57:654–666.

Haslberger, A. G. 2003. GM food: The risk assessment of immune hypersensitivity reactions covers more than allergenicity. *Food, Agriculture, and Environment* 1:42–45. Online at http://www.biotech-info.net/hypersensitivity.html.

Haub, Carl. 1987. Understanding population projections. *Population Bulletin* 42, no. 4.

Hayami, Yujiro, and Robert Herdt. 1977. Market price effects of technological change on income distribution in semisubsistence agriculture. *American Journal of Agricultural Economics* 69:245–256.

Hearts and Minds, Socially Responsible Food. 2003. Online at http://www.change.net/articles/foodiss.htm; accessed October 2003.

Heilbroner, Robert L. 1953. *The worldly philosophers*. New York: Simon & Schuster.

Herbert, Sandra. 1971. Darwin, Malthus and selection. *Journal of History of Biology* 4:209–217.

Herdt, Robert W. 1970. A disaggregate approach to aggregate supply. *American Journal of Agricultural Economics* 52:512–520.

———. 1983. Mechanization of rice production in developing Asian countries. In *Consequences of small-farm mechanization*, 1–13. Manila: International Rice Research Institute.

Herdt, Robert W., and Jock R. Anderson. 1987. The contribution of the CGIAR

Centers to world agricultural research. In *Policy for agricultural research*, ed. Vernon W. Ruttan and Carl E. Pray, 39–64. Boulder, Colo.: Westview.

Herdt, Robert W., and John W. Mellor. 1964. The contrasting response of rice to nitrogen—India and United States. *Journal of Farm Economics* 46:150–160.

Herring, Ronald J. 1983. *Land to the tiller: The political economy of agrarian reform in South Asia*. New Haven, Conn.: Yale University Press.

Hicks, L. E., R. A. Langham, and J. Takenaka. 1992. Cognitive and social measures following early nutritional supplementation: A sibling study. *American Journal of Public Health* 72.

Ho, M., T. Traavik, O. Olsvik, B. Tappeser, C. V. Howard, C. von Weizsacker, and G. C. McGavin. 1998. Gene technology and gene ecology of infectious diseases. *Microbial Ecology in Health and Disease* 10:33–59.

Ho, T. J. 1984. Economic status and nutrition in East Java. Washington, D.C.: World Bank Working Paper. Unpublished data from The East Java Nutrition Study sponsored by the University of Airlangga, Surabaya, the Provincial Health Services of East Java and the Royal Tropical Institute of Amsterdam.

Hopkins, Raymond F. 1988. Political calculations in subsidizing food. In *Food subsidies in developing countries*, ed. Per Pinstrup-Andersen, 107–125. Baltimore: Johns Hopkins University Press.

Hossain, Mahabub. 1988a. *Credit for alleviation of rural poverty: The Grameen Bank in Bangladesh*. Washington, D.C.: International Food Policy Research Institute. IFPRI Research Report 65.

———. 1988b. *Nature and impact of the green revolution in Bangladesh*. Washington, D.C.: International Food Policy Research Institute. IFPRI Research Report 67.

Houser, Daniel, and Barbara Sands. 2000. How centrally planned was China's great leap forward demographic disaster? University of Arizona Department of Economics Working Paper, June. Online at http://w3.arizona.edu/~econ/working_papers/china629.pdf.

Huang, Kuo W. 1985. *U.S. demand for food: A complete system of price and income effects*. Washington D.C.: USDA Technical Bulletin No. 1714.

Huddleston, Barbara. 1984a. *Briefs*. New York.: CARE.

———. 1984b. *Closing the cereals gap with trade and food aid*. Washington, D.C.: International Food Policy Research Institute. IFPRI Research Report 43.

Hull, T. H. 1978. Where credit is due: Policy implications of the recent rapid fertility decline in Bali. Paper presented at the annual meeting of the Population Association of America, Atlanta.

Hull, T. H., et al. 1977. Indonesia's family planning story: Success and challenge. *Population Bulletin* 32, no. 6.

Human Rights Watch. 1996. The small hands of slavery: Bonded child labor in India. Online at http://www.hrw.org/reports/1996/India3.htm, accessed 2003.

Hutabarat, Pos M. 1990. Proyeksi distribusi konsumsi kalorie menurut kelompok-kelompok pendapatan di Indonesia tahun 1990. [Projections of the distribution of caloric consumption by income groups in Indonesia in 1990.] Master's thesis, Bogor Agricultural University, Agricultural School.

Ibe, A. C., and L. F. Awosika. 1991. Sea level rise impact on African coastal zones. In *A change in the weather: African perspectives on climate change,* eds. S. H. Omide and C. Juma, 105–112. Nairobi, Kenya: African Centre for Technology Studies.

Imam, Izzedin I. 1979. *Peasant perceptions: Famine*. Dahka, Bangaladesh:

Bangladesh Rural Advancement Committee (July). In *People centered development—Contributions toward theory and planning frameworks*, ed. David C. Korten and Rudi Klauss, 152–155. West Hartford, Conn.: Kumarian Press, 1984.

Indonesia Oleh Direktorat Gizi Departemen Kesehatan R.I. 1979. *Daftar Komposisi Bahan Makanan*. Jakarta: Bhratara Karya Askara.

International Labor Organization (ILO). 1987. *Yearbook of Labor Statistics 1987*. Geneva: International Labor Office of the ILO.

———. 1988. *I.L.O. Information* Geneva: International Labor Office of the ILO. Vol. 16, no. 3 (August).

International Rice Research Institute (IRRI). 1989. Azolla helps organic farmer earn more. Manila: International Food Policy Research Institute. *The IRRI Reporter* (June).

———. 2002. Project summary and highlights, Project 3: Genetic enhancement for yield, grain quality, and stress resistance. Manila: IRRI. Online at http://www.irri.org/science/progsum/pdfs/dgreport2002/project%203.pdf.

ISRIC/UNEP. 1991. *World map of the status of human-induced soil degradation* (by L. R. Oldeman, R. T. A. Hakkeling, and W. G. Sombroek). Global Assessment of soil degradation, 2d ed. Niarobi: Wageningen.

Jackson, R., A. Ramsay, C. Christensen, S. Beaton, D. Hall, and I. Ramshaw. 2001. Expression of mourse interleukin-4 by a recombinant ectromelia virus supresses cytolytic lymphocyte responses and overcomes genetic resistance to mousepox. *Journal of Virology* 75:1205–1210.

Jackson, Tony, with Deborah Eade. 1982. *Against the grain: The dilemma of project food aid*. Oxford: OXFAM.

James, Clive. 2002. Preview: Status of commercialized trangenic crops: 2002. ISAAA Briefs, No. 27. Ithaca, N.Y.: ISAAA.

James, W.P.T., and E. C. Schofield. 1990. Human energy requirements: A manual for planner and nutritionists. Oxford: Oxford University Press.

Jamison, Dean T., et al., eds. 1993. *Disease control priorities in developing countries*. New York: Oxford University Press for the World Bank.

Jayne, T., L. Rubey, D. Tschirley, M. Mukumbu, M. Chisvo, A. Santos, M. Weber, and P. Diskin. 1995. Effects of market reform on access to food by low-income households: Evidence from four countries in eastern and southern Africa. International Development Paper 19. East Lansing: Michigan State University Press.

Jelliffe, D. B. 1966. *The assessment of the nutritional status of the community*. Geneva: WHO Monograph Series No. 53.

Jensen, H., and S. Robinson. 2002. General equilibrium measures of agricultural policy bias in fifteen developing countries. TMD Discussion Paper 105. Washington, D.C.: IFPRI.

Johnson, D. G. 1975. *World food problems and prospects*. Washington, D.C.: American Enterprise Institute.

Johnson, Stanley R., Zuhair A. Hassan, and Richard D. Green. 1984. *Demand systems estimation methods and applicaitons*. Ames: Iowa State University Press.

Joy, Leonard. 1973. Food and nutrition planning. *Journal of Agricultural Economics* 24:166–197.

Judd, M. Ann, James K. Boyce, and Robert E. Evenson. 1987. Investment in agricultural research and extension. In *Policy for agricultural research*, ed. Vernon Ruttan and Carl E. Pray, 7–38. Boulder, Colo.: Westview.

Kahkonen, S., and H. Leathers. 1997. Is there life after liberalization? Transaction costs analysis of maize and cotton marketing in Zambia and Tanzania. College Park: University of Maryland Press, IRIS Center.

Kakturskaya, M. 2003. Why aren't Russians having babies? *Argumenty I Fakty*, July 23. Reproduced in *World Press Review*, October.

Kakwani, Nanak 1987. Lorenz curve. In *The new Palgrave: A dictionary of economics*, vol. 3., ed. John Eatwell et al., 243–244. New York: Stockton Press.

Kamrin, M. No date. Environmental "hormones" pesticide information project. Michigan State University. Online at http://ace.ace.orst.edu/info/extoxnet/tics/env-horm.txt.

Karim, Rezaul, Manjur Majid, and F. James Levinson. 1984. The Bangladesh sorghum experiment. *Food Policy* 5:61–63.

Kates, Robert. 1996. Ending hunger: Current status and future prospects. *Consequences* 2, no. 2. Online at www.gcrio.org/consequences/vol2no2/article1.html.

Kates, Robert W., et al. 1988. *The hunger report: 1988*. Providence: Brown University Press, World Hunger Program.

Keilmann, A. A., and C. McCord. 1978. Weight-for-age as an index of death in children. *Lancet* (June):1247–1250.

Kendall, H. W., and D. Pimentel. 1994. Constraints on the expansion of the global food supply. *Ambio* 23:198–205.

Kendall, H. W., et al. 1997. Bioengineering of crops: Report of the World Bank panel on transgenic crops. Washington, D.C.: World Bank.

Kennedy, Eileen T. 1989. *The effects of sugar cane production on food security, health and nutrition in Kenya: A longitudinal study*. Washington, D.C.: International Food Policy Research Institute. Research Report No. 78.

Kennedy, Eileen T., and Bruce Cogill. 1987. *Income and nutritional effects of the commercialization of agriculture in southwestern Kenya*. Washington, D.C.: International Food Policy Research Institute. IFPRI Research Report 63.

Kennedy, Eileen T., and Odin Knudsen. 1985. A review of supplementary feeding programmes and recommendations on their design. In *Nutrition and development*, ed. Margaret Biswas and Per Pinstrup-Andersen, 77–96. Oxford: Oxford University Press.

Kennedy, Eileen T., P. Pinstrup-Andersen et al. 1983. *Nutrition-related policies and programs: Past performance and research needs*. Washington, D.C.: International Food Policy Research Institute (February).

Kenya Ministry of Planning and National Development. 1984. *Kenya contraceptive prevalence survey*. Nairobi: Central Bureau of Statistics.

Keys, Ancel, et al. 1950. *The biology of human starvation*. Minneapolis: University of Minnesota Press.

Kimbrell, Andrew. 2002. Seven deadly myths of industrial agriculture. In *Fatal harvest: The tragedy of industrial agriculture*, ed. Andrew Kimbrell. Washington, D.C.: Island Press.

Kinealy, Christine. 2002. *The great Irish famine*. New York: Palgrave.

Kluender, S. 2003. The Peace Corps in Zambia, personal website of a Peace Corps volunteer, online at http://peacecorpsonline.org/messages/messages/467/2018900.html.

Kostermans, Kees. 1994. *Assessing the quality of anthropometric data: Background and illustrated guidelines for survey managers*. Washington, D.C.: World Bank.

Krick, Jackie. 1988. Using the Z score as a descriptor of discrete changes in growth. *Nutritional Support Services* 6, no. 8 (August).

Krueger, Anne, Maurice Schiff, and Alberto Valdes. 1991. *The political economy of agricultural pricing policy.* Baltimore: Johns Hopkins University Press for the World Bank.

Kuznets, Simon. 1955. Economic growth and income inequality. *American Economic Review* 65:1–28.

Lakshmi, R. 2004. "Opening Files, Indians Find Scams," Washington Post, March 9, 2004, p. A-17.

Lancet editorial. 1995. Health effects of sanctions on Iraq. *Lancet* 346, no. 8988 (December 2):1439.

Landman, Lynn. 1983. China's one-child families—Girls need not apply. *RF Illustrated.* New York: The Rockefeller Foundation (December): 8–9.

Lappe, Frances Moore. 1971. *Diet for a small planet.* New York: Balantine.

———. 1992. *Diet for a small planet twentieth anniversary edition.* New York: Ballantine Books.

Lappe, Francis Moore, and Joseph Collins. 1977. *Food first.* Boston: Houghton Mifflin.

Lashof, D., and D. Tirpak. 1990. Policy options for stabilizing global climate. U.S. Environmental Protection Agency report. New York: Hemisphere.

Latham, Michael C. 1984. International nutrition problems and policies. In *World food issues,* ed. Matthew Drosdoff, 55–64. Ithaca, N.Y.: Cornell University Press, Center for the Analysis of World Food Issues, Program in International Agriculture.

Leclercq, Vincent. 1988. *Conditions et limites de l'insertion du Bresil dans les echanges mondiaux du soja.* Montpellier, France: INRA.

Lee, John E., and Gary C. Taylor. 1986. Agricultural research: Who pays and who benefits? *Research for tomorrow, 1986 yearbook of agriculture,* 14–21. Washington, D.C.: U.S. Department of Agriculture.

Lee, R. 1972. Population growth and the beginnings of sedentary life among the !Kung bushmen. In *Population growth: Anthropological implications,* ed. B. Spooner, 329–342. Cambridge, Mass.: MIT Press.

———. 1968a. Problems in the study of hunter gathers. In *Man the hunter,* ed. R. Lee and I. Devore, 3–12. Chicago: Aldine.

———. 1968b. What hunters do for a living, or how to make out on scarce resources. In *Symposium on man the hunter,* ed. R. B. Lee and Irven DeVore, 30–48. Chicago: Aldine.

———. 1969. !Kung bushmen subsistence: An input-output analysis. In *Environment and cultural behavior,* ed. A. Vayda, 47–49. Garden City, N.J.: Natural History Press.

Lele, Uma. J. [n.d.]. Overall flows of official development assistance to the MADIA countries. In *Aid to African agriculture: Lessons from two decades of donor experience,* ed. Uma Lele. World Bank discussion paper. (The discussion papers reflect only the views of their authors and should not be attributed to any other people or institutions.)

Lele, Uma J., and Arthur Goldsmith. 1989. The development of national agricultural research capacity: India's experience with the Rockefeller Foundation and its significance for Africa. *Economic Development and Cultural Change* 37:305–343.

Lele, Uma J., Bill H. Kinsey, and Antonia O. Obeya. 1989. Building agricultural research capacity in Africa: Policy lessons from the Madia countries. Unpublished working paper presented for the Joint TAC/CGIAR Center Directors Meeting, Rome, 1989.

Levine, R. E., et al. 1990. *Breastfeeding saves lives: An estimate of breastfeeding related infant survival.* Bethesda, Md.: Center to Prevent Childhood Malnutrition.

Levinger, Beryl. 1994. *Nutrition, health and education for all.* New York: United Nations Development Programme.

———. 1995. Critical transitions: Human capacity development across the lifespan. Online at http://www.edc.org/INT/HCD/.

Lewis, W. Arthur. 1954. Economic development with unlimited supplies of labor. *The Manchester School of Economic and Social Studies* (May):139–191.

Li, R., et al. 1994. Functional consequences of iron supplementation in iron-deficient female cotton mill workers in Beijing, China. *American Journal of Clinical Nutrition* 59, no. 4 (April):908–913.

Lin, Justin Yifu, and Dennis Tao Chang. 2000. Food availability, entitlements and the Chinese famine of 1959–61. *The Economic Journal* (January 2000):136–158.

Lin, Justin Yifu. 1990. Collectivization and China's agricultural crisis in 1959–1961. *Journal of political economy* (December):1228–1252.

Lipton, Michael. 1977. *Why poor people stay poor: Urban bias in world development.* Cambridge, Mass.: Harvard University Press.

Lipton, Michael, and Richard Longhurst. 1990. *New seeds and poor people.* Baltimore: Johns Hopkins University Press.

Lobine, E. 2000. Waterwar in Cochabamba, Bolvia. University of Greenwich, Public Services International Research Unit. Online at http://www.psiru.org/reports/Cochabamba.doc.

López, R. E. 1980. "The Structure of Production and the Derived Demand for Inputs in Canadian Agriculture," *American Journal of Agricultural Economics* 62:38–45.

Lorenz, Max C. 1905. Methods of measuring the concentration of wealth. *Publications of the American Statistical Association* 9:209–219.

Lutz, W., W. Sanderson, and S. Sherbov. 2001. The end of world population growth. *Nature* 412:543–545.

Lynn, R., and T. Vanhanen. 2002. *I.Q. and the wealth of nations.* New York: Praeger.

Mabbs-Zeno, C. C. 1987. *Where, if anywhere, is famine becoming more likely.* College Park, Md.: World Academy of Development and Cooperation (21 ISSN 0882-3235). Also available as an unpublished manuscript from ERS, USDA, Washington, D.C. 20005.

Mace, James. 1984. Historical introduction. In *Human life in Russia,* ed. E. Ammende, Cleveland: John T. Zubal Publishers.

Maddison, A. 1995. *Monitoring the world economy, 1820–1992.* Washington, D.C.: Organization for Economic Cooperation and Development.

Malthus, T. R. 1803–1826. *An essay on the principle of population or a view of its past and present effects on human happiness with an inquiry into our prospects respecting the future removal or mitigation of the evils which it occasions* (1st ed. 1803, 6th and last 1826). London: Ward, 1890.

Mamarbachi, D., et al. 1980. Observations on nutritional marasmus in a newly rich nation. *Ecology of Food and Nutrition* 9:43–54.

Mann, Charles. 1997. Reseeding the green revolution. *Science* 277 (August 22):1038–1043.

Martorell, Reynaldo. 1980. The impact of ordinary illnesses on the dietary intakes of malnourished children. *American Journal of Clinical Nutrition* 33:345–350.

————. 1988. Seminar at University of Maryland Nutrition Dept., December 12.

————. 1989. Body size, adaptation and function. *Human Organization* 48:15–20.

Masoro, E. J., B. P. Yu, and H. A. Bertrand. 1982. Action of food restriction in delaying the aging process (longevity/metabolic rate/lifetime caloric expenditure/life prolongation). *Proceedings, National Academy of Science* 79:4239–4241.

Maxwell, Bill. 2002. Slavery alive in Florida agricultural industry. *St. Petersburg Times*, July 3. Online at http://www.sptimes.com/2002/07/03/Columns/Slavery_alive_in_Flor.shtml; accessed 2003.

Maxwell, Simon J. 1978a. Food aid, food for work and public works. Brighton, England: University of Sussex. Institute of Development Studies, Discussion Paper 127 (March).

————. 1978b. Food aid for supplementary feeding programmes: An analysis. *Food Policy* 3:289–298.

Maxwell, Simon J., and H. W. Singer. 1979. Food aid to developing countries: A survey. *World Development* 7:225–247.

Mayer, Jean. 1976. The dimensions of human hunger. In *Food and Agriculture*, 14–23. San Francisco: Freeman.

Mazumdar, D. 1965. Size of farm and productivity: A problem of Indian peasant agriculture. *Economica* 32 (May):161–173.

————. 1975. The theory of sharecropping with labor market dualism. *Economica* 42 (August):261–271.

McFarland, William E., et al. 1974. *Demos, demographic-economic models of society—A computerized learning system*. Santa Barbara, Calif.: General Electric Tempo.

McGuire, Judy S. 1988. *Malnutrition—Opportunities and challenges for A.I.D.*, Resources for the Future, Washington, D.C. 20036 (November).

McKigney, John, and Hamish Munro, eds. 1976. *Nutrient requirements in adolescence*. Cambridge, Mass.: MIT Press.

McLaughlin, M. 1984. Interfaith action for economic justice (publisher unknown), p. 3.

Meier, G. 1979. Family planning in the banjars of Bali. *International Family Planning Perspectives* 5:63–66.

Mellor, John W. 1984. Food price policy and income distribution in low-income countries. In *Agricultural development in the third world*, ed. Carl K. Eicher and John M. Staatz. Baltimore: Johns Hopkins University Press.

————. 1985a. *Agricultural change and rural poverty*. Washington, D.C.: International Food Policy Research Institute. Food Policy Statement No. 3.

————. 1985b. *The role of government and new agricultural technologies*. Washington, D.C.: International Food Policy Research Institute. Food Policy Statement No. 4.

————. 1986a. *The new global context for agricultural research: Implications for policy*. Washington, D.C.: International Food Policy Research Institute. Food Policy Statement No. 6.

————. 1986b. Dealing with the uncertainty of growing food imbalances: International structures and national policies. In *Proceedings nineteenth international conference of agricultural economists*, 191–198. Brookfield, Vt.: Grower.

————. 1988. Global food balances and food security. *World Development* 16:997–1011.

Mellor, John W., and Bruce F. Johnston. 1984. The world food equation:

Interrelations among development, employment, and food consumption. *Journal of Economic Literature* 22:531–574.

Merrick, Thomas W., et al. 1986. World population in transition. *Population Bulletin* 41.

Miller, Gay Y., Joseph Rosenblatt, and Leroy Hushak. 1988. The effects of supply shifts on producer's surplus. *American Journal of Agricultural Economics* 70:886–891.

Mincer, Jacob. 1976. Unemployment effects of minimum wages. *Journal of Political Economy* 84, no. 4, part 2 (August):87–104.

Mintz, Sidney W. 1989. Food and culture: An anthropological view. In *Completing the food chain: Strategies for combating hunger and malnutrition*, ed. Paula M. Hirschoff and Neil G. Kolter, 114–121. Washington, D.C.: Smithsonian.

Mitchell, Donald O., Merlinda D. Ingco, and Ronald C. Duncan. 1997. *The world food outlook*. Cambridge: Cambridge University Press.

Mittal, Anuradha. 2002. The growing epidemic of hunger in a world of plenty. In *Fatal harvest: The tragedy of industrial agriculture*, ed. Andrew Kimbrell. Washington, D.C.: Island Press.

Mokyr, Joel. 1985. Why Ireland starved: A quantitative and analytical history of the Irish economy, 1800–1850, 2d ed. London: Allen and Unwin.

Mokyr, Joel, and Cormac Ó Gráda. 1999. Famine disease and famine mortality: Lessons from Ireland, 1845–1850. Northwestern University. Online at http://www.faculty.econ.northwestern.edu/faculty/mokyr/mogbeag.pdf.

Monto, A. S., and J. W. Koopman. 1980. The Tecumseh study XI, occurrence of acute enteric illness in the community. *American Journal of Epidemiology* 112:323–333.

Mundlak, Yair, Donald Larson, and Al Crego. 1996. *Agricultural development: Issues, evidence, and consequences*. Washington, D.C.: World Bank, International Economics Department.

Mwanaumo, A., P. Preckel, and P. Farris. 1994. Motivation for marketing system reform for the Zambian maize market. *Journal of International Food and Agribusiness Marketing* 5:29–49.

Myers, Robert G. 1988. *Programming for early child development and growth*. Paris: UNESCO-UNICEF Cooperative Program (June).

———. 1992. *The twelve who survive: Strengthening programmes of early childhood development in the third world*. London: Routledge .

Naiken, L. 1988. Comparison of the FAO and World Bank methodology for estimating the incidence of undernutrition. *FAO Quarterly Bulletin of Statistics* 1, no. 3:iii–v.

Nakajima, Hiroshi. 1989. *World health statistics annual*. Geneva: WHO.

National Academy of Science (NAS). 1989. Recommended dietary allowances, 10th ed. Washington, D.C.: NAS.

———. 2002. *Dietary reference intakes for energy, carbohydrates, fiber, fat, protein, and amino acids (macronutrients)*. Washington, D.C.: NAS.

———. 2003. *Dietary reference intakes: Applications in dietary planning*. Washington, D.C.: NAS.

National Research Council. 2000. *Beyond 6 billion: Forecasting the world's population*. Washington, D.C.: National Academies Press.

National Science and Technology Council. No date. *Biotechnology for the 21st century: New horizons*. Online at http://www.nal.usda.gov/bic/bio21/tablco.html.

Natsios, Andrew. 1999. The politics of famine in North Korea. United States Institute of Peace, Washington, D.C., August. Online at http://www.usip.org/pubs/specialreports/sr990802.html.

Neue, H. 1993. Methane emission from rice fields: Wetland rice fields may make a major contribution to global warming. *BioScience* 43, no. 7:466–473.

Newbery, D., and J. Stiglitz. 1981. *The theory of commodity price stabilization: A study in the economics of risk.* Oxford: Clarendon.

Nicol, Mark. 2003. Famine-struck North Koreans "eating children." *Telegraph,* June 9.

Nin, A., C. Arndt, T. Hertel, and P. Preckel. 2003. Bridging the gap between partial and total factor productivity measures using directional distance functions. *American Journal of Agricultural Economics* 85: 937–951.

Nord, M., M. Andrews, and S. Carlson. 2003. *Household Food Security in the United States, 2002.* Food and Rural Economics Division, Economic Research Service, U.S. Department of Agriculture, Food Assistance and Nutrition Research Report No. 35.

Notestein, Frank W. 1945. Population—The long view. In *Food for the world,* ed. Theodore W. Schultz. Chicago: University of Chicago Press.

O'Brien, Kevin. 2003. Aids and African armies. In *Headlines over the horizon,* Atlantic Monthly, July-August. Online at http://www.theatlantic.com/issues/2003/07/rand.htm; accessed July 2003.

Oram, Peter. 1995. *The potential of tehchnology to meet world food needs in 2020.* IFPRI 2020 Briefing Paper No. 13. Washington, D.C.: International Food Policy Research Institute.

Orwin, A. 1999. The privatization of water and wastewater utilties: An international survey. Online at http://www.environmentprobe.org/enviroprobe/pubs/ev542.html#South%20America.

Overpeck, M., H. Hoffman, and K. Prager. 1992. The lowest birth-weight infants and the U.S. infant mortality rate: NCHS 1983 linked birth/infant death data. *American Journal of Public Health* 82, no. 3:441–444.

Overton, M. 1996. Agricultural revolution in England: The transformation of the agrarian economy 1500–1850. Cambridge: Cambridge University Press.

Oxfam. 1997. Fighting famine in North Korea and Ethiopia, October. Online at http://www.caa.org.au/AWARE/1997/october-1997.html.

Paarlberg, D. 1988. *Toward a well-fed world.* Ames: Iowa State University Press.

Paglin, M. 1974. The measurement and trend of inequality: A basic revision. *American Economic Review* 65:598–609.

Pardey, P., and S. Beintema. 2001. Slow magic: Agricultural R&D a century after Mendel. Washington, D.C.: IFPRI.

Pardey, Philip G., and Julian M. Alston. 1995. Revamping agricultural R&D. Washington, D.C.: International Food Policy Research Institute. IFPRI 2020 Briefing Paper No. 24.

Parham, Walter. 2001. Degraded lands: South China's untapped resource. *FAS Public Interest Report* 54, no. 2, March-April. Online at http://www.fas.org/faspir/2001/v54n2/resource.htm.

Parizokova, Jana. 1977. *Body fat and physical fitness.* The Hague: Martinus Nijhoff, B. V./Medical Division.

Park, Robert Ezra. 1934. Forward. In *Shadow of the plantation,* ed. Charles Spurgen. Chicago: University of Chicago Press.

Parry, M. L., A. R. Magalhaes, and N. H. Nih. 1992. *The potential socio-economic effects of climate change: A summary of three regional assessments.* Nairobi, Kenya: United Nations Environment Programme (UNEP).

Payne, Philip R. 1985. The nature of malnutrition. In *Nutrition and development,* ed. Margaret Biswas and P. Pinstrup-Andersen. Oxford: Oxford University Press.

Pelletier, D. L., E. A. Frongillo Jr., and J. P. Habicht. 1993. Epidemiologic evidence for a potentiating effect of malnutrition on child mortality. *American Journal of Public Health* 83 (August):1130–1133.

———. 1995. The effects of malnutrition on child mortality in developing countries. *Bulletin of the World Health Organization* 73, no. 4:443–448.

Pellett, Peter L. 1977. Marasmus in a newly rich urbanized society. *Ecology of Food and Nutrition* 6:53–56.

———. 1987. Problems and pitfalls in the assessment of nutritional status. In *Food and evolution: Toward a theory of food habits,* ed. Marvin Harris and Erick B. Ross, 163–179. Philadelphia: Temple University Press.

Pelto, Gretl H. 1987. Cognitive performance and intake in preschoolers. Chapter 30 in *Cognitive performance and intake in preschoolers,* ed. Lindsay H. Allen, Adolfo Chavez, and Gretl H. Pelto. Mexico, D.F.: University of Connecticut and Instituto Nacional de la Nutricion, Final report, C.R.S.R. on food intake and human factors, Mexico Project.

Penning de Vries, F.W.T. , H. Van Keulen, R. Rabbinge, and J. C. Luyten. 1995. *Biophysical limits to global food production.* International Food Policy Research Institute 2020 Brief 18 (May). Washington, D.C.: IFPRI.

Perisse, J., F. Sizaret, and P. Francoise. 1969. The effect of income on the structure of the diet. *FAO Nutrition Newsletter* 7 (July-September):2.

Peterson, Willis L. 1979. International farm prices and the social cost of cheap food policies. *American Journal of Agricultural Economics* 61 (February):12–21.

Pfeifer, Karen. 1985. *Agrarian reform under state capitalism in Algeria.* Boulder, Colo.: Westview.

Philippines Journal of Nutrition. 1971. vol. 24:161.

Philippines Ministry of Agriculture. [1983] *National consumption patterns for major foods, 1977–1982.* Manila: Special Studies Division, Economic Research and Statistics Directorate, National Food Authority.

———. 1981. *Seasonal price indices of selected agricultural commodities.* Manila: National Policy Staff Paper: 81–2, Ministry of Agriculture.

———. 1981a. *Food consumption and nutrition.* Memo to Agricultural Minister Tanco. Manila: National Agricultural Policy Staff (September 8).

———. 1981b. *National agricultural policy staff memo.* Manila: National Agricultural Policy Staff (September 8).

Philippines National Economic Development Authority. 1983. 1987–1988 integrated survey of households (ISH), as quoted in *1983 economic and social indicators,* p. 157. Manila: National Economic Development Authority.

Philippines National Science and Technology Authority. 1983. Manila: FNRI Publication No. 82–ET-10 (February).

———. 1984. *Second nationwide nutrition survey: Philippines, 1982.* Manila: Food and Nutrition Research Institute (October).

Phillips, Marshall, and Albert Baetz, eds. 1980. *Diet and resistance to disease.* New York: Plenum Press.

Phipps, Tim T. 1984. Land prices and farm-based returns. *American Journal of Agricultural Economics* 66 (November):422–429.

Pike, Ruth L., and Myrtle Brown. 1984. *Nutrition: An integrated approach.* New York: John Wiley.

Pimentel, D. 1993. Climate changes and food supply. *Forum for Applied Research and Public Policy* 8, no 4:54–60. Online at http://www.ciesin.org/docs/ 004–138/004–138.html.

Pimentel, D., et al. 1994. Natural resources and an optimum human population. *Population and Environment* 15:347–369.

————. 1995. Environmental and economic costs of soil erosion and conservation benefits. *Science* 267:1117–1123.

————. 1996. Impact of population growth on food supplies and environmnet. Presented at AAAS annual meeting, February 9, in Baltimore.

Pimentel, David, and Mario Giampietro. 1994. Food, land, population and the U.S. economy. Washington, D.C.: Carrying Capacity Network.

Pingali, P. 1987. From hand tillage to animal traction: Causes and effects and the policy implications for sub-Saharan African agriculture. African Livestock Policy Analysis Network, Paper 15. Addis-Ababa: International Livestock Centre for Africa. Online at http://www.ilri.cgiar.org/InfoServ/Webpub/full-docs/X5509e/x5509e00.htm#Contents.

Pingali, P., and P. Heisey. 1999. Cereal crop productivity in developing countries: Past trends and future prospects. Economics Working Paper 99-03. Mexico, D.F.: CIMMYT.

Pinstrup-Andersen, P., R. Pandya-Lorch, and M. Rosegrant. 1998. *The world food situation: Recent developments, emerging issues, and long-term prospects.* Washington, D.C.: International Food Policy Research Institute.

Pinstrup-Andersen, Per, and Elizabeth Caicedo. 1978. The potential impact of changes in income distribution on food demand and human nutrition. *American Journal of Agricultural Economics* 60 (August):402–415.

Pinstrup-Andersen, Per, and Peter Hazell. 1985. The impact of the green revolution and prospects for the future. *Food Reviews International* 1, no. 1:11. (Also available from IFPRI as a reprint.)

Pinstrup-Andersen, Per, et al. 1976. The impact of increasing food supply on human nutrition: Implications for commodity priorities in agricultural research and policy. *American Journal of Agricultural Economics* 58:137–138.

Pinstrup-Anderson, Per, David Nygaard, and Annu Ratta. 1995. The right to food: Widely acknowledged and poorly protected. Washington, D.C.: International Food Policy Research Institute. IFPRI 2020 Briefing Paper No. 22.

Pollitt, E., K. Gorman, P. Engle, R. Martorell, and J. Rivera. 1993. Early supplementary feeding and cognition. *Monographs of the Society for Research in Child Development* 58, no. 235(7).

Pope John Paul II. 1996. *Message to Worldfood Summit, November 13, 1996.* Available online at www.fao.org/wfs/index_en.htm.

Population Information Program. 1985. Fertility and family planning surveys. *Population Reports.* Baltimore: Johns Hopkins University, Series M, No. 8 (September–October).

Population Reference Bureau. 1970. *1965 World population data sheet.* Washington D.C.: Population Reference Bureau.

————. 1987. *1987 World population data sheet.* Washington D.C.: Population Reference Bureau.

Posner, R. A. 1986. *Economic analysis of the law*, 3d ed. Boston: Little, Brown.

Postel, Sandra. 1997. Dividing the waters. *Technology Review* (April). Online at http://web.mit.edu/techreview/www/articles/apr97/toc.html.

Postel, Sandra, G. C. Daily, and P. R. Erlich. 1996. Human appropriation of renewable fresh water. *Science* 271:785–788.

Prentice, A. M., G. R. Goldberg, and Ann Prentice. 1994. Body mass index and lactation performance. *European Journal of Clinical Nutrition* 48, supp. 3 (November):78.

Pullum, Thomas W. 1983. Correlates of family-size desires. In *Determinants of fertility in developing countries,* vol. 1, *Supply and demand for children,* ed. Rudolfo A. Bulatao et al., 334–386. New York: Academic Press.

Pustilnik, Lev, and Gregory Yom Din. 2003. Influence of solar activitiy on state of wheat market in medieval England. Proceedings of the International Cosmic Ray Conference, p. 4131.

Qaim, M., and A. de Janvry. 2003. Adoption of BT cotton in Argentina. *American Journal of Agricultural Economics* 85:814–828.

Qaim, M., and D. Zilberman. 2003. Yield effects of genetically modified crops in developing countries. *Science* 299, no. 5608 (February 7):900–902.

Quandt, Sara A. 1987. Methods for determining dietary intake. In *Nutritional anthropology*, ed. Francis E. Johnson, 67–84. New York: Alan R. Liss.

Ramalingaswami, Vulimiri, Urban Jonsson, and John Rohde. 1996. Commentary: The Asian enigma. In *The progress of nations*. Washington, D.C.: United Nations International Children's Fund.

Ranade, C. G., and R. W. Herdt. 1978. Shares of farm earnings from rice production. In *Economic consequences of the new rice technology*, ed. R. Barker and Y. Hayami, 87–104. Los Banos, Philippines: International Rice Research Institute.

Rand, W., R. Uauy, and N. Scrimshaw. 1984. Protein-energy-requirement studies in developing countries: Results of international research. Food and Nutrition Bulletin Supplement No. 10. Tokyo: United Nations University Press. Online at http://www.unu.edu/unupress/unupbooks/80481e/80481E03.htm#5. %20Protein-energy%20interactions.

Rangarajan, C. 1982. *Agricultural growth and industrial performance in India.* Washington, D.C.: International Food Policy Research Institute. IFPRI Research Report 33.

Rask, Norman. 1986. Economic development and the dynamics of food needs. Unpublished paper delivered at College Park, University of Maryland Global Development Conference (September).

Ravallion, Martin. 1997. Famines and economics. *Journal of Economic Literature* 35 (September):1205–1242.

Ray, Anandarup. 1986. Trade and pricing policies in world agriculture. *Finance and Development* 23 (September):2–5.

Reardon, T., C. Barrett, V. Kelly, and S. Kimseyinga. 1999. Policy reforms and sustainable agricultural intensification in africa. *Development Policy Review* 17, no. 4: 375–395.

Rejesus, R., P. Heisey, and M. Smale. 1999. Sources of productivity growth in wheat: A review of recent performance and medium- to long-term prospects. Economics Working Paper 99-05. Mexico, D.F.: CIMMYT.

Repetto, Robert. 1985. *Paying the price: Pesticide subsidies in developing countries.* Washington, D.C.: World Resources Institute. Research Report No. 2 (December).

Reuters Information Service. 1996. *Tension in Jordan's Karak after bread riots* (August 16). Online at http://www.nando.net/newsroom/ntn/world/081696/ world7_23344.html.

Reutlinger, Schlomo, et al. 1986. *Poverty and hunger—Issues and options for food security in developing countries.* Washington D.C.: World Bank.

———. 1985. Food security and poverty in LDCs. *Finance and Development* 22 (December):7–11.

———. 1983. Policy implications of research on energy intake and activity levels with reference to the debate on the energy adequacy of existing diets in developing countries. Washington, D.C.: World Bank. Agriculture and Rural Development Department Research Unit Discussion Paper 7.

Reutlinger, Shlomo, and Marcelo Selowsky. 1976. *Malnutrition and poverty: Magnitude and policy options.* Washington D.C.: World Bank, Staff Occasional Paper No. 23.

Rivera, Juan, and Reynaldo Martorell. 1988. Nutrition, infection, and growth, Part I: Effects of infection on growth. *Clinical Nutrition* 7:156–162.

———. 1988. Nutrition, infection, and growth, Part II: Effects of malnutrition on infection and general conclusions. *Clinical Nutrition* 7:163–167.

Roberts, D. F. 1953. Body weight, race and climate. *American Journal of Physical Anthropology* 11:533–558.

Rogers, Beatrice Lorge. 1988a. Design and implementation considerations for consumer-oriented food subsidies. In *Food subsidies in developing countries*, ed. Per Pinstrup-Andersen, 127–146. Baltimore: Johns Hopkins University Press.

———. 1988b. *Economic perspectives on combating hunger.* Presentation at the Second Annual World Food Prize Celebration. Washington, D.C., Smithsonian, September 30. An edited version of this paper is available in *Completing the food chain: Strategies for combating hunger and malnutrition*, ed. Paula M. Hirschoff and Neil G. Kolter, 122–126. Washington, D.C.: Smithsonian, 1989.

———. 1988c. Pakistan's ration system: Distribution of costs and benefits. In *Food subsidies in developing countries*, ed. Per Pinstrup-Andersen, 242–252. Baltimore: Johns Hopkins University Press.

Rogers, J. E. Thorold. 1887. *Agriculture and prices in England*, vols. I–VIII. Oxford: Clarendon Press, reprinted by Kraus Reprint Ltd., 1963, Vaduz, Liechtenstein.

Rose, D., P. Strasberg, J. Jefe, and D. Tschirley. 1999. Higher calorie intakes related to higher incomes in northern Mozambique. *Flash* 17. Michigan State University, online at http://www.aec.msu.edu/agecon/FS2/Mozambique/flash17e.pdf.

Rose, Stephen, and David Fasentast. 1988. *Family incomes in the 1980s.* Washington, D.C.: Economic Policy Institute. Working Paper No. 103 (November).

Rosegrant, Mark W. 1986. Irrigation with equity in Southeast Asia. Washington, D.C.: International Food Policy Research Institute. *IFPRI Report* 8 (January):1, 4.

Rosegrant, M., R. Scheleyer, and S. Yadav. 1995. Water policy for efficient agricultural diversification: Market-based approaches. *Food Policy* 20:203–223.

Rosenzweig, C., and M. L. Parry. 1994. Potential impact of climate change on world food supply. *Nature* 367, no. 6459.

Rosenzweig, C., M. L. Parry, G. Fischer, and K. Frohberg. 1993. Climate change and world food supply. Research Report No. 3. Oxford: Oxford University, Environmental Change Unit.

Rosenzweig, Cynthia, and Daniel Hillel. 1995. Potential impacts of climate change on agriculture and food supply. *Consquences* (summer).

Rosset, P., J. Collins, and F. M. Lappe. 2000. Lessons from the green revolution. *Tikkun Magazine*, March 1. Online at http://www.foodfirst.org/media/printformat.php?id=148; accessed October 2003.

Rountree, John. 1985. Computations done at the University of Maryland from data provided by the Egyption Ministry of Agriculture, the Central Agency for Public Mobilization and Statistics, and the Ministry of Supply.

Royal Society. 1999. *Review of data on possible toxicity of GM potatoes.* London: Royal Society. Online at http://www.royalsoc.ac.uk/files/statfiles/document-29.pdf.

Runge, C. F., B. Senauer, P. Pardey, and M. Rosegrant. 2003. *Ending hunger in our lifetime: Food security and globalization.* Baltimore: Johns Hopkins University Press.

Rustein, Shea O. 1984. Infant and child mortality: Levels, trends and demographic differentials. Table 14 in *World fertility survey comparative studies no. 45,* rev. ed. Voorburg, Netherlands: International Statistical Institute.

Ryan, James G. 1977. *Human nutritional needs and crop breeding objectives in the Indian semi-arid tropics.* Huderabad, India: International Crops Research Institute for the Semi-Arid Tropics (ICRISAT).

Sahlins, Marshall. 1968. Notes on the original affluent society. In *Man the hunter,* ed. R. B. Lee and I. DeVore, 85–89. Chicago: Aldine.

Sahn, David E., ed. 1989. *Seasonal variability in third world agriculture—The consequences for food security.* Baltimore: Johns Hopkins University Press.

Sahn, David E., and Neville Edirisinghe. 1993. Politics of food policy in Sri Lanka: From basic human needs to an increased market orientation. In *The political economy of food and nutrition policy,* ed. Per Pinstrup-Andersen. Batimore: Johns Hopkins University Press, chapter 3.

Salaff, Janet W., and Arline Wong. 1983. *Incentives and disincentives in population policies.* Washington, D.C.: Draper World Population Fund Report No. 12 (August).

Sala-i-Martin, X. 2002. The world distribution of income (estimated from individual country distributions). Working Paper, May 1. New York: Columbia University. Online at http://www.econ.upf.es/deehome/what/wpapers/postscripts/615.pdf.

Sampath, R. 1992. Issues in irrigation pricing in developing countries. *World Development* 20:967–977.

Samuels, B. 1986. Infant mortality and low birth weight among minority groups in the United States: A review of the literature. In *Report of the secretary's task force on black and minority health,* Vol. 4: *Infant mortality and low birth weight.* Washington, D.C.: U.S. Department of Health and Human Services.

Sancoucy, R. 1995. Livestock: A driving force for food security and sustainable development. In *World animal review,* 84–85. Rome: FAO. Online at http://www.fao.org/docrep/V8180T/v8180T07.htm#livestock%20%20%20a%20driving%20force%20for%20food%20security%20and%20sustainable%20development.

Sandburg, Carl. 1936. *The people, yes.* New York: Harcourt, Brace and Co.

Santos-Villaneuva, P. 1966. The value of rural roads. In *Selected readings to accompany getting agriculture moving,* ed. Raymond E. Borton, 775–795. New York: Agricultural Development Council.

Sazawal, S., et al. 1995. Zinc supplementation in young children with acute diarrhea in India. *New England Journal of Medicine* 333, no. 13 (September):839–844.

Scandizzo, Pasquale L., and Colin Bruce. 1980. *Methodologies for measuring agricultural price intervention effects.* Washington, D.C.: World Bank. Staff Working Paper 394 (June).

Scandizzo, Pasquale L., and I. Tsakok. 1985. Food price policies and nutrition in developing countries. In *Nutrition and development,* ed. Margaret Biswas and Per Pinstrup-Andersen, 60–76. Oxford: Oxford University Press.

Schall, B. 2003. Biotechnology, biodiversity and the environment. Paper presented at the Conference on Biodiversity and Biotechnology and the Protection of Traditional Knowledge, Washington University School of Law, St. Louis, April. Online at http://ls.wustl.edu/centeris/Confpapers/.

Schemann, J. F., et al. 2003. "National Immunisation Days and Vitamin A Distribution in Mali: Has the Vitamin A Status of Pre-School Children Improved?" *Public Health and Nutrition* 6, no. 3: 233–244.

Scherr, Sara J., and Satya Yadav. 1997. Land degradation in the developing world: Issues and policy options for 2020. Washington, D.C.: International Food Policy Research Institute. IFPRI 2020 Brief No. 44 (June).

Schiff, Maurice, and Alberto Valdés. 1995. The plundering of agriculture in developing countries. *Finance & Development* (March). Washington, D.C.:World Bank.

Schnepf, Randall D., Erik Dohlman, and Christine Bolling. 2001. Agriculture in Brazil and Argentina: Developments and prospects for major field crops. Market and Trade Economics Division, Economic Research Service, U.S. Department of Agriculture, Agriculture and Trade Report. WRS-01-3, Washington, D.C.

Schroeder D. G., and K. H. Brown. 1994. Nutritional status as a predictor of child survival: Summarizing the association and quantifying its global impact. *Bulletin of the World Health Organization* 72, no. 4:569–579.

Schuh, G. Edward. 1988. Some issues associated with exchange rate realignments in developing countries. In *Macroeconomics, agriculture, and exchange rates,* ed. Philip L. Paarlberg and Robert G. Chambers, 231–240. Boulder, Colo.: Westview Press.

Schultz, T. P. 1999. Health and schooling investments in Africa. *Journal of Economic Perspectives* 13, no. 3:67–88.

Schultz, Theodore W. 1979. *The economics of research and agricultural productivity.* Arlington, Va.: International Agricultural Development Services Occasional Paper. As quoted in *Agricultural development in the third world,* ed. Carl K. Eicher and John M. Staatz, 335–347. Baltimore: Johns Hopkins University Press, 1984.

Scobie, Grant M. 1983. *Food subsidies in Egypt: Their impact on foreign exchange and trade.* Washington D.C.: International Food Policy Reserach Institute, IFPRI Research Report No. 40 (August).

Scobie, Grant M., and Rafael Posada T. 1984. The impact of technical change on income distribution: The case of rice in Colombia. In *Agricultural development in the third world,* ed. Carl K. Eicher and John M. Staatz, 378–388. Baltimore: Johns Hopkins University Press.

Scrimshaw, Nevin S. 1988. Completing the food chain: From production to consumption. Remarks presented at the Scond Annual World Food Price Celebration. Washington, D.C., Smithsonian, September 30. An edited version of this paper is available in *Completing the food chain: Strategies for combating hunger and malnutrition,* ed. Paula M. Hirschoff and Neil G. Kolter, 1–17. Washington, D.C.: Smithsonian, 1989.

Scrimshaw, Nevin S., and Vernon R. Young. 1976. The requirements of human nutrition. In *Food and agriculture,* ed. Scientific American, 26–40. San Francisco: Freeman.

Scrimshaw, Nevin S., Carl Taylor, and John Gordon. 1968. *Interactions of nutrition and infection.* Geneva: World Health Organization.

Scrimshaw, Susan. 1978. Infant mortality and behavior in the regulation of family size. *Population and Development Review* 4:383–403.

———. 1984. Infanticide in human populations: Societal and individual concerns. In *Infanticide: Comparative and evolutionary perspectives,* ed. Glen Hausfater and Sarah B. Hardy, 439–462. New York: Aldine.

Seckler, David. 1982. "Small but healthy": A basic hypothesis in the theory, measurement and policy of malnutrition. In *Newer concepts in nutrition and their implications for policy,* ed. P. V. Kukhtame, 127–137. Pune, India: Maharastra Association for the Cultivation of Science Research Institute, Law College Road.

Semba, R. D., et al. 1994. Maternal vitamin A deficiency and mother-to-child transmission of HIV-1. *Lancet* 343, no. 8913 (June 25):1593–1597.

Sen, Amartya K. 1981. *Poverty and famines.* Oxford: Clarendon Press.

———. 1987. *Hunger and entitlements.* Helsinki: World Institute for Development Economics Research.

———. 1990. Public action to remedy hunger: Tanco memorial lecture. London, The Hunger Project, August. Online at http://www.thp.org/reports/sen/sen890. htm#n1.

———. 1964. Size of holdings and productivity. *Economic and Political Weekly* (February).

———. 1966. Peasants and dualism with or without surplus labor. *Journal of Political Economy* 74:425–450.

———. 1973. *On economic inequality.* London: Oxford University Press.

———. 1981. *Poverty and famines: An essay on entitlement and deprivation.* Oxford: Clarendon Press.

Senauer, Benjamin, et al. 1988. Determinants of the intrahousehold allocation of food in the rural Philippines. *American Journal of Agricultural Economics* 70:170–180.

Shakir, A. 1975. The surveillance of protein-calorie malnutrition by simple and economic means (a report to UNICEF). *Journal of Tropical Pediatrics and Environmental Child Health* 21:69–85.

Shaw, A. 2000. Police, troops impose uneasy calm after food riots. Associated Press, October 19.

Shekar, Meera. 1991. *The Tamil Nadu Integrated Nutrition Project: A review of the project with special emphasis on the monitoring and information system.* Working Paper No. 14. Cornell Food and Nutrition Policy Program, Ithaca, N.Y.

Sherman, Adria R. 1986. Alterations in immunity related to nutritional status. *Nutrition Today* (July-August):7–13.

Sicat, Gerardo P. 1983. Toward a flexible interest rate policy, or losing interest in the usury law. In *Rural financial markets in developing countries: Their use and abuse,* ed. J. D. Von Pische et al., 373–386. Baltimore: Johns Hopkins University Press.

Simmons, George B., and Robert J. Lapham. 1987. The determinants of family planning program effectiveness. In *Organizing for effective family planning programs,* ed. Lampham and Simmons, 683–706. Washington, D.C.: National Academy Press.

Simon, Julian L. 1986. *Theory of population and economic growth.* New York: Blackwell.

———. 1996. *The ultimate resource.* Princeton, N.J.: Princeton University Press. Online at http://www.rhsmith.umd.edu/Faculty/JSimon/Ultimate_Resource/.

Simon, N., M. Cropper, A. Alberini, and S. Arora. 1999. Valuing mortality reductions in India: A study of compensating-wage differentials. World Bank Working Paper No. 2978. Washington, D.C.: World Bank.

Sinaga, R. S., and B. M. Sinaga. 1978. Comments on shares of farm earnings from rice production. In *Economic consequences of the new rice technology,* ed. R. Barker and Y. Hayami, 105–109. Los Banos, Philippines: International Rice Research Institute.

Smale, Melinda. 1997. The green revolution and wheat genetic diversity: Some unfounded assumptions. *World Development* 25, no. 8:1257–1269.

Snow, A. 2002. Transgenic crops—Why gene flow matters. *Nature biotechnology* 20:542.

Snyder, J. D., and M. H. Merson. 1982. The magnitude of the global problem of acute diarrhoeal disease: A review of active surveillance data. *Bulletin of the World Health Organization* 60:605–613.

Soliman, Ibrahim, and Shahla Shapouri. 1984. See U.S. Department of Agriculture, 1984.

Sommer, Alfred, et al. 1986. Impact of vitamin A supplementation on childhood mortality—A randomized controlled community trial. *Lancet* (May 24):1169–1173.

Sperduto, R. D., et al. 1993. The Linxian cataract studies: Two nutrition intervention trials. *Archives of Ophthalmology* 830, no. 111:1246–1253.

Spurr, G. B., M. Barac-Nieto, and M. G. Maksud. 1976. See U.S. Department of State, 1976.

Stackman, E. C., Richard Bradfield, and Paul C. Mangelsdorf. 1967. *Campaigns against hunger*. Boston: Bellknap Press of Harvard University Press.

Stanbury, John, ed. 1994. *The damaged brain of iodine deficiency: Cognitive, behavioral, neuromotor, educative aspects*. Port Washington, N.Y.: Cognizant Communication Corp.

Stein, A., H. Barnhart, M. Hickey, U. Ramakrishnan, D. Schroeder, and R. Martorell. 2003. Prospective study of protein-energy supplementation early in life and of growth in the sub-sequent generation in Guatemala. *American Journal of Clinical Nutrition* 78, no. 1:162–167.

Steindl, Josef. 1987. Pareto distribution. In *The new Palgrave: A dictionary of economics*, vol 3., ed. John Eatwell et al., 809–810. New York: Stockton Press.

Stephenson, Lani S., M. C. Latham, and A. Jansen. 1983. *A comparison of growth standards: Similarities between NCHS, Harvard, Denver and privileged African children and differences with Kenyan rural children*. Ithaca, N.Y.: Cornell International Nutrition Monograph Series No. 12.

Stevens, Robert D., and Cathy L. Jabara. 1988. *Agricultural development principles: Economic theory and empirical evidence*. Baltimore: Johns Hopkins University Press.

Stiglitz, J. 2002. *Globalization and its discontents*. New York: W. W. Norton.

———. 1986. *Economics of the public sector*. New York: W. W. Norton.

Stone, Bruce. 1985. *Fertilizer pricing policy and foodgrain production strategy*. Washington, D.C.: International Food Policy Research Institute. *IFPRI Report* 7 (May):1, 4.

Stout, B. A. 1998. Energy for agriculture in the twenty-first century. In *Feeding a world population of more than eight billion people: A challenge to science*, ed. J. C. Waterlow et al. Oxford: Oxford University Press.

Strategy Page. 2004. Korea, January 21. Online at http://www.strategypage. com//fyeo/qndguide/default.asp?target=korea.htm; accessed January 22, 2004.

Strauss, J. 1968. Estimating the Determinants of Food Consumption and Caloric Availability in Rural Sierra Leone. In eds. Singh, et al., *Agricultural Household Models: Extensions, Applications, and Policy*. Baltimore and London: Johns Hopkins University Press for the World Bank: 116–152.

Strauss, John, and Duncan Thomas. 1998. Health, nutrition, and economic development. *Journal of Economic Literature* 36:766–818.

Streeten, Paul. 1987. *What price food? Agricultural price policies in developing countries*. London: MacMillan.

Struck, Doug. 2001. North Korea food crisis intensifies. *Washington Post*, May 16, p. A-20.

Stuart, H., and S. Stevenson. 1950. Physical growth and development. In *Textbook of pediatrics*, ed. W. Nelson, 5th ed. Philadelphia: Saunders.

Subramanian, U., and M. Cropper. 1995. Public choices between lifesaving programs: How important are lives saved? World Bank Working Paper No. 1497. Washington, D.C.: World Bank.

Susser, E., et al. 1996. Schizophrenia after prenatal famine: Further evidence. *Archives of General Psychiatry* 53, no. 1 (January):25–31.

Sutton, John. 1989. See U.S. Department of Agriculture, 1989a.

Svedberg, P. 1999. 841 million undernourished? *World Development* 27:2081–2098.

Swindale, L. D. 1997. The globalization of agricultural research: A study of the control of the cassava mealybug in Africa. Consultative Group for International Agricultural Research. Online at ftp://ftp.cgiar.org/isnar/publicat/pdf/vision/swindale.pdf.

Tang, A. M., et al. 1993. Dietary micronutrient intake and risk of progression to acquired immunodeficiency syndrome (AIDS) in human immunodeficiency virus type 1 (HIV-1)-infected homosexual men. *American Journal of Epidemiology* 138, no. 11 (December 1):937–951.

Tanner, J. M. 1977. Human growth and constitution. In *Human biology—An introduction to human evolution, variation, growth and ecology*, by G. A. Harrison et al., 301–385. Oxford: Oxford University Press.

Tanner, J., R. Whitehouse, and M. Takaishi. 1966. Standards from birth to maturity for height, height velocity and weight velocity: British children I. *Archives of Disease in Childhood* 41:454.

Teshima, R., H. Akiyama, H. Okunuki, J. Sakushima, Y. Goda, H. Onodera, J. Sawada, and M. Toyoda. 2000. Effect of GM and non-GM soybeans on the immune system of BN rats and B10A mice. *Journal of the Food Hygenic Society of Japan* 41, no. 3:188–193.

Thomson-Wadsworth, Inc. 2003. 2002 dietary reference intakes (DRI). Online at http://www.newtexts.com/newtexts/nutrition%20tables.pdf.

Timmer, C. Peter. 1984. Choice of technique in rice milling on Java. In *Agricultural development in the third world*, ed. Carl K. Eicher and John M. Staatz, 278–288. Baltimore: Johns Hopkins University Press.

Timmer, C. Peter, Walter P. Falcon, and Scott R. Pearson. 1983. *Food policy analysis*. Baltimore: Johns Hopkins University Press.

Tinker, Anne, et al. 1994. *Women's health and nutrition: Making a difference*. Washington, D.C.: World Bank.

Todaro, Michael P. 1980. Internal migration in developing countries: A survey. In *Population and economic change in developing countries*, ed. Richard A. Easterlin, 361–402. Chicago: University of Chicago Press.

Transport for London. 2003. Congestion charging—Summary of week 6. Press release, April 1. Online at http://www.tfl.gov.uk/tfl/press_cc_news_latest.shtml.

Traub, James. 1988. Into the mouths of babes. *New York Times Magazine*, July 24, p. 18.

Trumbo, P., S. Schlicker, A. Yates, and M. Poos. 2002. Dietary reference intakes for energy, carbohydrate, fiber, fat, fatty acids, cholesterol, protein, and amino acids. *Journal of the American Dietetic Association* 102, no. 11 (November).

Tupasi, T. E. 1985. Nutritional and acute respiratory infection. In *Acute respiratory infections in childhood, Proceedings of an international workshop*, ed. R.

Douglas and E. Kerby-Eaton. Adelaide, Australia: University of Adelaide Press.

United Nations. 1991. *World population prospects 1990*. New York: United Nations. Population Study No. 120, Department of International Economic and Social Affairs.

UN Population Division. 2002a. World population prospects: Assumptions underlying the results of the 2002 revisions of the world population prospects. Online at http://esa.un.org/unpp/assumptions.html.

———. 2002b. World population prospects population database. Online at http://esa.un.org/unpp/.

UN, FAO. 1996. Backgrounder on plant genetic resources and plant breeding. Rome: FAO. Online at http://www.fao.org/FOCUS/e/96/06/02-e.htm.

UN, Population Information Network (POPIN). 1995. *Population and land degradation*. Vol. 2 of *Population and the environment: A review of issues and concepts for population programmes staff*. New York: United Nations.

UNAIDS. 2002. "Global reports: Estimates end of 2001." Online at http://www.unaids.org/html/pub/Global-Reports/Barcelona/TableEstimatesEnd2001_en_xls.xls.

UNAIDS/WHO Reference Group for Estimates, Modelling, and Projections. 2002. "Improving estimates and projections of HIV/AIDS." Online at http://www.epidem.org/Publications/Madrid%20report.pdf.

UNDP (United Nations Development Program). 2003. *Human development report 2003*. New York: UNDP. Online at http://www.undp.org/hdr2003/index.html.

UNEP (United Nations Environment Programme). 1990. *The impacts of climate change on agriculture*. United Nations Environment Programme Information Unit for Climate Change (IUCC) Fact Sheet 101. Nairobi, Kenya: UNEP.

UNICEF (United Nations International Children's Fund). 1982. *News* 113:9.

———. 1987. *ORT and much more—Developing whole CDD programmes*. CF/PD/PRO-1987–001, Memo to all field offices, January 15.

———. 1988. *State of the world's children, 1988*. New York: Oxford University Press.

———. 1996. *Progress of nations*. New York: United Nations. Online at http://www.unicef.org/pon96/.

———. 1998. *State of the world's children 1998*. New York: Oxford University Press.

———. 2003. *State of the world's children 2003*. New York: Oxford University Press.

University of California Food Task Force. 1974. *A hungry world: The challenge to agriculture, summary report*. Berkeley: Division of Agricultural Sciences.

Urban, Francis, and Arthur J. Dommen. 1989. See U.S. Department of Agriculture, 1989b.

U.S. Bureau of Census. 1961. *Historical statistics of the U.S. from colonial times to 1956*. Washington, D.C.: Bureau of Census.

———. 1987. *Statistical abstract of the United States: 1988*. Washington, D.C.: Bureau of Census.

———. 2003. Website. www.census.gov.

U.S. Congress, Office of Technology Assessment. 1986. *Technology, public policy, and the changing structure of American agriculture*. Washington, D.C.: Government Printing Office. OTA-F-285.

U.S. Congress. 1974. *National nutrition policy study—1974: Hearings before the Select Committee on Nutrition and Human Needs*, Part 3—*Nutrition and*

Special Groups. 93rd Congress, Washington, D.C.: Government Printing Office.

U.S. Department of Agriculture (USDA). 1917. *Geography of the world's agriculture,* by V. C. Finch and O. E. Baker, Office of Farm Management. Washington D.C.: USDA.

———. 1963. *Composition of foods, raw, processed, prepared.* Washington D.C.: Agricultural Handbook No. 8.

———. 1970. *Feed situation report* (November).

———. 1984. *The impact of wheat price policy change on nutritional status in Egypt,* by Soliman, Ibrahim and Shahla Shapouri. Washington, D.C.: USDA, ERS, International Economics Division (February).

———. 1985. *U.S. demand for food: A complete system of price and income effects,* by Kuw W. Huang. Washington, D.C.: USDA Technical Bulletin 1714.

———. 1988. *World food needs and availabilities, 1988–89: Summer.* Washington, D.C.: USDA, ERS (August).

———. 1989a. Environmental degradation and agriculture, by John Sutton. Washington, D.C.: USDA/ERS *World Agriculture Situation and Outlook Report* WAS-55 (June):35–41.

———. 1989b. *World agriculture,* by Francis Urban and Arthur J. Dommen. Washington, D.C.: USDA (June).

———. 1990. *U.S. government concessional exports, commodity by country and fiscal year.* Washington, D.C.: Unpublished database.

———. 1991. *Food cost reviews.* Washington, D.C.: USDA.

———. 1998. *Agricultural baseline projections to 2007.* Washington D.C.: USDA. Online at http://www.econ.ag.gov/Briefing/baseline/index98.htm.

USDA Agricultural Research Service. 2003. Research Q&A: Bt corn and monarch butterflies. Washington, D.C.: USDA. ARS online at http://www.ars.usda.gov/is/br/btcorn/.

U.S. Department of Energy (DOE). 2003. Residential energy consumption survey. Washington, D.C.: DOE. Online at http://www.eia.doe.gov/emeu/recs/recs2001/detail_tables.html.

U.S. Department of Health and Human Resources. 1981. *Height and weight of adults ages 18–74 years by socioeconomic and geographic variables, United States.* Hyattsville, Md.: National Center for Health Statistics, DHHS Publication No. (PHS) 81–1674. Data from the National Health Survey, Series 11, No. 224 (August).

U.S. Department of Health and Human Services. 1987. *Anthropometric reference data and prevalence of overweight, United States, 1976–80.* Hyattsville, Md.: National Center for Health Statistics, DHHS Publication No. (PHS) 87–1688 (October).

———. 1988. *The Surgeon General's report on nutriton and health, 1988.* Washington, D.C.: Public Health Service Publication No. 88–50210.

U.S. Department of Health, Education and Welfare. 1976. NCHS Growth Charts. *Monthly Vital Statistics Report* 25, no. 3, Supp. (HRA) 76–1120. Rockville, Md.: National Center for Health Statistics, Resources Administration (June).

———. 1979. *Weight by height and age for adults 18–74 years: United States, 1971–74.* Hyattsville, Md.: Public Health Service, Office of Health Research, Statistics and Technology, National Center for Health Statistics (NCHS), Vital and Health Statistics. Data from the National Health Survey, Series 11, Number 208.

U.S. Department of State. 1976. *Clinical and subclinical malnutrition and their influence on the capacity to do work,* by G. B. Spurr, M. Barac-Nieto, and M. G. Maksud. Washington D.C.: State Department, Project AID/CSD 2943, Final Report.

————. 1978. *Agricultural policies and rural malnutrition,* by Phillips Foster. Washington, D.C.: State Department, USAID Economics and Sector Planning Division, Office of Agriculture, Technical Assistance Bureau, Occasional Paper No. 8.

————. 1986a. *Development and spread of high yielding rice varieties in developing countries,* by Dana G. Dalrymple. Washington, D.C.: Agency for International Development.

————. 1986b. *Development and spread of high yielding wheat varieties in developing countries,* by Dana G. Dalrymple. Washington, D.C.: Agency for Internatonal Development.

U.S. Department of Transportation, Federal Highway Administration. 2002. *1999 status of the nation's highways, bridges, and transit: Conditions and performance report.* Washington D.C.: Government Printing Office. Online at: http://www.fhwa.dot.gov/policy/1999cpr/ch_10/cpm10_3.htm.

U.S. Environmental Protection Agency. 1999. *The benefits and costs of the Clean Air Act, 1990 to 2010.* Washington, D.C.: Government Printing Office. Online at: http://www.epa.gov/airprogm/oar/sect812/1990-2010/fullrept.pdf.

U.S. Federal Reserve System. Board of Governors. 1989. *Balance sheets for the U.S. economy, 1949–88.* Washington, D.C. (October).

U.S. National Academy of Sciences. 1974. *Recommendeed dietary allowances.* Washington, D.C.: National Academy of Sciences.

U.S. Water News Online. 2003. Massive groundwater supply found in arid northwestern China (February). Online at http://www.uswaternews.com/archives/arcglobal/3masgro2.html.

U.S. White House, Council of Economic Advisers. 1989. *Economic indicators.* Washington, D.C.: The White House (December).

U.S. White House, President's Science Advisory Committee. 1967. *The world food problem,* Vols. II and III: *Report of the panel on the world food supply.* Washington, D.C.: The White House.

Usher, R. 1996. The Cadillac that moos. *Time,* April 1, p. 25.

Uvin , Peter. 1993. State of world hunger. In *The hunger report 1993.* New York: Gordon and Breach.

Vergara, Benito S. 1979. *A farmer's primer on growing rice.* Los Banos, Philippines: International Rice Research Institute.

Viscusi, W. Kip. 1993. The value of risks to life and health. *Journal of Economic Literature* 31:1912–1946.

Viscusi, W. K., and T. Gayer. 2002. Safety at any price? *Regulation* 25, no. 3. Online at http://www.cato.org/pubs/regulation/regv25n3/regv25n3.html.

Von Braun, Joachim, and Eileen Kennedy. 1986. *Commercialization of subsistence agriculture: Income and nutritional effects in developing countries.* Washington, D.C.: International Food Policy Research Institute, Working Paper on Commercialization of Agriculture and Nutrition, No. 1.

Von Braun, Joachim, and Eileen Kennedy, eds. 1994. *Agricultural commercialization, economic development, and nutrition.* Baltimore: Johns Hopkins University Press, published for the International Food Policy Research Institute.

Von Braun, Joachim, et al. 1989. *Nontraditional export crops in Guatemala: Effects on production, income, and nutrition.* Washington, D.C.: International Food Policy Research Institute, IFPRI Research Report 73.

Walinsky, Louis. 1962. *Economic development in Burma, 1951–1960.* New York: Twentieth Century Fund.

Walker, Alexander, and Harry Stein. 1985. Growth of third world children. Chapter 20 in *Dietary fibre, fibre-depleted foods and disease,* ed. H. Trowell et al., 331–344. London: Academic Press.

Wallis, J.A.N. 1997. Brazil: The cerrados region. In *Intensified systems of farming in the tropics and subtropics,* 85–103. World Bank Discussion Paper No. 364. Washington, D.C.: World Bank.

Waterlow, J., R. Buzina, W. Keller, J. Lane, M. Nichaman, and J. Tanner. 1977. The presentation and use of height and weight data for comparing the nutritional status of groups of children under the age of ten years. *Bulletin of WHO* 55:489–498.

Weiner, J. S. 1977. Nutritional ecology. In *Human biology—An introduction to human evolution, variation, growth and ecology,* by A. G. Harrison et al., 400–423. Oxford: Oxford University Press.

Weiner, T. 2000. A farmer learns about Mexico's lack of the rule of law. *New York Times,* October 27.

Whitney, Eleanor N., and Eva Hamilton. 1977. *Understanding nutrition.* St. Paul, Minn.: West.

WHO (World Health Organization). 1985a. *Energy and protein requirements, Report of a joint FAO/WHO/UNU expert consultation.* Geneva: WHO, Technical Report Series 724.

———. 1985b. *Fourth programme report for control of diarrheal diseases 1983–1984.* Geneva: WHO, Program for Control of Diarrheal Diseases.

———. 1985c. *The management of diarrhoea and use of oral rehydration therapy.* Geneva: World Health Organization/UNICEF.

———. 1989. *Report on world health.* Washington, D.C.: WHO Regional Office for the Americas. Press release, September 25.

———. 1995a. *Physical status: The use and interpretation of anthropometry.* Report of a WHO Expert Committee. WHO Technical Report Series No. 854. Geneva: WHO.

———. 1995b. *World health report 1995: Bridging the gaps.* Geneva: WHO.

———. 1996a. *Investing in health research and development: Ad hoc committee on health research relating to future intervention options.* New York: United Nations.

———. 1996b. *State of the world's vaccines and immunization.* New York: United Nations. Online at http://www.who.ch/gpv/tEnglish/avail/sowvi.htm.

———. 1996c. *World health report, 1996.* Geneva: WHO.

———. 1997. *World health report, 1997.* Geneva: WHO.

———. 2002. Diet, nutrition and the prevention of chronic diseases. Technical Report 916. Geneva: WHO.

———. 2003a. Progress towards global immunization goals, 2001. Geneva: WHO. Online at http://www.who.int/vaccines-surveillance/documents/SlidesGlobalImmunization_2002update.

———. 2003b. Water supply, sanitation, and hygiene development. Online at http://www.who.int/water_sanitation_health/hygiene/en/.

WHO and UN. 1997. Micronutrient and trace element deficiencies: General information. Online at http://www.who.org/nut/micr/micrgen.htm.

Wild, Alan. 2003. Soils, land, and food: Managing the land during the twenty-first century. Cambridge: Cambridge University Press.

Williamson, J. 1990. What Washington means by policy reform. In *Latin American adjustment: How much has happened?* ed. J. Williamson. Washington, D.C.: Institute for International Economics.

Winick, M., K. Meyer, and R. Harris. 1973. Malnutrition and environmental enrichment by early adoption. *Science* 190 (December):1173–1175.

Winter, Roger P. 1988. In Sudan, both sides use food as a weapon. *Washington Post,* November 19, p. A-25.

Wittwer, Sylvan. 1995. *Food, climate, and carbon dioxide: The global environment and world food production.* New York: Lewis Publishers.

Wolfenbarger, L., and P. Phifer. 2000. The ecological risks and benefits of genetically engineered plants. *Science* 290:2088–2093.

World Bank and UNDP (United Nations Development Program). 1990. *A proposal for an internationally supported programme to enhance research in irrigation and drainage technology in developing countries,* vol. 2. Washington, D.C.: World Bank and UNDP.

World Bank. 1975. *Land reform sector policy paper* (May). Washington, D.C.: World Bank.

———. 1994. Enriching lives: Overcoming vitamin and mineral malnutrtion in developing countries. Washington, D.C.: World Bank.

———. 1997. Does better nutrition improve academic achievement? Yes. *World Bank Policy and Research Bulletin* 8, no. 2 (April-June).

———. 2001. Private-sector development strategy: Issues and options. Washington, D.C.: World Bank. Online at http://rru.worldbank.org/strategy/PSDstrategy-June1.pdf.

———. 2002. Globalization, growth, and poverty: Building an inclusive world economy. Washington, D.C.: World Bank. Online at http://econ.worldbank.org/prr/globalization/text-2857/.

———. 2003. Globalization, growth, and poverty: Building an inclusive world economy. Washington, D.C.: World Bank. Online at http://econ.worldbank.org/prr/globalization/text-2857/.

———. 2003. *World Development Indicators.* Available online at www.worldbank.org/data/wdi2003/worldview.htm

———. Various years. *World development report.* New York: Oxford University Press.

World Food Council. 1988. *The global state of hunger and malnutrition, 1988 report.* Nicosia, Cyprus: Secretariat, World Food Council (May).

World Food Programme. 1989. *Food aid works.* Rome: FAO, World Food Programme.

———. 2003. Online at http://www.wfp.org/country_brief/africa/zambia/brief/CFSAMZambia03.pdf.

World Resources Institute. 1997. *World resources 1996/96: The urban environment.* Washington, D.C.: World Resources Institute. Online at http://www.wri.org/wr-96–97.

WorldWatch Institute. 1996a. WorldWatch Institute urges World Bank and FAO to overhaul misleading food supply projections. Press release (May 1), Washington, D.C.

———. 1996b. Cropland Losses Threaten World Food Supplies. Press Release July 27, 1996. Available online at www.worldwatch.org/press/news/1996/07/27

Yao, Shujie. 1999. A note on causal factors of China's famine in 1959–61. *Journal of political economy*:1365–1372.

Ying, Yvonne. 1996. *Poverty and inequality in China*. Washington, D.C.: World Bank. Online at http://www.worldbank.org/html/prddr/trans/ja96/art2.htm.

Zaidi, S., and M. C. Fawzi. 1995. Health of Baghdad's children [letter], *Lancet* 346, no. 8988 (December 2):1485.

INDEX

ABOUT THE BOOK

Recognizing that millions of people in the less developed countries continue to go hungry while there is more than enough food in the world to feed them, the authors of *The World Food Problem* tackle the question of why—and what can be done about it.

Entirely new to the third edition are chapters on the history of famine, the basic economics of supply and demand, and economics and policy analyses. Throughout, data have been brought up-to-date and recent policy debates explored; the discussion is enriched with frequent examples of current problems and policies.

This highly readable and comprehensive text provides an accessible analysis of the state of world food supply and demand, as well as an assessment of prospects for the future.

Howard D. Leathers is associate professor of agriculture and resource economics, and **Phillips Foster** is professor emeritus of agriculture and resource economics, both at the University of Maryland, College Park.